AF581694

Dental Education

Dental Education

Editors

Jelena Dumančić
Božana Lončar Brzak

MDPI • Basel • Beijing • Wuhan • Barcelona • Belgrade • Manchester • Tokyo • Cluj • Tianjin

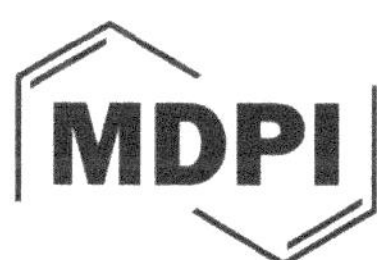

Editors

Jelena Dumančić
Department of Dental Anthropology
School of Dental Medicine
University of Zagreb
Zagreb
Croatia

Božana Lončar Brzak
Department of Oral Medicine
School of Dental Medicine
University of Zagreb
Zagreb
Croatia

Editorial Office
MDPI
St. Alban-Anlage 66
4052 Basel, Switzerland

This is a reprint of articles from the Special Issue published online in the open access journal *Dentistry Journal* (ISSN 2304-6767) (available at: www.mdpi.com/journal/dentistry/special_issues/Dental_Education).

For citation purposes, cite each article independently as indicated on the article page online and as indicated below:

LastName, A.A.; LastName, B.B.; LastName, C.C. Article Title. *Journal Name* **Year**, *Volume Number*, Page Range.

ISBN 978-3-0365-3111-3 (Hbk)
ISBN 978-3-0365-3110-6 (PDF)

Contents

Preface to "Dental Education"

The dental curriculum is like a living organism—it has developed through time, manifesting regional, cultural, and scientific heritage, and reflecting modern trends. The undergraduate dental curriculum is periodically rebuilt to ensure the harmonization of higher education systems between countries, especially in Europe. Structure, content, learning, and assessment in undergraduate and postgraduate dental education and auxiliary dental personnel training are shaped based on professional consensus. Constant updates on recent technological innovations and evidence-based best practice are necessary.

In modern times, ethical issues are raised more than ever. Can we teach our students how to be dedicated health professionals and manage a successful practice at the same time? Does the commercialization of our profession also affect the dental curriculum today?

The COVID-19 pandemic has imposed new challenges, moving us from lecture rooms and clinics to an online environment.

This Special Issue is dedicated to developing the understanding of dental education.

Jelena Dumančić, Božana Lončar Brzak
Editors

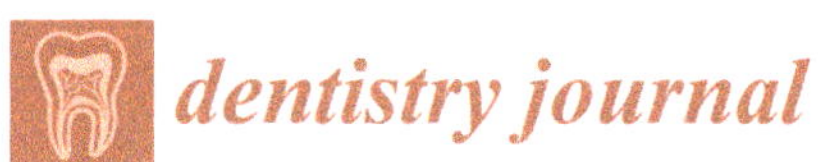

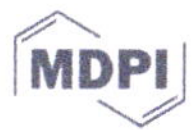

Article

Students' Perceptions of Educational Climate in a Spanish School of Dentistry Using the Dundee Ready Education Environment Measure: A Longitudinal Study

Alba María Hernández-Crespo [1], Paula Fernández-Riveiro [2,*], Óscar Rapado-González [1,3], Ángela Aneiros [1,4], Inmaculada Tomás [1,4,*] and María Mercedes Suárez-Cunqueiro [1,3,*]

1. Department of Surgery and Medical-Surgical Specialties, Medicine and Dentistry School, Universidade de Santiago de Compostela (USC), 15782 Santiago de Compostela, Spain; albahzcrespo@gmail.com (A.M.H.-C.); oscar.rapado@rai.usc.es (Ó.R.-G.); angela_aneiros@hotmail.com (Á.A.)
2. Department of Psychiatry, Radiology Public Health, Nursing and Medicine, Universidade de Santiago de Compostela (USC), 15782 Santiago de Compostela, Spain
3. Health Research Institute of Santiago (IDIS), 15782 Santiago de Compostela, Spain
4. Oral Sciences Research Group, Health Research Institute of Santiago (IDIS), 15782 Santiago de Compostela, Spain

* Correspondence: paula.fernandez.riveiro@usc.es (P.F.-R.); inmaculada.tomas@usc.es (I.T.); mariamercedes.suarez@usc.es (M.M.S.-C.); Tel.: +34-881-812-441 (P.F.-R.); +34-881-812-377 (I.T.); +34-881-812-437 (M.M.S.-C.)

Received: 30 October 2020; Accepted: 2 December 2020; Published: 7 December 2020

Abstract: Background: Educational Climate (EC) may determine teacher and student behaviour. Our aim was to evaluate EC longitudinally in a period of 'curricular transition' from traditional (teacher-centred learning) to Bologna curricula (interactive student-centred learning). Methods: The 'Dundee Ready Education Environment Measure' (DREEM) questionnaire was completed by 397 students from a Spanish School of Dentistry. Students' perception was assessed in different courses and academic years. Results: The overall EC scale average was 115.70 ± 20.20 (57.85%) and all domain values showed a percentage > 52%, which were interpreted as 'positive and acceptable'. The EC mean was: 118.02 ± 17.37 (59.01%) for 2010–2011; 116.46 ± 19.79 (58.23%) for 2013–2014; 115.60 ± 21.93 (57.80%) for 2014–2015; 112.02 ± 22.28 (56.01%) for 2015–2016, interpreted as 'more positive than negative EC'. The worst Learning domain scores corresponded to later academic years and may reflect the Bologna curriculum's more intensive clinical training involving greater responsibility and self-learning. Conclusions: EC and its domains were perceived more positively than negatively. The Social domain was the most positively evaluated, while the Learning domain was the worst.

Keywords: educational climate; dental students; DREEM scale; dental education; dentistry

1. Introduction

The educational environment is defined as students' perceptions of their influences and pressures, and how this perception is aligned with the curriculum's educational aims [1]. The perception of the educational environment is considered as the 'Educational Climate' (EC). The term EC has been described by Genn et al. [2] as "the expression of the educational environment and the academic curriculum". Thus, EC is considered "everything that is happening in the classroom, in a department, in the faculty or the university" [2]. Students' perceptions regarding EC are influenced by aspects such as learning outcomes, teacher skills, learning resources, learning and teaching approaches, assessment procedures, timetabling, student support, facilities, classrooms, group size, and atmosphere [3]. In addition, EC encourages teacher attitudes, and student achievements. Thus, EC has a significant impact on academic success, and on professional development [2–5] as well as being critical to students' personal and social well-being. Moreover, it is established the EC affects not only students, but also school staff, and even curriculum designers and administrative personnel [5]. The EC profile represents an opportunity to ascertain the strengths and weaknesses of an institution, thus enabling comparative analysis within or between institutions in order to foster change and improvement in the educational process. Universities should continuously evaluate the EC of their classes, departments, and schools to detect problems and implement corrective measures.

Several qualitative and quantitative methodologies have been used to evaluate students' perception of EC [6–9]. In academic healthcare institutions, one of the most widely used and reliable instruments is the 'Dundee Ready Educational Environment Measure' (DREEM) [10,11]. The DREEM was developed by a Delphi panel including 100 educators specializing in healthcare disciplines from 20 countries, and 1000 students. Currently, the DREEM questionnaire exists in different languages and has been widely used to assess EC in Dentistry Schools worldwide [9,12–17]. The DREEM scale is a universal tool, applicable regardless of national development level.

As a result of the Bologna reform process in the European Union [18], it was of great importance to determine student perception of EC during the 'curricular transition' period. The education reform derived from the European convergence process entailed an educational philosophy that focused more on the student being the learner, than the teacher being a person who teaches [19–21]. In other words, this educational reform involved a transition from traditional teacher-centred learning to interactive student-centred learning. Seeing as no scientific literature was available regarding this curricular transition in Dentistry Schools, we decided to measure EC using the DREEM to determine how students perceived this change and to detect problem areas. Thus, the purpose of this study was to longitudinally evaluate EC for undergraduate dental students in a period of 'curricular transition' brought on by the Bologna reform process.

2. Materials and Methods

2.1. Study Group

We carried out a prospective longitudinal study applying the DREEM questionnaire to undergraduate dental students from the Medicine and Dentistry School, Universidade de Santiago de Compostela (USC), Spain. Ethical approval for the study was obtained from the Universidade de Santiago de Compostela. The students in the sample were from 3rd, 4th, and 5th year courses. Before participating in the survey, students were informed regarding the data processing characteristics, the importance of voluntary participation, and the anonymity of the process. The average questionnaire completion time was approximately 7 min. Questionnaires were distributed to students at the end of several academic years (2010–2011, 2013–2014, 2014–2015, and 2015–2016), which had different curricular configurations: in the 2010–2011 academic year, all courses were taught using a teacher-centred approach, in the 2013–2014 academic year, the 3rd and 4th year courses used a student-centred approach, while 5th year courses used a teacher-centred approach. Finally, in the last two academic years (2014–2015, 2015–2016), all courses used a student-centred approach (Figure 1).

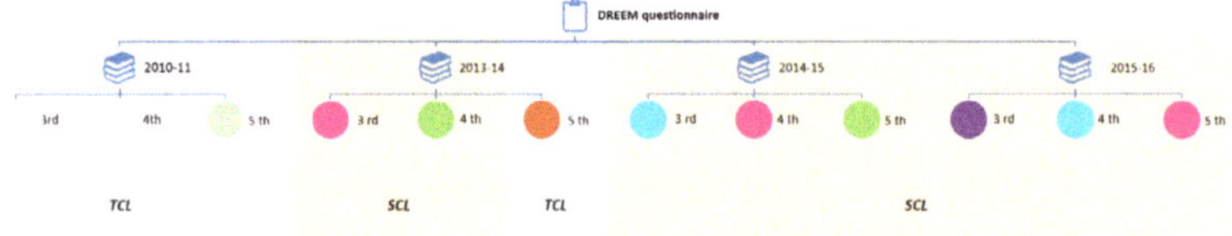

Figure 1. Workflow of study design showing the application of DREEM questionnaire on the different academic years and courses during 'curricular transition'. Each colour represents a different student's dental group indicating the same colour the study follow-up. Abbreviations: TCL, teacher-centred learning; SCL, student-centred learning.

2.2. Data Collection

The instrument used in this study was the DREEM questionnaire (Supplementary Table S1) which consists of 50 items, grouped into five domains: D1. Students' perception of learning (Learning), D2. Students' perception of teachers (Teachers), D3. Students' academic self-perception (Academic), D4. Students' perception of the atmosphere at the centre (Atmosphere) and D5. Students' social self-perception (Social). Each of these items was given a score based on a Likert scale with 5 options ranging from 4 to 0 (4 = strongly agree, 3 = agree, 2 = uncertain, 1 = disagree, 0 = strongly disagree). Nearly all DREEM items include positive statements, except items 4, 8, 9, 17, 25, 35, 39, 48, and 50, which are negative, thus their scores are reversed [10,17]. The mean scores for the different items, domains, and EC were interpreted according to the criteria established by McAleer and Roff et al. [10,22]. Therefore, the items with an average value of ≥3.50 were considered to be "educational aspects of excellence"; those between 3.01 and 3.49 were considered to be "positive educational aspects"; those with average values between 2.01 and 3.00 were considered to be "educational aspects that could be improved"; those ≤2.00 were defined as "problematic educational areas, which should be examined more exhaustively later". The DREEM questionnaire was validated for the Spanish language in 2014 by Tomas et al. [23].

The DREEM scale provides results for each item, for each domain (the sum of the scores of the corresponding items) and total EC score (the sum of the scores of each domain). The maximum possible scores for the different domains are: Learning Perception: 48; Teacher Perception: 44; Academic Perception: 32; Atmosphere Perception: 48 and Social: 28. The maximum score for EC is 200. The data can be expressed as percentages of maximum scores in the respective subscale or the overall scale. Therefore, in relation to the general interpretation of the scale, the higher the score (or percentage) obtained in the different parameters, the more positive perception about the aspect evaluated.

2.3. Statistical Analysis

The data obtained were processed with the PASW Statistics program (SPSS version 2.1) for Windows. The data in the overall assessment of EC, for each domain, and each questionnaire item were expressed as averages. The data in the overall assessment of the EC and for each domain were also expressed as percentages in relation to the maximum score [10]. Non-parametric tests, such as the Kruskal–Wallis test and the Mann–Whitney U test, were used for comparing ordinal EC variables, domains, and items between courses and academic years. Significance level was considered as $p \leq 0.05$. In the case of multiple comparisons between academic years, the Bonferroni correction was applied, establishing a value of $p < 0.008$ as significant. In the case of multiple comparisons between the teaching courses in different academic years, the Bonferroni correction was applied, establishing a p-value < 0.016 as significant.

3. Results

3.1. Description of the Study Group

A total of 397 (70%) dentistry students completed the DREEM questionnaire. There were one hundred and eighteen (29.7%) males and two hundred and seventy-five (69.3%) females (gender data were unavailable for four subjects). The average age was 23.19 ± 4.62 years. Regarding the different courses, there were 117 students in the 3rd course, 119 in the 4th course and 161 in the 5th course.

3.2. Global Analysis of 'Educational Climate'

The overall EC mean was 115.70 ± 20.20 (57.85%), which was interpreted as "more positive than negative EC". According to domain values, all were interpreted as "positive and acceptable". The mean obtained for Learning domain was 25.12 ± 6.04 (52.12%), for Teacher domain was 25.15 ± 5.79 (57.15%), for Academic domain was 19.65 ± 4.11 (61.40%), for Atmosphere domain was 28.44 ± 5.87 (59.25%) and for Social domain was 17.21 ± 3.59 (61.49%) (Table 1 and Figure 2). Social domain was the best-evaluated domain, within the range of "positive and acceptable". Learning domain was the worst-evaluated domain, within the range of "problematic educational aspect". Regarding the total of items derived from the four surveys of each academic year, with 50 items each (total of 200 items), 23.5% were within the range of "problematic educational aspects" (47 items), 68.5% in the range of "educational aspects that could be improved" (137 items) and 8% were "positive educational aspects" (16 items). None was found in the range of "educational aspects of excellence".

Table 1. Mean values (%) of the 'Educational Climate' and the domains of the Dundee Ready Education Environment Measure (DREEM) questionnaire based on academic years.

DREEM	Global Mean (%)	2010–2011 Mean (%)	2013–2014 Mean (%)	2014–2015 Mean (%)	2015–2016 Mean (%)	p-Value *
Educational Climate (EC)	115.70 (57.85%)	118.02 (59.01%)	116.46 (58.23%)	115.60 (57.80%)	112.02 (56.01%)	0.178
Learning (D1)	25.12 (52.12%)	25.94 (54.04%)	25.19 (52.47%)	26.00 (54.1%)	23.31 (48.56%)	0.013
Teachers (D2)	25.15 (57.15%)	26.15 (59.43%)	24.58 (57.07%)	25.09 (55.86%)	24.60 (56%)	0.154
Academic (D3)	19.65 (61.40%)	19.96 (62.37%)	19.82 (61.93%)	19.32 (60.37%)	19.29 (60.28%)	0.663
Atmosphere (D4)	28.44 (59.25%)	28.30 (59.00%)	28.89 (60.18%)	28.57 (59.52%)	28.01 (58.35%)	0.422
Social (D5)	17.21 (61.49%)	17.66 (63.07%)	17.49 (62.46%)	16.60 (59.28%)	16.78 (59.92%)	0.112

* The comparison of the mean values of the items between all academic years was performed by applying the Kruskal-Wallis test.

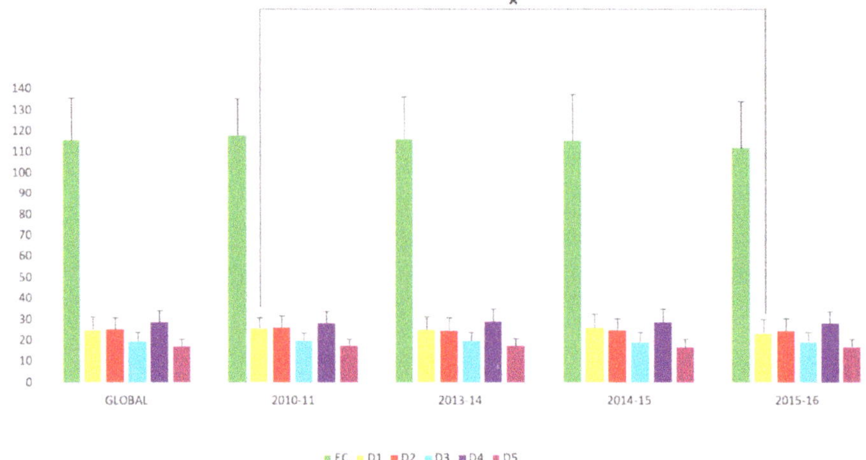

Figure 2. Means of scores and standard deviations for 'Educational Climate' and domains in the Dundee Ready Education Environment Measure (DREEM) questionnaire by academic years. * p-Value < 0.05.

3.3. Analysis of 'Educational Climate' by Academic Year

The mean EC by academic year were as follows: 118.02 ± 17.37 (59.01%) for 2010–2011; 116.46 ± 19.79 (58.23%) for 2013–2014; 115.60 ± 21.93 (57.8%) for 2014–2015; and 112.02 ± 22.28 (56.01%) for 2015–2016. In all academic years, the interpretation for EC was more positive than negative. Although we observed a decrease in EC mean value, the only significant difference was observed in 'Learning domain' ($p = 0.013$) when academic year 2015–2016 was compared to 2010–2011 ($p = 0.003$) and 2014–2015 ($p = 0.009$) (Table 1). The average results obtained for each item with respect to the academic years are shown in Tables 2 and 3. The following eight problematic items were common to all academic years (items 3, 4, 12, 13, 24, 25, 29, and 48): "There is a good support system for students who get stressed", "I am too tired to enjoy this course", "This school is well timetabled", "The teaching is student-centred", "The teaching time is put to good use", "The teaching over-emphasises factual learning", "The teachers are good at providing feedback to students", and "The teaching is too teacher-centred". On the other hand, only two positive items (15 and 46) were common to all academic years: "I have good friends at this school" and "My accommodation is pleasant". In addition, comparing the results among the different academic years, statistically significant differences were observed in 17 items. Three items (18%) belonged to Learning domain (items 1, 7, and 25); another three items (8%) to Teaching domain (items 9, 37, and 40); five items (29%) to Academic domain (items 5, 10, 21, 31 and 45); one item (6%) to Atmosphere domain (item 12) and five items (29%) to Social domain (items 3, 4, 14, 19 and 46). In addition, 47% of these items presented statistically significant differences between courses, with a value ≤ 2 (problematic items) (Supplementary Table S2).

Table 2. Mean values of the 50 items of the Dundee Ready Education Environment Measure (DREEM) questionnaire based on academic years.

Items	2010–2011 Mean	2013–2014 Mean	2014–2015 Mean	2015–2016 Mean
1. I am encouraged to participate in class	2.09	2.35	2.58	2.11
2. The teachers are knowledgeable	2.75	2.61	2.7	2.82
3. There is a good support system for students who get stressed	**0.94**	**1.14**	**1.42**	**0.9**
4. I am too tired to enjoy the course	**1.68**	**1.83**	**1.48**	**1.35**
5. Learning strategies which worked for me before continue to work for me now	2.58	2.54	2.19	2.56
6. The teachers are patient with patients	2.45	2.37	2.27	2.36
7. The teaching is often stimulating	2.22	**1.87**	2.16	**1.83**
8. The teachers ridicule the students	2.54	2.28	2.23	2.16
9. The teachers are authoritarian	**1.67**	**1.56**	2.01	**1.55**
10. I am confident about my passing this year	2.88	3.28	3.1	3.05
11. The atmosphere is relaxed during the ward teaching	2.33	2.23	2.3	2.14
12. This school is well timetabled	**1.13**	**1.67**	**1.55**	**1.19**
13. The teaching is student-centred	**1.77**	**1.74**	**1.71**	**1.57**
14. I am rarely bored on this course	2.27	**1.88**	2.18	**1.86**
15. I have good friends in this school	3.43	3.45	3.12	3.35
16. The teaching helps to develop my competence	2.72	2.75	2.62	2.62
17. Cheating is a problem in this school	2.78	2.48	2.74	2.52
18. The teachers have good communications skills with patients	2.74	2.81	2.53	2.56
19. My social life is good	3.17	3.02	2.75	3.14
20. The teaching is well focused	2.03	**1.96**	2.08	**1.72**
21. I feel I am being well prepared for my profession	**1.94**	**1.68**	2.01	**1.44**
22. The teaching helps to develop my confidence	2.19	2.06	2.18	**1.89**
23. The atmosphere is relaxed during lectures	2.42	2.45	2.44	2.3
24. The teaching time is put to good use	**1.78**	**1.9**	**1.95**	**1.64**
25. The teaching overemphasizes factual learning	**1.68**	**1.68**	**1.78**	**0.88**
26. Last year's work has been good preparation for this year's work	**1.9**	2.11	2.08	2.4
27. I am able to memorize all I need	2.39	2.3	2.41	2.4
28. I seldom feel lonely	2.77	2.71	2.55	2.79
29. The teachers are good at providing feedback to students	**1.93**	**1.93**	**2.00**	**1.7**
30. There are opportunities for me to develop interpersonal skills	2.36	2.55	2.34	2.6
31. I have learned a lot about empathy in my profession	2.71	2.92	2.53	2.7
32. The teachers provide constructive criticism here	2.42	2.21	2.21	2.05
33. I feel comfortable in class socially	2.94	3.03	2.82	3.16
34. The atmosphere is relaxed during seminars/tutorials	2.71	2.65	2.66	2.72
35. I find the experience disappointing	2.49	2.57	2.38	2.23
36. I am able to concentrate well	2.57	2.65	2.49	2.71
37. The teachers give clear examples	2.55	2.21	2.21	2.32
38. I am clear about the learning objectives of the course	2.72	2.57	2.42	2.7
39. The teachers get angry in class	2.17	2.06	2.18	2.07
40. The teachers are well prepared for their classes	2.49	2.21	2.22	2.57

Table 2. *Cont.*

Items	2010–2011 Mean	2013–2014 Mean	2014–2015 Mean	2015–2016 Mean
41. My problem-solving skills are being well developed here	2.63	2.47	2.59	2.38
42. The enjoyment outweighs the stress of the course	2.18	2.05	2.22	1.98
43. The atmosphere motivates me as a learner	2.27	2.27	2.44	2.11
44. The teaching encourages me to be an active learner	2.45	2.3	2.45	2.21
45. Much of what I have to learn seems relevant to a career in health care	2.93	2.61	2.41	2.76
46. My accommodation is pleasant	3.43	3.38	3.1	3.39
47. Long-term learning is emphasized over short term learning	2.68	2.42	2.48	2.6
48. The teaching is too teacher-centred	**1.62**	**1.46**	**1.59**	**1.54**
49. I feel able to ask the questions I want	2.13	2.34	2.19	2.35
50. The students irritate the teachers	2.45	2.21	2.53	2.43

The items (4, 8, 9, 17, 25, 35, 39, 48, and 50) in cursive are negative statements and their scores were reversed. Item with an average of ≤2 are in bold. Items with an average of >3 are underlined.

Table 3. Number, percentage (%) and interpretation of items on the Dundee Ready Education Environment Measure (DREEM) questionnaire by academic years.

Interpretation of Individual Items	2010–2011 (%)	2013–2014 (%)	2014–2015 (%)	2015–2016 (%)
≤2.00 = Educational problematic areas, which should be examined more exhaustively later	11 (22%)	13 (26%)	8 (16%)	15 (30%)
2.01–3.00 = Educational aspects that could be improved	36 (72%)	32 (64%)	39 (78%)	30 (60%)
3.01–3.49 = Positive educational aspects	3 (6%)	5 (10%)	3 (6%)	5 (10%)
≥3.50 = Educational aspects of excellence	0 (0%)	0 (0%)	0 (0%)	0 (0%)

3.4. Analysis of 'Educational Climate' by Teaching Courses

In the 4th course of the 2014–2015 academic year, lower values were observed in all domains (except in the Teaching domain) compared to previous years, although differences were not significant. In addition, this 4th course corresponded to 5th course in the 2015–2016 academic year, where all domains showed significantly lower values in Learning domain as compared to academic years 2010–2011 ($p = 0.001$), 2013–2014 ($p = 0.001$), and 2014–2015 ($p = 0.005$. The overall EC also showed a lower value, although it was not significant ($p = 0.057$) (Table 4).

Table 4. Mean values of the 'Educational Climate' and the domains of the Dundee Ready Education Environment Measure (DREEM) questionnaire of 3rd, 4th and 5th courses on the different academic years.

	2010–2011 Mean ± SD (%)	2013–2014 Mean ± SD (%)	2014–2015 Mean ± SD (%)	2015–2016 Mean ± SD (%)	*p*-Value *
			3rd course		
D1	26.38 ± 4.73 (62.80%)	24.12 ± 7.30 (50.25%)	28.24 ± 4.57 (58.83%)	24.85 ± 7.59 (51.77%)	0.097
D2	27.87 ± 4.84 (63.34%)	24.84 ± 7.18 (56.45%)	25.88 ± 5.33 (58.81%)	25.53 ± 5.46 (58.02%)	0.222
D3	19.38 ± 3.04 (60.58%)	19.51 ± 4.39 (60.96%)	19.72 ± 4.26 (61.62%)	18.14 ± 4.68 (56.68%)	0.588
D4	29.54 ± 5.38 (61.54%)	27.66 ± 6.87 (57.62%)	28.16 ± 5.24 (58.66%)	28.46 ± 6.17 (59.29%)	0.690
D5	17.80 ± 3.19 (63.57%)	16.87 ± 3.49 (60.25%)	16.08 ± 3.49 (57.42%)	16.53 ± 4.25 (59.03%)	0.300
EC	121.00 ± 15.95 (60.50%)	115.06 ± 21.41 (57.53%)	118.08 ± 19.93 (59.04%)	113.53 ± 24.39 (56.76%)	0.481
			4th course		
D1	25.19 ± 4.66 (52.47%)	24.33 ± 5.83 (50.68%)	22.20 ± 7.09 (46.25%)	24.28 ± 4.90 (50.58%)	0.325
D2	26.10 ± 5.21 (59.31%)	23.46 ± 4.93 (53.31%)	25.45 ± 5.05 (55.56%)	26.14 ± 5.75 (59.40%)	0.181
D3	19.50 ± 3.2 (60.93%)	18.86 ± 4.58 (58.93%)	17.10 ± 4.06 (53.43%)	19.28 ± 4.30 (60.25%)	0.116

Table 4. *Cont.*

	2010–2011 Mean ± SD (%)	2013–2014 Mean ± SD (%)	2014–2015 Mean ± SD (%)	2015–2016 Mean ± SD (%)	p-Value *
D4	27.32 ± 5.5 (56.91%)	28.22 ± 6.09 (58.79%)	26.35 ± 6.81 (54.89%)	28.47 ± 5.14 (59.31%)	0682
D5	17.17 ± 3.45 (61.31%)	16.36 ± 4.23 (58.42%)	16.00 ± 3.30 (57.14%)	17.19 ± 2.89 (61.39%)	0.631
EC	115.30 ± 17.15 (57.65%)	112.00 ± 20.72 (60.00%)	107.10 ± 20.58 (53.55%)	115.38 ± 18.40 (57.69%)	0.558
			5th course		
D1	26.41 ± 4.90 (55.02%)	26.59 ± 5.20 (55.39%)	26.71 ± 6.07 (55.64%)	21.77 ± 6.94 (45.35%)	0.001 **
D2	24.95 ± 5.87 (5670%)	25.13 ± 6.46 (57.11%)	24.14 ± 5.5 (54.86%)	23.40 ± 5.8 (53.18%)	0.464
D3	20.88 ± 3.60 (65.25%)	20.68 ± 3.63 (64.62%)	20.57 ± 4.8 (64.28%)	19.95 ± 4.4 (62.34%)	0.566
D4	28.44 ± 5.53 (59.25%)	30.26 ± 5.24 (63.04%)	30.53 ± 6.57 (63.60%)	27.43 ± 5.77 (57.14%)	0.064
D5	18.09 ± 2.74 (64.60%)	18.65 ± 3.09 (66.60%)	17.50 ± 4.54 (62.50%)	16.65 ± 3.75 (59.46%)	0.123
EC	118.79 ± 18.53 (59.39%)	120.68 ± 17.3 (60.34%)	119.46 ± 23.6 (59.73%)	109.22 ± 22.9 (53.61%)	0.057

* The comparison of the mean values of the items between all academic years was performed by applying the Kruskal–Wallis test. ** p-Value < 0.05.

4. Discussion

To the best of our knowledge, the present study represents the first longitudinal analysis of EC, in a period of 'curricular transition' in Dentistry. EC is considered the expression and manifestation of the curriculum. It represents a critical element of the analysis of the quality of the teaching-learning process [2,24]. Our analysis of EC in different academic years and courses facilitates the detection of strengths and weaknesses from the student perspective and may contribute to strategies for educational improvement.

Although the DREEM survey evaluates the perception of teaching in five aspects of learning, it is not designed to analyse specific clinical or laboratory lessons, nor type of dental treatments performed by the students during their training. According to Miles et al. [25] the assessment of student percentages in the DREEM questionnaire provides a different analytical approach to comparing mean scores for overall scale, domains, and items. Keeping this in mind, we have expressed the results as both mean values and percentages. Most Health Science studies have reported EC values between 101–140 (51–70%) [4,9,26–29]. In the dental field, Zamzuri et al. [30] were the first to analyse EC for Dental Assistant and Dental Prosthesis Students from a Dental Training Institute in Malaysia, reporting 62.5% (125/200) and 59% (118/200), respectively. Subsequently, in a study involving 126 students from the Dentistry School of Manipal (India), Thomas et al. [16] found an EC mean of 57% (115/200). In our study, the result obtained for EC was 58% (115.70/200), which is interpreted by other authors as a more positive than negative perception [9,13,16,30,31]. However, higher EC values have been reported in studies conducted in New Zealand, Australia, and Germany [15,32,33]. This positive perception is in accordance with findings reported by members of our team in a multicenter study [17] performed at nine Spanish Public Schools of Dentistry. Our team performed a psychometric validation of the DREEM Spanish-language version involving 1391 students at the same Dentistry Schools. Results from this validation revealed that the Spanish version of the DREEM is a reliable and valid instrument for analysing the EC for dental students. These findings indicate that the DREEM is culturally independent [23].

In the present study, all domain values showed a percentage >52%, which were interpreted as "positive and acceptable". The best score was for Social domain. However, Edgren et al. [34] stated that obtaining optimal results in the general perception of EC and its domains or subscales could mask the existence of specific problems. For this reason, it is very important to analyse the individual values of each questionnaire item [34,35]. We found four items scoring ≥3 in almost every academic year and interpreted as positive: item 15 (I have good friends in this school), item 46 (My accommodation is pleasant), item 10 (I am confident about my passing this year) and item 19 (My social life is good). Our findings are in line with Thomas et al. [16] for item 10 and with Kang et al. [14] for item 15. In our study, most of the positive items were associated with aspects of students' social life. Like other authors [13,15,36,37], we found no excellent items, indicating that improvement measures must continue to be applied to our curriculum and educational environment. A total of forty-seven items (23.5%) were associated with problematic educational areas. The worst score was detected for item 3 ("There is a good support system for students who get stressed"), suggesting that a solution is needed, since stress may lead to worse academic outcomes [16]. In fact, in the study by Tomás et al. [38], item 3 was found to be a problematic aspect for both teachers and students in Spanish Schools of Dentistry. According to a number of studies, the lack of leisure time and anxiety associated with exams could be factors involved in stress [39–42]. It is widely observed that dental studies present high levels of stress associated with manifestations such as insomnia, eating disorders, inability to concentrate, hostility, and depression [43–45]. To improve this educational problem, Avalos et al. [46] proposed the implementation of a more individualized tutoring system and a student 'mentoring' program. Whittle et al. [47] advised the wider promotion and dissemination of existing university student support systems. At present, and in line with the educational reforms associated with the Bologna Process, these measures are being implemented in Spanish Schools of Dentistry. Apart from stress, we found another three negative items: "This school is well timetabled" (item 12), "The teaching over emphasizes factual learning" (item 25) and "The teaching is too teacher-centred" (item 48), which also received negative scores in the study by Ostapczuk et al. [32].

We found students' perceptions of EC to be higher (59.01%) in the traditional curriculum (2010–2011) compared to the Bologna curriculum (2015–2016) (56.01%), although differences were not significant. This means that the development of the new curriculum did not have a significant negative impact on CE in its early years. Only Learning domain showed significant differences between 2010–2011 and 2015–2016 academic years. A higher percentage (30%) of items were identified as 'problematic educational areas' in the 2015–2016 academic year. While Tomás et al. [17] found a lower number of problematic items (14%), other authors reported problematic scores in 28% of items in the later academic years [16]. Of the fifteen total problematic items, eight (items 3, 4, 12, 13, 24, 25, 29, and 48) were present in all academic years and have also been reported by numerous other authors [13,15,36,37]. Unlike various studies [12–15], we did not find item 27 to be problematic, probably due to better memorization methods and more effective task management by students. Considering the problematic items present in all academic years, 50% were involved in the Learning domain (items 13, 24, 25, and 48). This tendency was also reported by Ahmad et al. [36].

With respect to courses and academic years, all domains presented higher values in the academic year 2010–2011. Interestingly, the Learning domain presented a value of 46.25% in the 4th course of the 2014–2015 academic year and 45.35% in the 5th course of the 2015–2016 academic year, reflecting a negative perception of the learning process in courses adapted to the Bologna education reform. Moreover, this domain was the only one that showed statistically significant differences between the 5th course in different academic years. Student perception in the final course is in line with the findings reported by other authors [33,37]. It may be related to the greater responsibility and need for self-learning associated with intensive clinical work.

One of the notable strengths of this study was its prospective longitudinal design. Nevertheless, the limitation that it was conducted at a single institution with a limited sample size should be kept in mind. This study was designed to reveal the problematic educational areas related to the idiosyncrasy of our own institution in order to improve several curricular aspects.

5. Conclusions

Overall, EC and its domains were perceived more positively than negatively by dental students during a period of 'curricular transition'. The Social domain was the most positively evaluated, while the Learning domain was the worst. Our analysis revealed problematic educational areas during the transition from traditional to Bologna curricula, especially related to the Learning domain. The identification of problematic educational areas through the DREEM scale has potential for assessing the educational needs of higher education students to develop strategies for enhancing the teaching-learning process.

Supplementary Materials: The following are available online at http://www.mdpi.com/2304-6767/8/4/133/s1, Table S1: Dundee Ready Education Environment (DREEM) questionnaire (50 items). Table S2: Mean values of the items with statistically significant differences with respect to the academic years.

Author Contributions: Conceptualization, I.T.; methodology, I.T.; formal analysis, I.T.; investigation, A.M.H.-C., I.T., Á.A., Ó.R.-G., and M.M.S.-C.; data curation, A.M.H.-C., I.T., and Á.A.; writing—original draft preparation, Ó.R.-G., M.M.S.-C., and A.M.H.-C.; writing—review and editing, Ó.R.-G. and M.M.S.-C.; visualization, I.T. and P.F.-R.; supervision, M.M.S.-C. and I.T.; project administration, M.M.S.-C. and I.T.; funding acquisition, P.F.-R. All authors have read and agreed to the published version of the manuscript.

Funding: This research received no external funding.

Acknowledgments: The authors wish to thank all participants who completed the questionnaire.

Conflicts of Interest: The authors declare no conflict of interest.

References

1. Rothman, A.I.; Ayoade, F. The development of a learning environment: A questionnaire for use in curriculum evaluation. *J. Med. Educ.* **1970**, *45*, 754–759. [CrossRef] [PubMed]
2. Genn, J.M. AMEE Medical Education Guide No. 23 (Part 1): Curriculum, environment, climate, quality and change in medical education–a unifying perspective. *Med. Teach.* **2001**, *23*, 337–344. [CrossRef] [PubMed]
3. Roff, S.; McAleer, S. What is educational climate? *Med. Teach.* **2001**, *23*, 333–334. [PubMed]
4. Mayya, S.S.; Roff, S. Students' perceptions of educational environment: A comparison of academic achievers and under-achievers at Kasturba Medical College, India. *Educ. Health* **2004**, *17*, 280–291. [CrossRef] [PubMed]
5. Zaini, R. The use of DREEM as curriculum need analysis tool. *Med. Teach.* **2005**, *27*, 385.
6. Denz-Penhey, H.; Murdoch, J.C. A comparison between findings from the DREEM questionnaire and that from qualitative interviews. *Med. Teach.* **2009**, *31*, e449–e453. [CrossRef]
7. Marshall, R.E. Measuring the Medical School learning environment. *Acad. Med.* **1978**, *53*, 98–104. [CrossRef]
8. Gerzina, T.M.; McLean, T.; Fairley, J. Dental clinical teaching: Perceptions of students and teachers. *J. Dent. Educ.* **2005**, *69*, 1377–1384. [CrossRef]
9. Ali, K.; McHarg, J.; Kay, E.; Moles, D.; Tredwin, C.; Coombes, L.; Heffernan, E. Academic environment in a newly established dental school with an enquiry-based curriculum: Perceptions of students from the inaugural cohorts. *Eur. J. Dent. Educ.* **2012**, *16*, 102–109. [CrossRef]
10. Roff, S.; McAleer, S.; Harden, R.; Al-Qahtani, M. Development and validation of the Dundee Ready Education Environment Measure (DREEM). *Med. Teach.* **1977**, *19*, 295–299. [CrossRef]
11. Chan, C.Y.W.; Sum, M.Y.; Tan, G.M.Y.; Tor, P.C.; Sim, K. Adoption and correlates of the Dundee Ready Educational Environment Measure (DREEM) in the evaluation of undergraduate learning environments—A systematic review. *Med. Teach.* **2018**, *40*, 1240–1247. [CrossRef] [PubMed]
12. Ali, K.; Raja, M.; Watson, G.; Coombes, L.; Heffernan, E. The dental school learning milieu: Students' perceptions at five academic dental institutions in Pakistan. *J. Dent. Educ.* **2012**, *76*, 487–494. [CrossRef] [PubMed]
13. Kossioni, A.E.; Varela, R.; Ekonomu, I.; Lyrakos, G.; Dimoliatis, I.D.K. Students' perceptions of the educational environment in a Greek Dental School, as measured by DREEM. *Eur. J. Dent. Educ.* **2012**, *16*, e73–e78. [CrossRef] [PubMed]
14. Kang, I.; Foster Page, L.A.; Anderson, V.R.; Thomson, W.M.; Broadbent, J.M. Changes in students' perceptions of their dental education environment. *Eur. J. Dent. Educ.* **2015**, *19*, 122–130. [CrossRef]
15. Foster Page, L.A.; Kang, M.; Anderson, V.; Thomson, W.M. Appraisal of the Dundee Ready Educational Environment Measure in the New Zealand dental educational environment. *Eur. J. Dent. Educ.* **2012**, *16*, 78–85. [CrossRef]
16. Thomas, B.S.; Abraham, R.R.; Alexander, M.; Ramnarayan, K. Students' perceptions regarding educational environment in an Indian Dental School. *Med. Teach.* **2009**, *31*, e185–e186. [CrossRef]
17. Tomás, I.; Millán, U.; Casares, M.A.; Abad, M.; Ceballos, L.; Gómez-Moreno, G.; Hidalgo, J.J.; Llena, C.; López-Jornet, P.; Machuca, M.C.; et al. Analysis of the 'educational climate' in Spanish public schools of dentistry using the Dundee Ready Education Environment Measure: A multicenter study. *Eur. J. Dent. Educ.* **2013**, *17*, 159–168. [CrossRef]

18. Oliver, R.; Sanz, M. The Bologna Process and health science education: Times are changing. *Med. Educ.* **2007**, *41*, 309–317. [CrossRef]
19. Rich, S.K.; Keim, R.G.; Shuler, C.F. Problem-based learning versus a traditional educational methodology: A comparison of preclinical and clinical periodontics performance. *J. Dent. Educ.* **2005**, *69*, 649–662. [CrossRef]
20. Shanley, D.B. Dental education and dentistry in Europe. *J. Am. Coll. Dent.* **2007**, *74*, 4–8.
21. Plasschaert, A.J.M.; Manogue, M.; Lindh, C.; McLoughlin, J.; Murtomaa, H.; Nattestad, A.; Sanz, M. Curriculum content, structure and ECTS for European Dental Schools. Part II: Methods of learning and teaching, assessment procedures and performance criteria. *Eur. J. Dent. Educ.* **2007**, *11*, 125–136. [CrossRef] [PubMed]
22. McAleer, S.; Roff, S. A practical guide to using the Dundee Ready Education Environment Measure (DREEM). AMEE Medical Education Guide No. 23. *Med. Teach.* **2001**, *23*, 29–33.
23. Tomás, I.; Casares-De-Cal, M.A.; Aneiros, A.; Abad, M.; Ceballos, L.; Gómez-Moreno, G.; Hidalgo, J.J.; Llena, C.; López-Jornet, P.; Machuca, M.C.; et al. Psychometric validation of the Spanish version of the Dundee Ready Education Environment Measure applied to dental students. *Eur. J. Dent. Educ.* **2014**, *18*, 162–169. [CrossRef] [PubMed]
24. Harden, R.M. The learning environment and the curriculum. *Med. Teach.* **2001**, *23*, 335–336. [CrossRef]
25. Miles, S.; Leinster, S.J. Comparing staff and student perceptions of the student experience at a new Medical School. *Med. Teach.* **2009**, *31*, 539–546. [CrossRef] [PubMed]
26. Al-Mohaimeed, A. Perceptions of the educational environment of a new Medical School, Saudi Arabia. *Int. J. Health Sci.* **2013**, *7*, 150–159. [CrossRef] [PubMed]
27. Vaughan, B.; Carter, A.; Macfarlane, C.; Morrison, T. The DREEM, part 1: Measurement of the educational environment in an osteopathy teaching program. *BMC Med. Educ.* **2014**, *14*, 99. [CrossRef]
28. Jiffry, M.T.M.; McAleer, S.; Fernando, S.; Marasinghe, R.B. Using the DREEM questionnaire to gather baseline information on an evolving Medical School in Sri Lanka. *Med. Teach.* **2005**, *27*, 348–352. [CrossRef]
29. Ousey, K.; Stephenson, J.; Brown, T.; Garside, J. Investigating perceptions of the academic educational environment across six undergraduate health care courses in the United Kingdom. *Nurse Educ. Pract.* **2014**, *14*, 24–29. [CrossRef]
30. Zamzuri, A.T.; Azli, N.A.; Roff, S.; McAleer, S. How do students at dental training college Malaysia perceived their educational environment? *Malays. Dent. J.* **2004**, *25*, 15–26.
31. Stratulat, S.I.; Candel, O.S.; Tăbîrţă, A.; Checheriţă, L.E.; Costan, V.V. The perception of the educational environment in multinational students from a dental medicine faculty in Romania. *Eur. J. Dent. Educ.* **2019**, *24*, 193–198. [CrossRef] [PubMed]
32. Ostapczuk, M.S.; Hugger, A.; de Bruin, J.; Ritz-Timme, S.; Rotthoff, T. DREEM on, dentists! Students' perceptions of the educational environment in a German Dental School as measured by the Dundee Ready Education Environment Measure. *Eur. J. Dent. Educ.* **2012**, *16*, 67–77. [CrossRef] [PubMed]
33. Stormon, N.; Ford, P.J.; Eley, D.S. DREEM-ing of dentistry: Students' perception of the academic learning environment in Australia. *Eur. J. Dent. Educ.* **2019**, *23*, 35–41. [CrossRef] [PubMed]
34. Edgren, G.; Haffling, A.C.; Jakobsson, U.; Mcaleer, S.; Danielsen, N. Comparing the educational environment (as measured by DREEM) at two different stages of curriculum reform. *Med. Teach.* **2010**, *32*, e233–e238. [CrossRef]
35. Herrera, C.; Pacheco, J.; Rosso, F.; Cisterna, C.; Aichele, D.; Becker, S.; Padilla, O.; Riquelme, A. Evaluation of the undergraduate educational environment in six Medical Schools in Chile. *Rev. Med. Chile* **2010**, *138*, 677–684.
36. Ahmad, M.S.; Bhayat, A.; Fadel, H.T.; Mahrous, M.S. Comparing dental students perceptions of their educational environment in Northwestern Saudi Arabia. *Saudi Med. J.* **2015**, *36*, 477–483. [CrossRef]
37. Doshi, D.; Srikanth Reddy, B.; Karunakar, P.; Deshpande, K. Evaluating student's perceptions of the learning environment in an indian dental school. *J. Clin. Diagn. Res.* **2014**, *8*, ZC43–ZC47. [CrossRef]
38. Tomás, I.; Aneiros, A.; Casares-de-Cal, M.A.; Quintas, V.; Prada-López, I.; Balsa-Castro, C.; Ceballos, L.; Gómez-Moreno, G.; Llena, C.; López-Jornet, P.; et al. Comparing student and staff perceptions of the 'Educational Climate' in Spanish Dental Schools using the Dundee Ready Education Environment Measure. *Eur. J. Dent. Educ.* **2017**, *22*, e131–e141. [CrossRef]
39. Rajab, L. Perceived sources of stress among dental students at the University of Jordan. *J. Dent. Educ.* **2001**, *65*, 232–241. [CrossRef]

40. Bradley, I.; Clark, D.; Eisner, J.; De Gruchy, K.; Singer, D.; Hinkleman, K.; Gelskey, S.; Wood, W. The student survey of problems in the academic environment in Canadian Dental Faculties. *J. Dent. Educ.* **1989**, *53*, 126–131. [CrossRef]
41. Sanders, A.E.; Lushington, K. Sources of stress for Australian dental students. *J. Dent. Educ.* **1999**, *63*, 688–697. [CrossRef] [PubMed]
42. Schaufeli, W.B.; Salanova, M. Efficacy or inefficacy, that's the question: Burnout and work engagement, and their relationships with efficacy beliefs. *Anxiety Stress. Coping* **2007**, *20*, 177–196. [CrossRef] [PubMed]
43. Morse, Z.; Dravo, U. Stress levels of dental students at the Fiji School of Medicine. *Eur. J. Dent. Educ.* **2007**, *11*, 99–103. [CrossRef] [PubMed]
44. Polychronopoulou, A.; Divaris, K. A longitudinal study of Greek dental students' perceived sources of stress. *J. Dent. Educ.* **2010**, *74*, 524–530. [CrossRef] [PubMed]
45. Pau, A.K.H.; Croucher, R. Emotional intelligence and perceived stress in dental undergraduates. *J. Dent. Educ.* **2003**, *67*, 1023–1028. [CrossRef] [PubMed]
46. Avalos, G.; Dunne, F.; Freeman, C. Determining the quality of the medical educational environment at an Irish Medical School using the DREEM inventory. *Ir. Med. J.* **2007**, *100*, 522–530.
47. Whittle, S.R.; Whelan, B.; Murdoch-Eaton, D.G. DREEM and beyond; studies of the educational environment as a means for its enhancement. *Educ. Health* **2007**, *20*, 7.

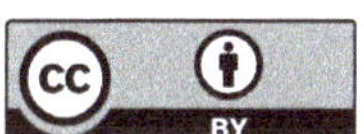

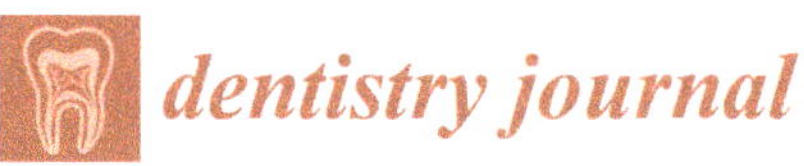

MDPI

Article

Improvement of the Working Environment and Daily Work-Related Tasks of Dental Hygienists Working in Private Dental Offices from the Japan Dental Hygienists' Association Survey 2019

Yoshiaki Nomura [1,*], Yuki Ohara [2,3], Yuko Yamamoto [4], Ayako Okada [5], Noriyasu Hosoya [4], Nobuhiro Hanada [1] and Noriko Takei [2]

1 Department of Translational Research, Tsurumi University School of Dental Medicine, Yokohama 230-8501, Japan; hanada-n@tsurumi-u.ac.jp
2 Japan Dental Hygienists' Association, Tokyo 169-0071, Japan; yohara@tmig.or.jp (Y.O.); nori@pm-ms.tepm.jp (N.T.)
3 Tokyo Metropolitan Institute of Gerontology, Tokyo 173-0015, Japan
4 Department of Endodontology, Tsurumi University School of Dental Medicine, Yokohama 230-8501, Japan; yamamoto-y@tsurumi-u.ac.jp (Y.Y.); hosoya-n@tsurumi-u.ac.jp (N.H.)
5 Department of Operative Dentistry, Tsurumi University School of Dental Medicine, Yokohama 230-8501, Japan; okada-a@tsurumi-u.ac.jp
* Correspondence: nomura-y@tsurumi-u.ac.jp

Citation: Nomura, Y.; Ohara, Y.; Yamamoto, Y.; Okada, A.; Hosoya, N.; Hanada, N.; Takei, N. Improvement of the Working Environment and Daily Work-Related Tasks of Dental Hygienists Working in Private Dental Offices from the Japan Dental Hygienists' Association Survey 2019. *Dent. J.* **2021**, *9*, 22. https://doi.org/10.3390/dj9020022

Academic Editors: Jelena Dumancic and Božana Lončar Brzak

Received: 19 January 2021
Accepted: 17 February 2021
Published: 19 February 2021

Publisher's Note: MDPI stays neutral with regard to jurisdictional claims in published maps and institutional affiliations.

Abstract: A dental hygienist performs various daily work-related tasks. The aim of this study was to elucidate the daily work-related tasks of Japanese dental hygienists and construct groups to understand the relationships between daily work-related tasks, the attractiveness of dental hygienist work, and the improvement of the working environment. The Japan Dental Hygienists' Association has conducted a postal survey on the employment status of dental hygienists in Japan every five years since 1981. The data on the implementation of 74 daily work-related tasks in dental offices were analyzed from the survey carried out in 2019. The questionnaires were distributed to 16,722 dental hygienists and 8932 were returned (collection rate: 53.4%). The 3796 dental hygienists working at dental clinics were clearly classified into nine groups. Full-time workers requested a reduced workload. Part-time workers requested better treatment rather than reducing the workload. Salary and human relationships were common problems with the working environment. Full-time workers felt that job security was an attractive feature of the dental hygienist role. The data presented in this study may help with the improvement of working conditions for dental hygienists.

Keywords: dental hygienists; job satisfaction; work assignments; workplace environment; Japan

1. Introduction

Dental hygienists play an important role in promoting oral health [1–8]. The demand has increased for dental hygienists. Even though the laws of each country regulate the range of work completed by dental hygienists, various skills are required for daily work-related tasks. The demand for dental hygienists has expanded in Japan. For example, the evaluation and improvement of oral health has been introduced in the Japanese national insurance system [9]. Dental hygienists need to have a medical team approach for the improvement of oral hygiene of compromised patients [10–14].

The Japanese law on dental hygienists declares that their main task is the improvement of oral health nationwide. The scope of the work of dental hygienists is oral care and oral health guidance under the supervision of a dentist, cleaning teeth, the mechanical removal of deposits on the tooth surface over the gingival margin, and assistance with dental treatment. Their assistance with dental treatment has been expanded. Therefore, there is a need to understand the situation of dental hygienists. This information is useful to promote a medical team approach for the medical and dental treatment of patients with compromised health. It also available for utilizing limited social capital and influencing policymaking. This information is available for many countries other than Japan. However, gathering information on the real work-related tasks of dental hygienists is not enough.

The Japan Dental Hygienists' Association conducts a survey of dental hygienists every five years, assessing a wide range of items [15]. In 2019, for dental hygienists working in dental clinics, 74 kinds of daily work-related tasks and requests for an improved working environment were included in the questionnaire. Through these items, the daily working tasks of dental hygienists were elucidated. In addition to descriptive statistics, summarizing the information by statistical modeling is effective for understanding the various daily work-related tasks of dental hygienists.

The aim of this study was to elucidate the daily work-related tasks of Japanese's dental hygienists and present the information effectively by clustering. There has been no report that has analyzed almost all of the daily work-related tasks of dental hygienists. In addition, requests for improvement of the working environment and the attractiveness of dental hygienists' work were analyzed. The results of this study may be useful for the improvement of working conditions of dental hygienists and could have an effect on the policymaking process.

2. Materials and Methods

2.1. Survey Method

The Japan Dental Hygienists' Association has conducted a postal survey on the employment status of dental hygienists in Japan every five years since 1981 [15]. As this survey was supported by the Japanese government, it conformed to the national survey guidelines. On 1 October 2019, the questionnaire, including a stamped envelope for return, was distributed to all 16,722 members of the Japan Dental Hygienists' Association by mail. The return date was set for 11 November.

2.2. Questionnaire

The questionnaire used in this study consisted of 104 major items related to demographic factors, employment status, daily work-related tasks, willingness to work, etc. The questionnaire consisted of 40 common major items for all dental hygienists, including requests for the improvement of working conditions and the attractiveness of work of dental hygienists, and 11 major items for the dental hygienists working at dental clinics, including implementation of 74 daily work-related tasks in dental offices. In this study, data on dental hygienists working in dental clinics were analyzed. A total of 74 daily work-related tasks were classified into 3 major categories: preventive dental treatment, assistance work, and dental office management. Preventive dental treatment consisted of 3 items and dental office management consisted of 7 items. Assistance work was subcategorized into 10 categories: medical interviews (5), examinations (11), periodontal treatment (4), oral function (2), restorative procedures (9), orthodontic treatment (7), dental implants (5), medical treatment (5), special care dentistry (9), and health instructions (7). Numbers indicated the items for daily work-related tasks. These tasks are listed with the descriptive statistics in Table S1.

The attractiveness of dental hygienists' work consisted of 7 items: national license, highly specialized occupation, stable employment, stable income, contribution to people and society, maintaining health and life, and directly helping people. Requests for the improvement of working conditions consisted of 13 items: a rise in salary, reducing workload, working relationships, reduced working hours, flexibility in terms of days off and vacation, improvement of parenting support, improvement of nursing care support, valuing of professionalism, opportunities for improving skills, flexibility in terms of work and working hours, improving medical safety systems, ensuring employment stability, and improvement of the employee benefits system.

2.3. Statistical Analysis

2.3.1. IRT Analysis

A three-parameter logistic model with item response theory (IRT) analysis was applied to calculate the item discriminations, item difficulties, and item guesses for the work-related tasks [15]. Item response and item information curves were presented for each work-related task. The analyses were carried out in R ver. 3.50 software with the LTR and irtoys packages using the following formula:

$$P_i(\theta) = \frac{(1 - c_i)}{1 + e^{-Da_i(\theta - b_i)}}$$

2.3.2. Ordination Analysis

For the classification of daily work-related tasks, we applied t-distributed stochastic neighbor embedding (tSNE) analysis. Scatter plots of each dental hygienist were illustrated by 2 dimensions, obtained by tSNE analysis. Using this scatter plot, classification was carried out and the clusters were named groups. To find the rules of classification, we carried out decision analyses by Quick, Unbiased and Efficient Statistical Tree (QUEST). tSNE analysis was performed by R software ver. 3.50 with vegan, and Rtsne package. Decision analysis was carried out by SPSS v. 24.0 (IBM, Tokyo, Japan).

2.3.3. Correspondence Analysis

A dataset of cross-tabulation for the prevalence of dental caries was used for network plot and correspondence analysis. Network plot was performed by SPSS Modeler Ver.18.0 (IBM, Tokyo, Japan), and correspondence analysis was performed by SPSS Statistics Ver 24.0 (IBM, Tokyo, Japan).

2.4. Ethical Approval and Consent to Participate

This study was approved by the Ethics Committee of the Tsurumi University School of Dental Medicine (approval number: 1837) and conducted in accordance with the Declaration of Helsinki. Informed written consent was obtained from all participants.

3. Results

3.1. Characteristic of the Subjects Analyzed in This Study

From 8932 dental hygienists, responses were returned (collection rate: 8932/16,722, 53.4%). Their working places were dental clinic—3796 (42.5%), hospital—1307 (14.6%), government—913 (10.2%), nursing home—367 (4.1%), leaving jobs—1063 (11.9%), and other—1486 (16.6%). Their educational backgrounds were graduated from university—6811 (76.3%), master's course—108 (1.2%), doctoral course—59 (0.7%), junior college—1245 (14.0%), dental hygienist school—6881 (77.1%), and no answer—83 (0.9%). Among the 3796 dental hygienists working at dental clinics, the mean age and career length were 45.3 ± 12.2 years old, median: 47.0 (25th–75th: 37–54), and 19.2 ± 11.3 years, median: 20 (25th–75th: 10–27), respectively. Age and carrier were not normally distributed by Kolmogorov–Smirnov test. Among them, the number of full-time workers was 2064 (54.4%) and the number of part-time workers was 1732 (45.6%). Descriptive statistics of the items analyzed in this study are presented in Tables S1 and S2.

3.2. Analysis of Daily Tasks by Item Response Theory

The daily work-related tasks of dental hygienists were analyzed independently by item response theory by the categories presented in Section 2.2. The item response curves that had the highest item information of each category are shown in Figure 1. The item response and item information curves of prevention and assistant works are shown in Figure S1. By the item response theory, we calculated the abilities of the dental hygienists and used them for the following analysis. Models by IRT are shown in Table S3.

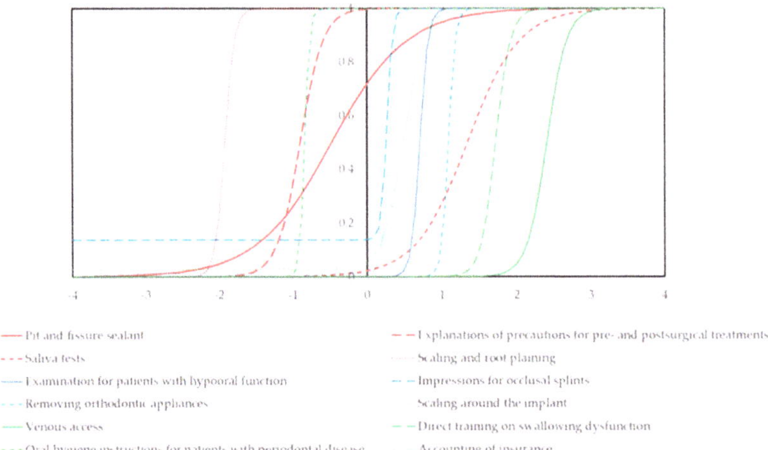

Figure 1. Item response curve of representative dental hygienists' daily tasks. From all dental hygienists' daily work-related tasks, the items that had the highest item information in each category are presented. All of the item response and information curves of the daily work-related tasks are shown in Figure S1.

3.3. Classification of Daily Tasks by the SNE Analysis

By using the ability of each job category calculated by IRT analysis, we classified the dental hygienists. For the classification, t-distributed stochastic neighbor embedding (tSNE) analysis was applied. The results are shown in Figure 2. Each dental hygienist was clearly classified by the tSNE analysis. Cross-tabulation of groups and 74 kinds of daily work-related tasks are shown in Table S4. For each group, the mean and median of the ability calculated by IRT analysis are shown in Table S3. In this table, each group is characterized (Table 1). Additionally, the rules of each group were analyzed by Quick, Unbiased and Efficient Statistical Tree (QUEST) analysis. The results are shown in Figure S2 and were consistent with the results shown in Table 1.

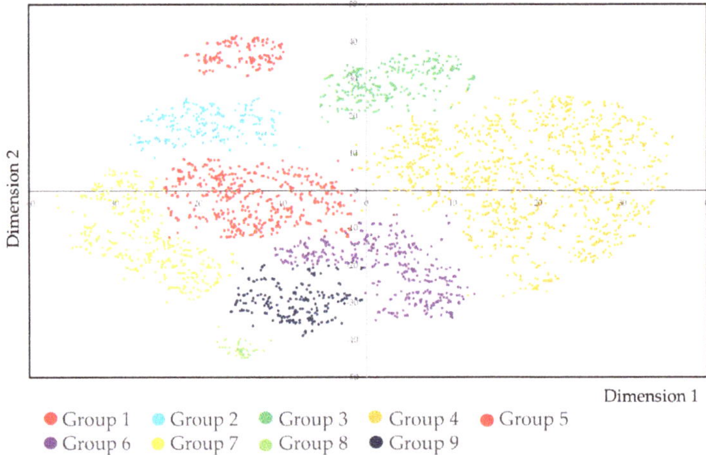

Figure 2. t-distributed stochastic neighbor embedding (tSNE) plot by ability, calculated by item response theory (IRT) analysis of the daily work-related tasks of dental hygienists. Ability indicates the weighted number of implemented daily work-related tasks. Dental hygienists participating in this study were clearly classified by the implementation of daily work-related tasks. tSNE: t-distributed stochastic neighbor embedding.

Table 1. Characteristics of the groups by tSNE analysis.

		Group 1	Group 2	Group 3	Group 4	Group 5	Group 6	Group 7	Group 8	Group 9
		$n = 156$	$n = 264$	$n = 299$	$n = 1381$	$n = 529$	$n = 449$	$n = 428$	$n = 55$	$n = 235$
Preventive dental care		+	+	+	+	+	+			
Assistance work	Periodontal treatment	+	+	+	+	+		+		
	Medical treatment	+								
	Special care dentistry	+								
	Orthodontic treatment		+	+					+	
	Dental implants	+		+						
	Health instructions	+	+	+	+					

The "+" show that the median of ability exceeded the 75th percentile of ability calculated for the whole sample. This indicates that dental hygienists in each group implemented the daily work-related tasks more frequently than the third quartile. Group 9 had no characteristic tasks. Median and mean values of all daily work-related tasks are shown in Table S3.

The characteristic daily work-related tasks implemented in each group were as follows:
Group 1: Medical treatment, special care dentistry, and dental implants;
Group 2: Orthodontic treatment, preventive dental care, and periodontal treatment;
Group 3: Dental implants, orthodontic treatment, preventive dental care, and periodontal treatment;
Group 4: Health instructions, preventive dental care, and periodontal treatment;
Group 5: Preventive dental care and periodontal treatment;
Group 6: Preventive dental care;
Group 7: Periodontal treatment;
Group 8: Specialized orthodontic treatment;
Group 9: No specific tasks.

Cross-tabulation of the group and employment status is shown in Table S5. The proportion of part-time workers was higher in groups 4, 5, 6, 7, and 9.

3.4. The Contribution of Daily Tasks to the Attractiveness of Dental Hygienists' Work, and Improvement of Working Environment

3.4.1. Contribution of Daily Tasks to the Improvement of the Working Environment

The questionnaire asked about requested improvements of the working environment and the attractiveness of dental hygienists' work, with 14 and 7 items, respectively. For these items, cross-tabulations were constructed against the groups. The results are shown in Table S5. To visualize the results, we carried out a correspondence analysis. The results of requested improvements to the working environment are shown in Figure 3.

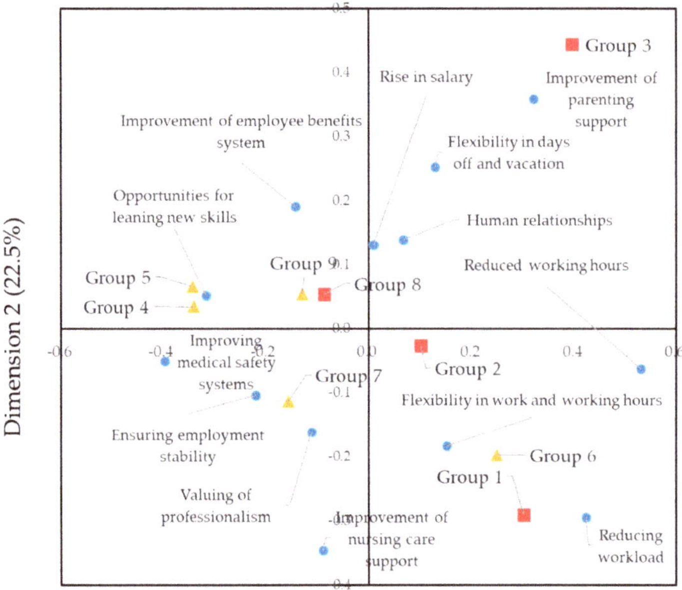

Figure 3. Biplot of groups by daily tasks and requests for improvement of the working environment. The results of the corresponding analysis are graphically illustrated as a biplot. Items with similar characteristics are plotted closely and the smaller the angle in relation to a given point, the stronger the relation. Blue circles indicate requested improvements of the working conditions. Red squares indicate groups in which the proportion of full-time workers is high. Yellow triangles indicate groups in which the proportion of part-time workers is high. The contribution ratio of dimension 1 was 67.8% and for dimension 2 it was 22.5%.

Groups 1 and 6 were surrounded by reduced working hours, reduced workload, and flexibility of work and working hours. The angle between flexibility of work in groups 1 and 6 were smaller than in group 2. This indicated that the correlations flexibility of work in groups 1 and 6 were stronger than group 2. Group 1, in which the proportion of full-time workers was high, was located near the reduced working load. The opportunity to improve one's skills was located near groups 4 and 5, in which the proportion of part-time workers was high. Ensuring employment stability and a rise in salary were located near groups 8 and 9. The correlations between ensuring employment stability in group 7 was stronger than in groups 8 and 9.

3.4.2. Contribution of Daily Tasks to the Attractiveness of Dental Hygienists' Work

A biplot of the groups and the attractiveness of dental hygienists' work is shown in Figure 4. Stable income and stable employment were in the negative direction. When focused on dimension 1, groups 1, 2, and 8, in which the proportion of full-time workers was high, were located in the negative direction. Associations between stable income and employment with these groups were higher than other groups. These results indicated that the values of the regular employee were different from part-time workers.

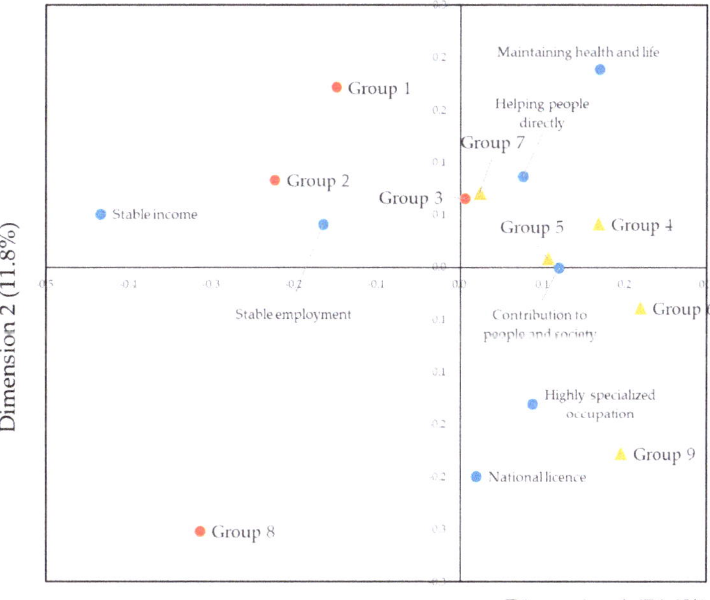

Figure 4. Biplot of groups by daily tasks and the attractiveness of dental hygienists' work. Blue circles indicate the attractiveness of dental hygienists' work. Red squares indicate groups in which the proportion of full-time workers were high. Yellow triangles indicate groups in which the proportion of part-time workers were high. The contribution ratio of dimension 1 was 76.4% and that of dimension 2 was 11.8%.

4. Discussion

In this study, 74 of Japanese dental hygienists' daily work-related tasks were analyzed by statistical modeling. Dental hygienists were clustered by the implementation of these tasks.

The role of a dental hygienist covers both clinical and health promotion responsibilities. The clinical practices allowed by law vary between countries. In the USA, the work performed by dental hygienists differs between states. Most states allow scaling, fluoride application, and pit and fissure sealants. Some states allow X-ray exposure. In the UK, scaling, tooth cleaning, pit and fissure sealants, impressions, X-ray exposure, and administering a local anesthetic are allowed. In Japan, fit and fissure sealants, X-ray exposure, impressions, and administering a local anesthetic are not allowed. Only assisting a dentist with these procedures is allowed. Therefore, in order to extrapolate the results of this study to countries other than Japan, one may refer to Figure S1 as a useful tool. All of the tasks, including assisting dentists, were analyzed by IRT.

Professional and personal life, income and job security, and quality of service are all important factors affecting the job satisfaction of dental hygienists [16]. The characteristics of the groups in terms of the attractiveness of the job and requests for improvements of the working environment were investigated. The item response and item information curves presented in Figure S1 provide valuable information beyond simple descriptive statistics.

Item information curves located in the negative direction and with high item information were "prophylactic calculus removal" (Figure S1A), "scaling and root planing" (Figure S1D), and "oral hygiene instruction for patients with periodontal disease" (Figure S1K). The frequencies of these tasks were 3593 (94.7%), 3681 (97.0%), and 3258 (92.8%), respectively. These results indicated that most dental hygienists implemented these tasks. Initially, dental hygienists performed prophylaxis [17]. If dental hygienists implemented these tasks, they also implemented other tasks within the preventive dental treatment, periodontal treatment, and medical and dental guidance. Consistent with previous study, these tasks were common in the groups presented in Table 1.

In contrast to these tasks, item response and item information curves were located in the forward direction for "examination" (Figure S1C), "orthodontic treatment" (Figure S1G), "medical treatment" (Figure S1I), and "special care dentistry" (Figure S1J). These tasks were implemented by a limited number of dental hygienists. When dental hygienists implemented the tasks with high item information, they implemented other tasks within the groups of tasks.

In addition to these tasks, dental hygienists implemented dental office management. "Sterilization and disinfection of dental equipment" was implemented by 3353 (88.3%) of dental hygienists and "management and ordering of drugs and dental equipment" by 2930 (77.1%). These tasks are not necessarily specialties of dental hygienists. Division of labor is necessary to reduce the workload of dental hygienists.

From the tSNE analysis, we found that dental hygienists were clearly classified. For the groups and requests for improvement of working conditions, full-time workers were located in the forward direction and part-time workers were located in the negative direction when we focused on dimension 1. Reducing working hours and reducing workload were located in the forward direction. The results indicated that full-time dental hygienists work too hard and thus reducing the workload is necessary. A previous report had shown that 68% of dental hygienists experience unmanageable workloads [18]. In this study, 1625 (42.9%) dental hygienists answered "Yes" to the question about "reducing workload." The difference may be derived from the difference in proportion of part-time workers. The part-time workers requested "opportunities for improving one's skills," "improvement of employee benefits system," "ensuring employment stability," and "valuing professionalism." Dental hygienists sought to expand their activities [19]. Dental hygienists actively participated in continuing education after career breaks and engaged as part-time workers [20]. These results suggest that, for part-time workers, better treatment was more important than reducing their workload. It was related to the job satisfaction of dental hygienists [18]. Dental hygienists' workplace satisfaction was associated with their salary [18,20]. A rise in salary was located in the center of dimension 1. This indicates that getting a raise is a common problem, independent of the groups classified by the tSNE analysis. Psychosocial health is important for dental hygienists [21,22]. Human relationships were located near the center, indicating that they represent a common problem for dental hygienists [23]. The results were consistent with previous studies.

In terms of the attractiveness of dental hygienists' work and groups, full-time workers were located in the negative direction and part-time workers in the forward direction. "Stable income" and "stable employment" were located in the negative direction. Full-time workers felt that job security was an attractive feature of dental hygienists' work. In contrast, "maintaining health and life," "contribution to people and society," and "helping people directly" were located in the forward direction. Part-time workers felt the work was more attractive than full-time workers.

There are several limitations of this study. The response rate was not high, and the sample only included members of the Japan Dental Hygienists' Association. The members of the Japan Dental Hygienists' Association are dental hygienists who are willing to study and improve their skills. This included a small number of dental hygienists who had lost their willingness to work. However, this may be the first report to analyze the daily work-related tasks of dental hygienists and their association with job satisfaction. The work-related tasks of dental hygienists vary between countries. The results of each task are applicable to countries other than Japan.

5. Conclusions

The attractiveness of dental hygienists' work and requests for improvement of the working environment largely depend on the daily work-related tasks and working style. To improve the job satisfaction of dental hygienists, there must be an improvement in working conditions corresponding to the daily work-related tasks and working style. The groups constructed by daily work-related tasks may help with the effective improvement of working conditions of dental hygienists.

Supplementary Materials: The following are available online at https://www.mdpi.com/2304-6767/9/2/22/s1, Figure S1: Item response and item information curves of daily tasks of dental hygienists. Figure S2: Decision tree to find out the groups classified by tSNE analysis. Table S1: Cross-tabulation of groups and 74 dental hygienists' daily work-related tasks in dental offices. Table S2: Cross-tabulation of items related to the attractiveness of dental hygienists' work, and the improvement of working conditions. Table S3: Results of three parameter logistic models for daily work-related tasks. Table S4: Mean and median of the ability calculated by IRT analysis of each group. Table S5: Employment status in each group.

Author Contributions: Conceptualization, methodology, validation, and investigation, Y.N., Y.O., and N.T.; software, formal analysis, writing—original draft preparation, writing—review and editing, and visualization, Y.N.; resources, project administration, and funding acquisition, Y.O. and N.T.; data curation, Y.Y. and A.O.; supervision, N.H. (Noriyasu Hosoya), N.H. (Nobuhiro Hanada), and N.T. All authors have read and agreed to the published version of the manuscript.

Funding: This research was funded by JSPS KAKENHI (grant numbers 17K12030 and 20K10303), SECOM Science and Technology Foundation, and the annual fund of the Japan Dental Hygienists' Association. None of the funders played a role in the design of the study, data collection, analysis, interpretation of the results, or writing of the manuscript.

Institutional Review Board Statement: This study was approved by the ethics committee of the Tsurumi University School of Dental Medicine (approval number: 1837) and conducted in accordance with the Declaration of Helsinki. Informed written consent was obtained from all participants.

Informed Consent Statement: Informed consent was obtained from all subjects involved in the study.

Data Availability Statement: Data are available from the corresponding author upon reasonable request.

Conflicts of Interest: The authors declare no conflict of interest.

References

1. Mishler, S.K.; Inglehart, M.R.; McComas, M.J.; Kinch, C.A.; Kinney, J.S. General Dentists' Perceptions of Dental Hygienists' Professional Role: A Survey. *J. Dent. Hyg.* **2018**, *92*, 30–39.
2. Watson, R. How does the "new" definition of Oral health and the recent World Oral Health survey impact dental hygienists? *Int. J. Dent. Hyg.* **2017**, *15*, 163. [CrossRef]

3. Howell, G.J.C.; Hicks, M. Dental hygienists' role in patient assessments and clinical examinations in U.S. dental practices: A review of the literature. *J. Allied Health* **2010**, *39*, e1–e6.
4. McCombs, G.B.; Amyot, G.C.C.; Wilder, R.S.; Skaff, K.O.; Green, L.M. Dental hygienists' contributions to improving the nation's oral health through school-based initiatives from 1970 through 1999: A historical review. *J. Dent. Hyg.* **2007**, *81*, 52.
5. Adams, T.L. Inter-professional conflict and professionalization: Dentistry and dental hygiene in Ontario. *Soc. Sci. Med.* **2004**, *58*, 2243–2252. [CrossRef]
6. Lautar, C.; Kirby, D.M. Towards the professional status of dental hygiene in Alberta. *Probe* **1996**, *30*, 93–98.
7. Lautar, C. Is dental hygiene a profession? A literature review. *Probe* **1995**, *29*, 127–132.
8. Walsh, M.M. The economic contribution of dental hygienists' activities to dental practice: Review of the literature. *J. Public Health Dent.* **1987**, *47*, 193–197. [CrossRef]
9. Nomura, Y.; Tsutsumi, I.; Nagasaki, M.; Tsuda, H.; Koga, F.; Kashima, N.; Uraguchi, M.; Okada, A.; Kakuta, E.; Hanada, N. Supplied Food Consistency and Oral Functions of Institutionalized Elderly. *Int. J. Dent.* **2020**, *2020*, 3463056. [CrossRef]
10. Nakajima, N. Challenges of dental hygienists in a multidisciplinary team approach during palliative care for patients with advanced cancer: A nationwide study. *Am. J. Hosp. Palliat. Med.* **2020**. [CrossRef]
11. Nawata, W.; Umezaki, Y.; Yamaguchi, M.; Nakajima, M.; Makino, M.; Yoneda, M.; Hirofuji, T.; Yamano, T.; Ooboshi, H.; Morita, H. Continuous Professional Oral Health Care Intervention Improves Severe Aspiration Pneumonia. *Case Rep. Dent.* **2019**, *2019*, 4945921. [CrossRef] [PubMed]
12. Obana, M.; Furuya, J.; Matsubara, C.; Tohara, H.; Inaji, M.; Miki, K.; Numasawa, Y.; Minakuchi, S.; Maehara, T. Effect of a collaborative transdisciplinary team approach on oral health status in acute stroke patients. *J. Oral Rehabil.* **2019**, *46*, 1170–1176. [CrossRef] [PubMed]
13. Macey, R.; Glenny, A.M.; Brocklehurst, P. Feasibility study: Assessing the efficacy and social acceptability of using dental hygienist-therapists as front-line clinicians. *Br. Dent. J.* **2016**, *221*, 717–721. [CrossRef] [PubMed]
14. Braun, P.A.; Cusick, A. Collaboration between Medical Providers and Dental Hygienists in Pediatric Health Care. *J. Evid. Based Dent. Pract.* **2016**, *16*, S59–S67. [CrossRef]
15. Nomura, Y.; Kakuta, E.; Okada, A.; Yamamoto, Y.; Tomonari, H.; Hosoya, N.; Hanada, N.; Yoshida, N.; Takei, N. Prioritization of the Skills to Be Mastered for the Daily Jobs of Japanese Dental Hygienists. *Int. J. Dent.* **2020**, *2020*, 4297646. [CrossRef]
16. Hamasha, A.A.; Alturki, A.; Alghofaili, N.; Alhomaied, A.; Alsanee, F.; Aljaghwani, F.; Alhamdan, M.; El-Metwally, A. Predictors and Level of Job Satisfaction among the Dental Workforce in National Guard Health Affairs. *J. Int. Soc. Prev. Community Dent.* **2019**, *9*, 89–93. [CrossRef]
17. Hach, M.; Aaberg, K.B.; Lempert, S.M.; Danielsen, B. Work assignments, delegation of tasks and job satisfaction among Danish dental hygienists. *Int. J. Dent. Hyg.* **2017**, *15*, 229–235. [CrossRef]
18. McCombs, G.B.; Tolle, S.L.; Newcomb, T.L.; Bruhn, A.M.; Hunt, A.W.; Stafford, L.K. Workplace Bullying: A survey of Virginia dental hygienists. *J. Dent. Hyg.* **2018**, *92*, 22–29.
19. Loretto, N.R.; Caldas, A.F., Jr.; Junior, C.L.G. Job satisfaction among dental assistants in Brazil. *Braz. Dent. J.* **2013**, *24*, 53–58. [CrossRef]
20. Ayers, K.; Meldrum, A.M.; Thomson, W.M.; Newton, J.T. The working practices and job satisfaction of dental hygienists in New Zealand. *J. Public Health Dent.* **2006**, *66*, 186–191. [CrossRef]
21. Malkawi, Z.A. Career satisfaction of Jordanian dental hygienists. *Int. J. Dent. Hyg.* **2016**, *14*, 243–248. [CrossRef] [PubMed]
22. Berthelsen, H.; Westerlund, H.; Hakanen, J.J.; Kristensen, T.S. It is not just about occupation, but also about where you work. *Community Dent. Oral Epidemiol.* **2017**, *45*, 372–379. [CrossRef] [PubMed]
23. Lindmark, U.; Wagman, P.; Wåhlin, C.; Rolander, B. Workplace health in dental care—A salutogenic approach. *Int. J. Dent. Hyg.* **2018**, *16*, 103–113. [CrossRef] [PubMed]

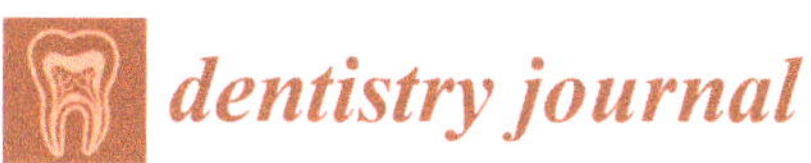

MDPI

Article

Assessment of Health-Promoting Lifestyle among Dental Students in Zagreb, Croatia

Larisa Musić [1], Tonći Mašina [2], Ivan Puhar [1], Laura Plančak [3], Valentina Kostrić [4], Mihaela Kobale [4] and Ana Badovinac [1,*]

1 Department of Periodontology, School of Dental Medicine, University of Zagreb, HR-10000 Zagreb, Croatia; lmusic@sfzg.hr (L.M.); puhar@sfzg.hr (I.P.)
2 Department of Physical Education, School of Medicine Zagreb, University of Zagreb, HR-10000 Zagreb, Croatia; tonci.masina@mef.hr
3 School of Dental Medicine, University of Zagreb, HR-10000 Zagreb, Croatia; lplancak@sfzg.hr
4 Private Dental Practice, HR-10000 Zagreb, Croatia; kostricvalentina@gmail.com (V.K.); kobale.mihaela@gmail.com (M.K.)
* Correspondence: badovinac@sfzg.hr; Tel.: +385-1-4802155

Abstract: As future healthcare professionals, dental medicine students are expected to exhibit healthy lifestyle behaviors. This study aims to assess the health-promoting behaviors among undergraduate dental medicine students of all six academic study years at the University of Zagreb, and determine their predictors. Students were invited to complete a two-part survey, consisting of a self-reported sociodemographic questionnaire and the Health-Promoting Lifestyle Profile II (HPLP II). Three hundred and forty-nine students completed the survey; the response rate was 60.3%. The total mean HPLP II score was 2.64 ± 0.34. Students in the second academic study year scored the lowest (2.50 ± 0.33), and students in the sixth academic study year scored the highest (2.77 ± 0.32). Health responsibility was the overall lowest scored subcategory, while interpersonal relations was scored the highest. Female students reported lower spiritual growth and stress management than male students. Higher body mass index (BMI) was related to lower health responsibility. Smoking, place of residence and the age of participants did not seem to have an impact on health-promoting behaviors. Dental students at our faculty exhibit moderate health-promoting behaviors, even in the absence of a formal health-promoting course in the existing curriculum.

Keywords: dental education; dental students; healthy lifestyle; surveys and questionnaires; health behavior; health promotion; school health services

Citation: Music, L.; Mašina, T.; Puhar, I.; Plančak, L.; Kostrić, V.; Kobale, M.; Badovinac, A. Assessment of Health-Promoting Lifestyle among Dental Students in Zagreb, Croatia. *Dent. J.* **2021**, *9*, 28. https://doi.org/10.3390/dj9030028

Academic Editor: Guglielmo Campus

Received: 9 February 2021
Accepted: 2 March 2021
Published: 6 March 2021

1. Introduction

As defined by the World Health Organization, a healthy lifestyle entails living in a manner that lowers the risk of severe illness or early death [1]. Behavioral risk factors such as smoking, poor nutrition, and physical inactivity increase the risk of chronic, non-communicable diseases, which cumulatively led to an estimated 71% of all deaths globally, as reported by the latest available data from the year 2016 [2]. As these risk factors are modifiable, through their control, many non-communicable diseases may be avoided, if not prevented [3].

Indeed, a longitudinal US population-based study including more than 120,000 subjects reported that people who exhibited low-risk lifestyle habits (e.g., non-smoking, healthy weight (BMI < 25 kg/m^2), ≥30 min/day of moderate to vigorous physical activity, moderate alcohol intake, and a high diet quality score) enjoyed significantly longer lives than those who exhibited none [4].

Poor health behaviors and habits, such as poor nutrition and, consequently, obesity [5,6], physical activity, and sedentary behavior [7], seem likely to persist into a person's adulthood. Thus, while healthy lifestyle behaviors are essential in all periods of life, the adoption of correct habits and attitudes is preferable during youth and adolescence [8,9].

The beginning of university education represents a significant turning point in an individual's life [10]. A large body of evidence suggests that in this period, many students face challenges in the maintenance of and adherence to healthy lifestyle behaviors, in terms of physical activity [11,12], nutrition, substance use [13,14], social connections, personal behaviors [15], and sleeping habits [16,17].

Health promotion and health-promoting behaviors are complementary to a healthy lifestyle and include actions, attitudes, and beliefs which individuals enforce to stay healthy, maintain good physical fitness, prevent disease. They also enable individuals to increase control over and to improve their health [1,18].

Students of biomedical disciplines are expected to grow into the role of health behavior promoters. To facilitate this growth, an educational framework should be set in order to raise awareness, educate, and motivate students to adopt and maintain a healthy lifestyle. In the curriculum of the integrated study program at our faculty, however, there is no course dedicated to this subject. In 2018, an interdisciplinary promotion-preventive initiative under the name of "Healthy University" was founded at the University of Zagreb.

A number of studies have assessed health-promoting behaviors in student populations around the world [19–24] using the Health-Promoting Lifestyle Profile II (HPLP II), first described by Walker et al. [18]. In Croatia, health-promoting lifestyles have previously been assessed among medical students [25,26]. However, such data for the population of dental students is missing.

Thus, we conducted the present study with the primary objective of evaluating the health-promoting behaviors among students of dental medicine in Croatia and observing possible differences related to the year of their academic study. Furthermore, the secondary objective was to elucidate the possible predictors of such behaviors. The findings of this study may be implemented in tailored programs and activities, aiming to improve and promote healthy lifestyles.

2. Materials and Methods

This cross-sectional study was conducted on the population of undergraduate students of the School of Dental Medicine, University of Zagreb, during February and March 2019. The Ethics Committee of the School of Dental Medicine approved the study (No: 05-PA-30-11/2018). The study was performed in accordance with the Declaration of Helsinki.

The Croatian version of the HPLP II questionnaire was prepared in Google Form and shared for online access. The questionnaire was anonymous and voluntary. Participant information was provided in written form before students moved forward with the survey. They were informed about the type and the purpose of the survey and the ability for withdrawal at any point in time.

The survey consisted of two parts. The first part was a self-reported questionnaire on seven sociodemographic items (age, gender, weight, height, year of study, place of residence, and smoking status). The body mass index (BMI) of participants was calculated [27]. The second part of the survey was a Croatian version of the HPLP II questionnaire examining attitudes toward health, healthy lifestyles, and the psychosocial aspects of respondents, previously translated by Mašina et al. [25]. The HPLP II questionnaire consists of 52 questions divided into two main categories and six subcategories. The category of positive health behavior includes the following subcategories: health responsibility, physical activity, and nutritional habits, and the psychosocial value category includes spiritual growth, interpersonal relations, and stress management. Health responsibility covers nine questions about an individual's attitude to their health. The physical activity subcategory has eight questions related to regular exercise and activity. Nine questions in the subcategory nutritional habits refer to the choice of meal-type and nutritional value. The subcategories of spiritual growth and interpersonal relationships also have nine questions related to the relationships with oneself and others. Stress management has eight questions that include stress recognition and actions to control it. Possible answers follow a four-point scale ranging from 1 (never) to 4 (routinely). The total HPLP II score and scores of the individual subcategories of the HPLP II questionnaire were calculated according to the available scoring instructions [18], by calculating the mean of the individual's responses. A higher HPLP II score indicates a better health-promoting lifestyle.

The value of the Cronbach alpha coefficient of the Croatian version of HPLP II questionnaire completed by the students of Dental Medicine was 0.91, and ranged from 0.66 to 0.84 for subcategories.

Data Analysis

The data were organized into a Microsoft Excel spreadsheet (Microsoft Inc., Redmond, WA, USA), and the statistical analyses were performed using IBM SPSS® Statistics version 25.0 for Windows (IBM Corp., Armonk, NY, USA). The normality of the distribution for continuous variables was analyzed by the Kolmogorov–Smirnov test, and for further statistical analyses, parametric tests were used. Differences between the years of study, with respect to the value of individual domains of the HPLP II questionnaire, as well as the total value of the HPLP II questionnaire, were analyzed by one-way ANOVA and post hoc test. Multiple regression analysis was used to examine predictors for the overall HPLP II score and for the scores of six health-promoting lifestyle subscales. The significance level was set at 5%.

3. Results

3.1. Demographic Data

A total of 578 students from year 1 to 6 were enrolled in the academic program in the year 2018/2019 at the School of Dental Medicine, University of Zagreb. Three hundred and forty-nine of these students took part and completed the survey, with the response rate being 60.3%. Among those who completed the survey, 14.6% of the participants were male, and 85.4% were female, and the mean age of the students was 22.3 ± 1.03. The percentage of male students was lowest in the fifth year (7.0%) and highest in the second year (21.2%). The response rate of the students was highest in the first year (71.8%), while the lowest response rate was in the fifth year (54.8%). The distribution of the students by academic year, gender, and age, as well as the response rate, are shown in Table 1.

Table 1. Response rate and distribution of students by academic year, gender, and age.

Academic Year	Total Number *N* (%)	Male *N* (%)	Female *N* (%)	Participating Students *N* (%)	Participants' Mean Age ± *SD*
Year 1	74 (21.2%)	11 (14.9%)	63 (85.1%)	74 (71.8%)	19.1 ± 0.6
Year 2	52 (14.9%)	11 (21.2%)	41 (78.8%)	52 (55.3%)	20.3 ± 0.7
Year 3	54 (15.5%)	10 (18.5%)	44 (81.5%)	54 (58.1%)	22.7 ± 0.7
Year 4	56 (16.0%)	7 (12.5%)	49 (87.5%)	56 (59.6%)	22.5 ± 1.3
Year 5	57 (16.3%)	4 (7.0%)	53 (93.0%)	57 (54.8%)	23.5 ± 0.9
Year 6	56 (16.0%)	8 (14.3%)	48 (85.7%)	56 (62.2%)	24.5 ± 0.9
Total	349 (100%)	51 (14.6%)	298 (85.4%)	349 (60.3%)	22.3 ± 10.3

SD: standard deviation.

Among those who completed the survey, 37.0% of the participants lived in their family home, 16.9% lived in a student dormitory, 28.4% lived in a rented apartment, and 17.8% lived elsewhere. Furthermore, the majority of the participants were non-smokers (80.5%), 13.5% of the participants were smokers, and the remaining 6.0% were former smokers (Table 2).

Table 2. Place of residence and smoking status by academic year.

		Academic Year						
		1	2	3	4	5	6	Total
		N (%)	N (%)	N (%)	N (%)	N (%)	N (%)	N (%)
Place of Residence	Family Home	28 (37.8%)	22 (42.3%)	20 (37.0%)	21 (37.5%)	17 (29.8%)	21 (37.5%)	129 (37.0%)
	Dorm	15 (20.3%)	11 (21.2%)	12 (22.2%)	12 (21.4%)	4 (7.0%)	5 (8.9%)	59 (16.9%)
	Rented Apartment	22 (29.7%)	11 (21.2%)	11 (20.4%)	15 (26.8%)	24 (42.1%)	16 (28.6%)	99 (28.4%)
	Other	9 (12.2%)	8 (15.4%)	11 (20.4%)	8 (14.3%)	12 (21.1%)	14 (25.0%)	62 (17.8%)
Smoking	Yes	7 (9.5%)	9 (17.3%)	5 (9.3%)	7 (12.5%)	12 (21.1%)	7 (12.5%)	47 (13.5%)
	No	65 (87.8%)	38 (73.1%)	45 (83.3%)	46 (82.1%)	42 (73.7%)	45 (80.4%)	281 (80.5%)
	Former	2 (2.7%)	5 (9.6%)	4 (7.4%)	3 (5.4%)	3 (5.3%)	4 (7.1%)	21 (6.0%)

3.2. HPLP II Overall Score and Subcategories Score by Academic year

The overall mean HPLP II score was 2.64 ± 0.34, ranging 1.73–3.50. The sixth-year students had the highest scores of 2.77 ± 0.32, while second-year students showed the lowest scores of 2.50 ± 0.33 ($p < 0.001$). When analyzing the total mean scores of the subcategories of the HPLP II questionnaire, the students scored the highest score on interpersonal relations (3.30 ± 0.39), followed by spiritual growth (2.95 ± 0.47), nutrition (2.72 ± 0.41), stress management (2.37 ± 0.46), and physical activity (2.23 ± 0.65), while scoring the lowest in the subcategory of health responsibility (2.17 ± 0.57).

The results of the mean scores in the HPLP II subcategories showed that sixth-year students achieved higher values than their colleagues in lower years of study (first to fifth) in the subcategories of physical activity (2.46 ± 0.66), nutrition (2.85 ± 0.46), interpersonal relations (3.42 ± 0.31), stress management (2.53 ± 0.41), and spiritual growth (3.06 ± 0.50), and the fifth-year students achieved the highest values (2.27 ± 0.51) in the domain of health responsibility. Second-year students achieved the worst results in all subcategories compared to students in other years of study (Table 3).

Table 3. Health-Promoting Lifestyle Profile II (HPLP II) scores according to the academic year.

Year	Overall HPLP II	Health Responsibility	Physical Activity	Nutrition	Spiritual Growth	Interpersonal Relations	Stress Management
Year 1	2.58 ± 0.31 ^{f}	2.17 ± 0.54	2.15 ± 0.59 ^{f}	2.63 ± 0.45 ^{cdf}	2.89 ± 0.44	3.29 ± 0.35	2.29 ± 0.43 ^{ef}
Year 2	2.50 ± 0.33 ^{cdef}	2.01 ± 0.50	1.99 ± 0.59 ^{def}	2.57 ± 0.37 ^{cdf}	2.89 ± 0.51	3.26 ± 0.47	2.17 ± 0.42 ^{cdef}
Year 3	2.65 ± 0.34 ^{b}	2.11 ± 0.71	2.22 ± 0.66 ^{f}	2.78 ± 0.36 ^{ab}	2.99 ± 0.38	3.33 ± 0.33	2.38 ± 0.42 ^{b}
Year 4	2.66 ± 0.38 ^{b}	2.22 ± 0.61	2.28 ± 0.78 ^{b}	2.79 ± 0.34 ^{ab}	2.90 ± 0.48	3.27 ± 0.45	2.41 ± 0.55 ^{b}
Year 5	2.67 ± 0.33 ^{b}	2.27 ± 0.51	2.30 ± 0.52 ^{b}	2.72 ± 0.40 ^{f}	2.96 ± 0.51	3.27 ± 0.42	2.46 ± 0.46 ^{ab}
Year 6	2.77 ± 0.32 ^{ab}	2.22 ± 0.53	2.46 ± 0.66 ^{abc}	2.85 ± 0.46 ^{ab}	3.06 ± 0.50	3.42 ± 0.31	2.53 ± 0.41 ^{abde}
All Students	2.64 ± 0.34	2.17 ± 0.57	2.23 ± 0.65	2.72 ± 0.41	2.95 ± 0.47	3.30 ± 0.39	2.37 ± 0.46
p Value	0.001 *	0.216	0.006 *	0.002 *	0.308	0.221	0.001 *

The values are expressed as means ± SD; * One-way ANOVA test was conducted, and $p < 0.05$ values are bold; Post hoc tests were done between the years of study: [a] Difference is statistically significant from Year 1 ($p < 0.05$). [b] Difference is statistically significant from Year 2 ($p < 0.05$). [c] Difference is statistically significant from Year 3 ($p < 0.05$). [d] Difference is statistically significant from Year 4 ($p < 0.05$). [e] Difference is statistically significant from Year 5 ($p < 0.05$). [f] Difference is statistically significant from Year 6 ($p < 0.05$).

One-way ANOVA assessed that differences in overall HPLP II mean score according to the year of study were statistically significant ($p = 0.001$). Likewise, significant differences were observed according to the year of study for the mean scores of HPLP II subcategories physical activity ($p = 0.006$), nutrition ($p = 0.002$), and stress management ($p = 0.001$). In order to establish the differences between the year of study, and the statistically significantly different subcategories (physical activity, nutrition, and stress management), as well as the overall HPLP II mean scores, a post hoc test was carried out. The results of one-way ANOVA and post hoc comparisons are shown in Table 3.

Multiple regression analysis of the demographic variables (age, gender, BMI, year of study, place of residence, and smoking habit) with the overall HPLP II score and score of six subcategories was performed to determine the predictors of a healthy lifestyle in the participants. A higher year of study was shown to be a predictor for a higher total score of HPLP II ($\beta = 0.207$, $p < 0.001$). In the subcategory of health responsibility, higher BMI was related to lower health responsibility ($\beta = -0.149$, $p = 0.009$), and a higher year of study was a predictor for better health responsibility ($\beta = 0.108$, $p = 0.049$). Higher BMI and higher year of study were predictors for better nutrition ($\beta = 0.124$, $p = 0.028$ and $\beta = 0.177$, $p = 0.001$, respectively), while age was shown to be a predictor for higher spiritual growth and female gender for lower spiritual growth ($\beta = 0.113$, $p = 0.040$ and $\beta = -0.137$, $p = 0.016$, respectively). A higher year of study was shown to be a predictor for better stress management ($\beta = 0.218$, $p < 0.001$), and female students seemed to have weaker stress management than male students ($\beta = -0.171$, $p = 0.002$) (Table 4). No predictors could be found for the subcategories of interpersonal relations and physical activity, and demographic variables smoking and place of residence did not show any significant effect on the health-promoting lifestyle (data not shown). Generally, the multiple regression analysis that was performed to determine predictors of a healthy lifestyle explained only 5–8% of the variance.

Table 4. Multiple regression analysis of predictors for the overall HPLP II score and certain HPLP II subcategories.

		Unstandardized Coefficients		Standardized Coefficients			
Dependent Variable	**Predictor**	**B**	**Std. Error**	**Beta**	***t* Value**	***p* Value**	**R^2**
Health Responsibility	Intercept	2.634	0.410		6.423	0.000	0.05
	BMI	−0.033	0.013	−0.149	−2.638	0.009	
	Academic year	0.035	0.018	0.108	1.975	0.049	
Nutrition	Intercept	1.935	0.294		6.576	0.000	0.07
	BMI	0.020	0.009	0.124	2.201	0.028	
	Academic year	0.041	0.013	0.177	3.261	0.001	
Spiritual Growth	Intercept	2.798	0.336		8.323	0.000	0.05
	Age	0.005	0.002	0.113	2.066	0.040	
	Female gender	−0.182	0.075	−0.137	−2.417	0.016	
Stress Management	Intercept	2.393	0.324		7.384	0.000	0.08
	Female gender	−0.224	0.073	−0.171	−3.082	0.002	
	Academic year	0.057	0.014	0.218	4.077	<0.001	
Overall HPLP II Score	Intercept	2.527	0.244		10.343	0.000	0.05
	Academic year	0.040	0.011	0.207	3.800	<0.001	

Note: Only statistically significant ($p < 0.05$) predictors from the regression analysis are shown. BMI: body mass index.

4. Discussion

This study has assessed, for the first time, the health-promoting behavior of dental medicine students in Croatia. The overall mean HPLP II scores (2.64 ± 0.34) among dental students at the School of Dental Medicine in Zagreb highlights their moderate health-promoting lifestyle. The results of our study are consistent with previously reported data on a Croatian population of medical students [25]. Moreover, similar findings were highlighted by other international studies conducted on a population of dental students (2.49 ± 0.32) [20], medical students [19], nursing students [28], and mixed faculty students [22].

When assessing the results according to the year of the academic study, the sixth-year students scored the highest results, whereas the second-year students engaged least frequently in health-promoting behavior. Moreover, the year of study was highlighted as a predictor for a higher total score of HPLP II. As of yet, there is no official educational health-promoting framework at our faculty. Thus, we can only speculate that sixth-year students' awareness and motivation for health-promoting behavior is progressively stimulated and grown throughout the course of their healthcare education. The lowest scores of the second-year students were closely followed by the first-year students, with no statistically significant difference in scores between the two. While there is no clear explanation for this observation, it could be attributed to the high academic pressure experienced within the first two years, also reflected in our faculty's 6-year study program's lowest pass rates. Due to an overwhelming time schedule, studying, and social challenges, it is possible that the students pay less attention to healthy behaviors in this period of their education. However, published data on age and years of study as predictors of health awareness and engagement in healthy behaviors seem to be quite inconsistent and contradictory. Similar to our results, several studies in various settings reported lower HPLP II scores in younger students and those early in their academic education [28–31]. Conversely, studies on Turkish and Japanese student populations reported a negative correlation between HPLP II scores and the year of university study [19,21].

Overall, students scored highest in the subscales of nutrition, spiritual growth, and particularly interpersonal relationships. Subcategories pertaining to the psychosocial value category (spiritual growth and interpersonal relations) were also scored highest among medical students in Turkey and Croatia and university students in Japan [19,21]. Cultural differences between European and Asian students have already been reported regarding their attitudes towards oral health behavior [32]. Interestingly, it seems that these culturally-based differences cannot be observed among students in relation to their health-promoting lifestyle. The highest scores in the subcategory of interpersonal relationships among Croatian dental students could be attributed to being cultural-specific. Croatians are generally considered to be sociable and to frequently interact with both their primary (i.e., family) and secondary (i.e., friends) spheres of sociability, as reported by a study on sociability patterns [33].

Surprisingly, the students scored lowest in the subcategory of health responsibility, which is similar to their Turkish, Iranian, and Japanese colleagues [20,21]. As initially described by Walker et al. [18], this subcategory assesses whether the individual is paying attention and taking responsibility for their health, being educated about health, and seeking timely help when necessary. Individuals at that age are generally of good health and may not perceive it to be necessary to pay much attention to health responsibility. As shown by the multiple regression analysis in our study, a higher BMI seemed to be a predictor of lower health responsibility. However, as reported by Harrington et al., BMI may not be a definite predictor of health behavior. Their findings suggest that both obese and overweight students, as well as students of a healthy weight, may be at risk for poor health behaviors, such as inadequate nutrition and physical inactivity [34].

In this study, physical activity was among the overall lowest scored subcategories. When assessing the data in relation to the year of study, it seems that sixth-year students engaged in physical activities the most, as they scored highest in this subcategory. As suggested by the published data, sedentary lifestyle and physical inactivity seem to be a source of concern among college students. A meta-analysis by Keating et al. reported that 40% to 50% of college students are physically inactive [12]. A significant decrease in physical activity seems to follow college enrollment, with time restriction among the most frequently reported reasons for this phenomenon [35]. Croatian population-based studies have highlighted that the lowest physical activity is reported in the 15–24 age group [36], and that 28% of university students are insufficiently physically active [37]. Similar findings on low physical activity scores were also reported by Wei et al. and Lee at al. [21,38]. While in Japan, physical education is not a compulsory course at most universities [21], in Croatia, it is, albeit mostly only in the first year of academic studies. Based on the evidence, it seems that through the university curriculum and development of extracurricular programs, there should be significantly more promotion of physical activity among students.

The results of multiple regression analysis highlighted interesting data on the predictors of stress management. Students of higher year of study and male gender seem to be correlated with better management of stress. The latter was also observed among Croatian medical students [25]. As reported by the dental literature, dental students experience a considerable amount of stress during their education [39,40], more so than their medical counterparts [41]. Stress management training proved to be beneficial when provided to different student populations [42,43], and as such, the implementation of stress management training is warranted in the dental curriculum. In our study, other demographic data, such as smoking and place of residence, did not seem to be good predictors of health-promoting behaviors. Although our multiple regression analysis showed statistically significant correlations between several predictors of a healthy lifestyle and observed dependent variables, the results should be interpreted with caution because of the high-variability data according to the low R-squared values (0.05–0.08). This clearly indicates that there are many other factors to consider and explore in future research that definitely influence health-promoting lifestyles for our participants.

The present study has certain limitations. The study was of cross-sectional design, hence reporting data at a specific point in time and not allowing for the analysis of potential changes in the health-promoting behaviors of the studied student population over time. Furthermore, there was a significant difference between the number of students of male and female gender participating in the study, though expected due to the continuous feminization of the dental profession [44,45]. Thus, data regarding differences between the genders should be interpreted with caution. The impact of uncontrolled socially desirable response bias, as often reported in questionnaire-type studies, should also be taken into consideration [46].

At present, the formal education of students on health-promoting behaviors at our faculty is not well defined. Only recently, Zagreb University developed a preventive–promotional framework, educating and supporting students in a healthy lifestyle. Some universities and campuses in the UK [47] and the US [48] have already recognized the importance of health and wellbeing-building environments. As highlighted by Holt et al. [49], these initiatives should be planned and organized to meet the specific needs of their students. This study, along with the data previously published by one of the co-authors [32], provides valuable information on the health-behavior of our faculty's students, and this information is being used to construct a new health-promoting elective course that is tailored to addressing their particular requirements.

Future research should focus on the assessment of changes in measures of health-promoting lifestyles in the same observed population over a period of time, and more importantly, following a health-promoting intervention. As biomedical students are seen as future health-lifestyle promoters, a significant number of studies are conducted on these populations. However, data on student populations that may not be traditionally associated with health promotion, such as technical faculties, would be of high value. As previously highlighted, tailored health-promoting courses and programs could thus be built around the needs of a specific student population.

5. Conclusions

In conclusion, this study highlights that a moderate health-promoting lifestyle can be observed among dental students in Zagreb, Croatia, even in the absence of an official health-promoting educational framework. While students of biomedical faculties exhibit overall favorable health-promoting behaviors, differences among the subcategories may be attributed to specific predictors that have yet to be fully elucidated among different countries and cultures. The development and implementation of promotive and preventive health programs is highly warranted.

Author Contributions: Conceptualization: L.M. and A.B.; methodology: L.M. and A.B.; statistical analysis: T.M.; investigation and preparation of documentation: L.P., M.K., and V.K.; writing—original draft preparation: L.M. and A.B.; writing—review and editing: I.P.; visualization: L.M. and A.B.; supervision: A.B. All authors have read and agreed to the published version of the manuscript.

Funding: This research received no external funding.

Institutional Review Board Statement: The study was conducted according to the guidelines of the Declaration of Helsinki, and approved by the Ethics Committee of the School of Dental Medicine, University of Zagreb (No: 05-PA-30-11/2018; Date of approval: 6 December 2018).

Informed Consent Statement: Participant information was provided in written form before students moved forward with the survey. Participants were informed about the type and the purpose of the survey and the ability for withdrawal at any point in time.

Data Availability Statement: Not applicable.

Acknowledgments: The authors would like to thank the undergraduate students of the School of Dental Medicine, University of Zagreb, for participation in this study.

Conflicts of Interest: The authors declare no conflict of interest.

References

1. World Health Organization. Regional Office for Healthy Living: What Is a Healthy Lifestyle? Available online: https://apps.who.int/iris/handle/10665/108180 (accessed on 25 August 2020).
2. Bennett, J.E.; Stevens, G.A.; Mathers, C.D.; Bonita, R.; Rehm, J.; Kruk, M.E.; Riley, L.M.; Dain, K.; Kengne, A.P.; Chalkidou, K.; et al. NCD Countdown 2030 collaborators NCD Countdown 2030: Worldwide Trends in Non-Communicable Disease Mortality and Progress towards Sustainable Development Goal Target 3.4. *Lancet Lond. Engl.* **2018**, *392*, 1072–1088. [CrossRef]
3. Peters, R.; Ee, N.; Peters, J.; Beckett, N.; Booth, A.; Rockwood, K.; Anstey, K.J. Common Risk Factors for Major Noncommunicable Disease, a Systematic Overview of Reviews and Commentary: The Implied Potential for Targeted Risk Reduction. *Ther. Adv. Chronic Dis.* **2019**, *10*. [CrossRef] [PubMed]
4. Li, Y.; Pan, A.; Wang, D.D.; Liu, X.; Dhana, K.; Franco, O.H.; Kaptoge, S.; Di Angelantonio, E.; Stampfer, M.; Willett, W.C.; et al. Impact of Healthy Lifestyle Factors on Life Expectancies in the US Population. *Circulation* **2018**, *138*, 345–355. [CrossRef]
5. Simmonds, M.; Burch, J.; Llewellyn, A.; Griffiths, C.; Yang, H.; Owen, C.; Duffy, S.; Woolacott, N.; Simmonds, M.; Burch, J.; et al. The Use of Measures of Obesity in Childhood for Predicting Obesity and the Development of Obesity-Related Diseases in Adulthood: A Systematic Review and Meta-Analysis. *Health Technol. Assess.* **2015**, *19*, 1–336. [CrossRef]
6. Craigie, A.M.; Lake, A.A.; Kelly, S.A.; Adamson, A.J.; Mathers, J.C. Tracking of Obesity-Related Behaviours from Childhood to Adulthood: A Systematic Review. *Maturitas* **2011**, *70*, 266–284. [CrossRef]
7. Biddle, S.J.H.; Pearson, N.; Ross, G.M.; Braithwaite, R. Tracking of Sedentary Behaviours of Young People: A Systematic Review. *Prev. Med.* **2010**, *51*, 345–351. [CrossRef] [PubMed]
8. Healthy Active Living for Children and Youth. *Paediatr. Child Health* **2002**, *7*, 339–345.
9. Roura, E.; Milà-Villarroel, R.; Lucía Pareja, S.; Adot Caballero, A. Assessment of Eating Habits and Physical Activity among Spanish Adolescents. The "Cooking and Active Leisure" TAS Program. *PLoS ONE* **2016**, *11*, e0159962. [CrossRef] [PubMed]
10. Assaf, I.; Brieteh, F.; Tfaily, M.; El-Baida, M.; Kadry, S.; Balusamy, B. Students University Healthy Lifestyle Practice: Quantitative Analysis. *Health Inf. Sci. Syst.* **2019**, *7*, 7. [CrossRef] [PubMed]
11. Racette, S.B.; Deusinger, S.S.; Strube, M.J.; Highstein, G.R.; Deusinger, R.H. Changes in Weight and Health Behaviors from Freshman through Senior Year of College. *J. Nutr. Educ. Behav.* **2008**, *40*, 39–42. [CrossRef] [PubMed]
12. Keating, X.D.; Guan, J.; Piñero, J.C.; Bridges, D.M. A Meta-Analysis of College Students' Physical Activity Behaviors. *J. Am. Coll. Health* **2005**, *54*, 116–126. [CrossRef]
13. Douglas, K.A.; Collins, J.L.; Warren, C.; Kann, L.; Gold, R.; Clayton, S.; Ross, J.G.; Kolbe, L.J. Results From the 1995 National College Health Risk Behavior Survey. *J. Am. Coll. Health* **1997**, *46*, 55–67. [CrossRef]
14. Cockroft, M.C.; Bartlett, T.R.; Wallace, D.C. Sleep, Nutrition, Disordered Eating, Problematic Tobacco and Alcohol Use, and Exercise in College Students With and Without Diabetes. *J. Psychosoc. Nurs. Ment. Health Serv.* **2019**, *57*, 23–32. [CrossRef]
15. Allgöwer, A.; Wardle, J.; Steptoe, A. Depressive Symptoms, Social Support, and Personal Health Behaviors in Young Men and Women. *Health Psychol.* **2001**, *20*, 223–227. [CrossRef] [PubMed]
16. Schlarb, A.A.; Friedrich, A.; Claßen, M. Sleep Problems in University Students—An Intervention. *Neuropsychiatr. Dis. Treat.* **2017**, *13*, 1989–2001. [CrossRef]
17. Taylor, D.J.; Bramoweth, A.D.; Grieser, E.A.; Tatum, J.I.; Roane, B.M. Epidemiology of Insomnia in College Students: Relationship with Mental Health, Quality of Life, and Substance Use Difficulties. *Behav. Ther.* **2013**, *44*, 339–348. [CrossRef] [PubMed]
18. Walker, S.N.; Sechrist, K.R.; Pender, N.J. The Health-Promoting Lifestyle Profile: Development and Psychometric Characteristics. *Nurs. Res.* **1987**, *36*, 76–81. [CrossRef]

19. Nacar, M.; Baykan, Z.; Cetinkaya, F.; Arslantas, D.; Ozer, A.; Coskun, O.; Bati, H.; Karaoglu, N.; Elmali, F.; Yilmaze, G. Health Promoting Lifestyle Behaviour in Medical Students: A Multicentre Study from Turkey. *Asian Pac. J. Cancer Prev.* **2014**, *15*, 8969–8974. [CrossRef]
20. Peker, K.; Bermek, G. Predictors of Health-Promoting Behaviors Among Freshman Dental Students at Istanbul University. *J. Dent. Educ.* **2011**, *75*, 413–420. [CrossRef]
21. Wei, C.-N.; Harada, K.; Ueda, K.; Fukumoto, K.; Minamoto, K.; Ueda, A. Assessment of Health-Promoting Lifestyle Profile in Japanese University Students. *Environ. Health Prev. Med.* **2012**, *17*, 222–227. [CrossRef] [PubMed]
22. Lolokote, S.; Hidru, T.H.; Li, X. Do Socio-Cultural Factors Influence College Students' Self-Rated Health Status and Health-Promoting Lifestyles? A Cross-Sectional Multicenter Study in Dalian, China. *BMC Public Health* **2017**, *17*, 478. [CrossRef] [PubMed]
23. Bi, J.; Huang, Y.; Xiao, Y.; Cheng, J.; Li, F.; Wang, T.; Chen, J.; Wu, L.; Liu, Y.; Luo, R.; et al. Association of Lifestyle Factors and Suboptimal Health Status: A Cross-Sectional Study of Chinese Students. *BMJ Open* **2014**, *4*, e005156. [CrossRef] [PubMed]
24. Tol, A.; Tavassoli, E.; Shariferad, G.R.; Shojaeezadeh, D. Health-Promoting Lifestyle and Quality of Life among Undergraduate Students at School of Health, Isfahan University of Medical Sciences. *J. Educ. Health Promot.* **2013**, *2*. [CrossRef]
25. Mašina, T.; Madžar, T.; Musil, V.; Milošević, M. Differences in Health-Promoting Lifestyle Profile Among Croatian Medical Students According to Gender and Year of Study. *Acta Clin. Croat.* **2017**, *56*, 84–91. [CrossRef] [PubMed]
26. Mašina, T. Physical Activity and Health-Promoting Lifestyle of First and Second Year Medical Students. *Paediatr. Today* **2016**, *12*, 160–168. [CrossRef]
27. Weir, C.B.; Jan, A. BMI Classification Percentile and Cut Off Points. In *StatPearls*; StatPearls Publishing: Treasure Island, FL, USA, 2020.
28. Al-Kandari, F.; Vidal, V.L. Correlation of the Health-Promoting Lifestyle, Enrollment Level, and Academic Performance of College of Nursing Students in Kuwait. *Nurs. Health Sci.* **2007**, *9*, 112–119. [CrossRef]
29. Naçar, M.; Çetinkaya, F.; Baykan, Z.; Zararsiz, G.; Yilmazel, G.; Sağiroğlu, M. Health Related Lifestyle Behaviors among Students at a Vocational Education Center in Turkey. *Health* **2015**, *7*, 1536–1544. [CrossRef]
30. Ay, S.; Yanikkerem, E.; Calim, S.I.; Yazici, M. Health-Promoting Lifestyle Behaviour for Cancer Prevention: A Survey of Turkish University Students. *Asian Pac. J. Cancer Prev.* **2012**, *13*, 2269–2277. [CrossRef]
31. Kreutz, G.; Ginsborg, J.; Williamon, A. Health-Promoting Behaviours in Conservatoire Students. *Psychol. Music* **2008**. [CrossRef]
32. Badovinac, A.; Božić, D.; Vučinac, I.; Vešligaj, J.; Vražić, D.; Plančak, D. Oral Health Attitudes and Behavior of Dental Students at the University of Zagreb, Croatia. *J. Dent. Educ.* **2013**, *77*, 1171–1178. [CrossRef]
33. Dobrotić, I.; Laklija, M. Obrasci društvenosti i percepcija izvora neformalne socijalne podrške u Hrvatskoj. *Drustvena Istraz.* **2012**, *21*, 39–58. [CrossRef]
34. Harrington, M.R.; Ickes, M.J. Differences in Health Behaviors of Overweight or Obese College Students Compared to Healthy Weight Students. *Am. J. Health Educ.* **2016**, *47*, 32–41. [CrossRef]
35. Alkhateeb, S.A.; Alkhameesi, N.F.; Lamfon, G.N.; Khawandanh, S.Z.; Kurdi, L.K.; Faran, M.Y.; Khoja, A.A.; Bukhari, L.M.; Aljahdali, H.R.; Ashour, N.A.; et al. Pattern of Physical Exercise Practice among University Students in the Kingdom of Saudi Arabia (before Beginning and during College): A Cross-Sectional Study. *BMC Public Health* **2019**, *19*, 1716. [CrossRef] [PubMed]
36. Pedišić, Ž.; Rakovac, M.; Bennie, J.; Jurakić, D.; Bauman, A.E. Levels and Correlates of Domain-Specific Physical Activity in University Students: Cross-Sectional Findings from Croatia. *Kinesiology* **2014**, *46*, 12–22.
37. Jurakić, D.; Pedišić, Ž.; Andrijašević, M. Physical Activity of Croatian Population: Cross-Sectional Study Using International Physical Activity Questionnaire. *Croat. Med. J.* **2009**, *50*, 165–173. [CrossRef]
38. Lee, R.L.T.; Loke, A.J.T.Y. Health-Promoting Behaviors and Psychosocial Well-Being of University Students in Hong Kong. *Public Health Nurs. Boston Mass* **2005**, *22*, 209–220. [CrossRef] [PubMed]
39. Abu-Ghazaleh, S.B.; Rajab, L.D.; Sonbol, H.N. Psychological Stress Among Dental Students at the University of Jordan. *J. Dent. Educ.* **2011**, *75*, 1107–1114. [CrossRef] [PubMed]
40. Elani, H.W.; Allison, P.J.; Kumar, R.A.; Mancini, L.; Lambrou, A.; Bedos, C. A Systematic Review of Stress in Dental Students. *J. Dent. Educ.* **2014**, *78*, 226–242. [CrossRef]
41. Murphy, R.J.; Gray, S.A.; Sterling, G.; Reeves, K.; DuCette, J. A Comparative Study of Professional Student Stress. *J. Dent. Educ.* **2009**, *73*, 328–337. [CrossRef]
42. Tisdelle, D.A.; Hansen, D.J.; St Lawrence, J.S.; Brown, J.C. Stress Management Training for Dental Students. *J. Dent. Educ.* **1984**, *48*, 196–202. [CrossRef]
43. Kang, Y.S.; Choi, S.Y.; Ryu, E. The Effectiveness of a Stress Coping Program Based on Mindfulness Meditation on the Stress, Anxiety, and Depression Experienced by Nursing Students in Korea. *Nurse Educ. Today* **2009**, *29*, 538–543. [CrossRef] [PubMed]
44. Barac Furtinger, V.; Alyeva, R.; Maximovskaya, L.N. Is European Dentistry Becoming a Female Profession? *Acta Stomatol. Croat.* **2013**, *47*, 51–57. [CrossRef]
45. McKay, J.C.; Quiñonez, C.R. The Feminization of Dentistry: Implications for the Profession. *J. Can. Dent. Assoc.* **2012**, *78*, 7.
46. Paulhus, D.L. Measurement and Control of Response Bias. In *Measures of Personality and Social Psychological Attitudes*; Elsevier: Amsterdam, The Netherlands, 1991; pp. 17–59. ISBN 978-0-12-590241-0.
47. UK Healthy Universities Network Healthy Universities. Available online: https://healthyuniversities.ac.uk/ (accessed on 27 August 2020).

48. Healthier Campus Initiative. Available online: https://www.ahealthieramerica.org/articles/healthier-campus-initiative-146 (accessed on 26 August 2020).
49. Holt, M.; Powell, S. Healthy Universities: A Guiding Framework for Universities to Examine the Distinctive Health Needs of Its Own Student Population. *Perspect. Public Health* **2017**, *137*, 53–58. [CrossRef] [PubMed]

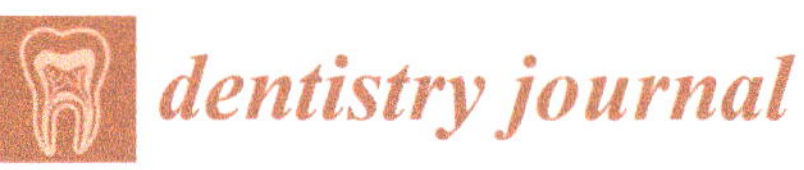

MDPI

Article

Maintenance of Dental Records and Forensic Odontology Awareness: A Survey of Croatian Dentists with Implications for Dental Education

Ivana Savić Pavičin [1], Ana Jonjić [2], Ivana Maretić [3], Jelena Dumančić [1,4,*] and Ajla Zymber Çeshko [5]

1 Department of Dental Anthropology, School of Dental Medicine, University of Zagreb, 10000 Zagreb, Croatia; savic@sfzg.hr
2 School of Dental Medicine, University of Zagreb, 10000 Zagreb, Croatia; ana.jonjic94@gmail.com
3 Private Dental Polyclinic Vinica, 42000 Varaždin, Croatia; s.mareticivana@gmail.com
4 Department of Dental Medicine, University Hospital Centre Zagreb, 10000 Zagreb, Croatia
5 School of Dentistry, FAMA College, 10000 Prishtina, Kosovo; ajlazymber1@icloud.com
* Correspondence: dumancic@sfzg.hr; Tel.: +385-1-4802-146

Abstract: Forensic odontology is the application of dentistry within the criminal justice system. Forensic expertise, including dental identification, mostly relies on dental records. We explored the practice of maintaining dental records among Croatian dentists, as well as their knowledge of legal regulations and the application of dental records in forensic odontology. In all, 145 dentists participated in an online survey. Questions covered general information on dentists, maintenance of dental records, and knowledge of legal requirements and forensic odontology. Overall, 70% of dentists obtain and archive written informed consents, while 87% record dental status. Generally, non-carious dental lesions and developmental dental anomalies were not recorded. About 72% of dentists record filling material and surfaces. Only 32% of dentists know the legal requirements for keeping records, whereas 21% have no knowledge of forensic odontology and its purpose. The survey revealed different practices in the maintenance of dental records, including significant flaws and lack of awareness of its forensic importance. This obvious need for additional education on proper maintenance of dental records could be met by including forensic odontology in compulsory undergraduate courses and postgraduate dental education. Establishing national and international standards in dental charting would comply with contemporary trends in health care and the requirements of forensic expertise.

Keywords: dental record; record keeping; documentation; forensic odontology; dental education; Croatia

Citation: Savić Pavičin, I.; Jonjić, A.; Maretić, I.; Dumančić, J.; Zymber Çeshko, A. Maintenance of Dental Records and Forensic Odontology Awareness: A Survey of Croatian Dentists with Implications for Dental Education. *Dent. J.* **2021**, *9*, 37. https://doi.org/10.3390/dj9040037

Academic Editor: Hans S. Malmstrom

Received: 9 February 2021
Accepted: 22 March 2021
Published: 25 March 2021

1. Introduction

Forensic odontology is a branch of dentistry that applies dental science in order to provide evidence in the interest of the law [1]. It includes dental identification, bitemark analysis, age estimation, and expertise in civil litigation cases related to dental malpractice and injuries [2]. Besides dental identification, other forensic odontology methods can be utilized in personal identification, such as lip prints (cheiloscopy) and palatal rugae patterns (rugoscopy) [3,4]. Most of these procedures rely on dental documentation, which is a source regarding an individual's antemortem dental information. It consists of their dental record with a status chart, intraoral and extraoral X-rays, photographs, dental casts, medical history, and written consent [5]. Numerous qualitative and quantitative characteristics of teeth make dental identification a high-value forensic procedure. Its advantages are the ease of utilizing such resources as well as minor technological and financial requirements. Dental identification is especially useful in cases where teeth are the only remaining preserved parts of a human body: fires, mass graves, plane crashes, or natural disasters such as floods and avalanches [5–8]. However, for dental identification to be successful, dentists must conscientiously keep dental documentation on their patients. Additionally, the importance of maintaining and keeping dental records in terms of legal requirements should also be emphasized, where such records demonstrate the quality and thoroughness of dental care when presented in court proceedings and when providing forensic expertise [5]. Maintaining and keeping dental records are legal obligations for all dentists [9].

In Croatia, the use of dental identification began in the 1970s, when mass casualties occurred in two traffic accidents. Later, another significant development was during and after the Croatian War of Independence 1991–1995, when a need to identify victims from mass graves emerged [10].

The lack of data on the current practice of maintaining dental records has led us to investigate the thoroughness and comprehensiveness of practices in maintaining dental records, including knowledge and awareness among dentists of the legal importance and possibilities of using such records for forensic purposes.

2. Materials and Methods

This research was conducted using an online questionnaire (Google Forms) and titled "Questionnaire on Practices and Quality of Maintaining Dental Records in the Republic of Croatia and Possibility of its Use for Forensic Purposes". Prior to its use, it received approval from the Ethics Committee of the School of Dental Medicine, University of Zagreb. In 2019, the questionnaire was sent to 197 email addresses, available publicly or through social media. In all, 145 dentists participated in the survey, giving a response rate of 74%.

The survey consisted of 40 questions with single, multiple choice, and open-ended questions.

Given below is an outline of the organization of the questions into five sections.

2.1. General Information on Dentists

The first group of questions was formulated to obtain information on gender, age, years of work experience, and the location of the respondent's dental practice. This included questions on the school of basic dental degree and type of employment covering options such as public dental service at a health center, private practice under contract with the Croatian Health Insurance Fund (CHIF), exclusively private practice, or working in a clinic or polyclinic.

2.2. Data on Dental Documentation

The questions focused on the practice of taking the general patient information such as gender, date of birth, contact number, and address, as well as the maiden name for female patients, names of other dentists the patient has visited, and name of their general practitioner.

Questions also covered recording medical history and entering dental status in the patient's records. This also included information on trauma, anomalies in tooth number, position and morphology, and developmental changes in dentitions. The issue of using abbreviations in documentation and treatment codes as stipulated by the CHIF was also addressed. The frequency of the routine use of X-rays and photographs was also examined.

2.3. Information on Dental Documentation Keeping

Questions posed in this section addressed the format of dental documentation, including all relevant components and the duration of storing dental documentation as stipulated in the Dental Medicine Act of the Republic of Croatia [9]. A question was also asked as to what dentists considered a barrier to better management of dental documentation in their everyday work

2.4. Knowledge of Legal Aspects of Dental Practice

Respondents were given the opportunity to answer questions on obtaining written consents, archiving them, and their knowledge of the right of patients to dispose of personal dental records.

2.5. Awareness of Forensic Odontology

This section enquired about the level of awareness among dentists and their acquired education in forensic odontology.

A statistical analysis was performed using IBM SPSS Statistics (Version 25.0. Armonk, NY, USA: IBM Corp.). A chi-square test was used to assess differences in categorical variables except in cases when there were less than 10 participants per cell, when Fisher's exact test was used. The statistical significance level was set at $p < 0.05$.

3. Results

3.1. General Information on Dentists

The largest number of respondents belonged to the age group of 25 to 45 years, possessed 5 to 20 years of work experience, and were employed in a public health center, respectively. Most of the respondents were graduates of the School of Dental Medicine, University of Zagreb, and were employed in cities across Central Croatia. (Table 1).

Table 1. General information on dentists (number, percentage (%)).

Gender	Female	116 (80.0)
	Male	29 (20.0)
Age	25–45 years	102 (70.3)
	45–65 years	43 (29.7)
Work experience	<5 years	33 (22.8)
	5–20 years	78 (53.8)
	20< years	34 (23.5)
School of basic dental degree	School of Dental Medicine University of Zagreb	118 (81.4)
	Study of Dental Medicine University of Rijeka	16 (11.0)
	Study of Dental Medicine University of Split	7 (4.8)
	Other	4 (2.8)
Practice location, region	Central Croatia	68 (46.9)
	Istria and Croatian Littoral	18 (12.4)
	Slavonia	23 (15.9)
	Dalmatia	36 (24.8)
Type of employment	Public health center	49 (33.8)
	Private practice with CHIF * contract	42 (29.0)
	Private practice	31 (21.4)
	Clinic/polyclinic	23 (15.9)

* Croatian Health Insurance Fund.

3.2. Data on Dental Documentation

Statistical analysis shows that 86.9% of dentists record dental status at first visit, and this routine is more prevalent among dentists in health centers and private practices operating under a CHIF contract than those operating exclusively in private practices ($p < 0.05$). (Table 2).

Table 2. Dental documentation: data items recorded/retained (number, percentage (%)).

Record patients' basic personal data		145 (100.0)
Record patients' additional personal details (maiden name, name of general practitioner, name of another dentist)		67 (46.2)
Medical history	Record	135 (93.1)
	Record and update with each visit	93 (64.1)
Full dental status	Record on first visit	126 (86.9)
	Update with each visit	45 (31.0)
	Update twice a year	41 (28.3)
Record additional data on dentition	Changes in dentitions	80 (55.2)
	Trauma data	119 (82.1)
	Dental anomalies	
	Number	87 (60.4)
	Position	48 (33.1)
	Shape	16 (11.0)
	Diastema	19 (13.1)
	Non-carious lesions	51 (35.2)
	Occlusion, Angle's classification	29 (20.0)
Record details for restorative treatment	Filling surface	104 (71.7)
	Filling material	104 (71.7)
	Other (color, Black's classification, type of preparation)	87 (60.0)
Use abbreviations/codes for recording treatment		101 (69.7)
Store past list of codes for treatment stipulated by the CHIF after they have been changed		43 (29.7)
Use of tooth coding	FDI system	104 (71.7)
	Palmer–Zsigmondy system	28 (19.3)
	ADA Universal system	20 (13.8)
Routinely take X-rays	Orthopantomogram	137 (94.5)
	Periapical radiograph	101 (69.7)
	Bitewing radiograph	45 (31.0)
	Do not routinely take X-rays	5 (3.4)
Take intraoral or extraoral (facial) photographs		89 (61.4)

The practice of updating dental status data is less common for male than female dentists ($p < 0.05$). Dentists in Istria collect significantly more additional data on patients compared with dentists in Dalmatia ($p < 0.05$). In collecting additional data on patients, dentists employed in clinics or polyclinics are more up to date than employees in private practices ($p < 0.05$). When recording details for restorative treatment, such as the color of a material, Black's classification, or the type of preparation, female dentists recorded more details than their male counterparts ($p < 0.05$). The analysis also shows that dentists employed in health centers more often keep old codes for treatment as stipulated by the CHIF than doctors employed in private practices operating under a CHIF contract ($p < 0.05$).

Extraoral and intraoral photographs are more often used by doctors in Central Croatia and Istria than by doctors in Slavonia ($p < 0.05$). Also, photos are used more often in private surgeries, whether operating under a CHIF contract or not, and in clinics, than in health centers ($p < 0.05$).

3.3. Data on Dental Documentation Keeping

The largest number of respondents answered that they keep dental records for a period of five to ten years (33%) while a further 45% keep such records for even longer.

The analysis shows that documentation was kept longer by doctors in Istria and the Croatian Littoral (northern coastal region) than in Dalmatia (southern coastal region) and Slavonia ($p < 0.05$). The same practice is observed in doctors employed in clinics and polyclinics compared with dentists employed in health centers or private practices operating under a CHIF contract ($p < 0.05$). Statistical analysis shows that dentists in health centers kept X-rays for a significantly shorter period (less than five years) compared with employees in private practices operating under a CHIF contract ($p < 0.05$). On the other hand, it is evident that doctors in private surgeries, regardless of whether operating under a CHIF contract or not, keep X-rays for significantly longer (more than 20 years) compared with those in health centers ($p < 0.05$). (Table 3).

Table 3. Practice and duration of dental documentation keeping, and barriers to good practice (number, percentage (%)).

Format of dental records	Digital form	135 (93.1)
	Digital form with backup	99 (68.3)
	Paper form	73 (50.3)
X-ray format	Analog	63 (43.4)
	Digital	137 (94.5)
Duration of X-ray keeping	<5 years	18 (12.4)
	5–10 years	54 (37.2)
	11–15 years	34 (23.4)
	16–20 years	9 (6.2)
	>20 years	30 (20.7)
Other documentation keeping up to 10 years	Dental casts	137 (94.5)
	Temporary works	141 (97.2)
	Implant serial number	88 (60.7)
Barriers to good practice of record keeping	Lack of time	110 (75.9)
	Lack of education	43 (29.7)
	Lack of storage space	51 (35.2)
	Do not consider it important	5 (3.4)

3.4. *Knowledge of Legal Aspects of Dental Practice*

In all, 69% of dentists seek written consents prior to treatment, with a significantly larger number in Istria than those in Dalmatia ($p < 0.05$). Depending on the type of dental practice, the analysis showed that doctors employed in clinics and polyclinics are more likely to obtain written consents than doctors employed in health centers and private practices ($p < 0.05$). (Table 4).

Table 4. Knowledge of legal aspects of dental practice (number, percentage (%)).

Know the law on record retention for 10 years		47 (32.4)
Obtain written consent before treatment		100 (69.0)
Retain informed consent		102 (70.3)
Consider the patient's rights in access to information	Right to the original records	33 (22.8)
	Right to a copy of records	102 (70.3)
	No rights	10 (6.9)

3.5. *Awareness of Forensic Odontology*

Respondents who obtained their degree in dentistry outside of Croatia more often answered that they have no education or training in forensic odontology ($p < 0.05$). (Table 5).

Table 5. Awareness of forensic odontology (number, percentage (%)).

Recognize the scope of forensic odontology in:	Identification of the deceased in unidentified cases	138 (95.2)
	Identification of the perpetrator by bitemark analysis	109 (75.2)
	Other legal proceedings	97 (66.9)
Familiarity with forensic odontology gained in:	Undergraduate study	104 (72.2)
	Specialist study	5 (3.4)
	Professional continuing education	19 (13.1)
	Doctoral study	12 (8.3)
	No knowledge	32 (22.1)

4. Discussion

The total number of collected responses to the questionnaire was 145, equivalent to a response rate of 74%. Accordingly, the survey sampled 2.86% of the total number of currently active dentists in the Republic of Croatia, according to data from the Croatian Dental Chamber [11]. Although it is a low proportion of the total target population, the number is consistent with responses in similar studies [1,12,13]. Our study is the first study on the manner and quality (suitability) of maintaining dental records in the Republic of Croatia. Dentists from all parts of Croatia participated in the survey, with the highest response coming from Central Croatia, followed by Dalmatia. This is due to the larger population of cities in those areas, especially Zagreb as the Croatian capital and Split. The largest number of respondents coming from the 25 to 45 age group can be explained by the higher digital literacy of the younger generation of dentists.

Table 6 lists the current legal requirements for dental documentation maintenance in Croatia. Based on the results obtained in this study, it is evident that Croatian dentists keep dental records in line with statutory requirements and record basic patient data, such as gender, date of birth, address, and contact phone number. About 46% of respondents regularly entered additional data, which can be useful in forensic procedures. This was the case significantly more often for dentists in Istria and the Croatian Littoral as well as those working in clinics and polyclinics. This may be due to greater development of dental tourism in Istria and the Littoral, where foreign patients are treated [14], and possibly a greater awareness among dentists of the need to establish protective measures against potential lawsuits.

Dental charting, handwritten or electronic, should provide an up-to-date insight into the status of a patient's dentition, i.e., the number of existing natural teeth, detected caries lesions, fixed or mobile prosthetic works, fillings, and extractions. During a patient's first visit, dental status is taken by 87% of respondents, more often dentists working in health centers and private practices under a CHIF contract, compared with exclusively private practices ($p < 0.05$). A possible reason for this may be the fact that patients visit public or private surgeries operating under a CHIF contract over a longer period of time, and also when requiring conservative treatment, which is mainly covered by the CHIF, whereas patients visit private dental practice only for specific treatment or procedures, which are usually not covered by the CHIF. The second reason is that the CHIF supervises and controls the work of contracted practices.

Table 6. Legal requirements for dental documentation maintenance in Croatia.

Requirement	Law/Regulation
Patients' basic personal data to be registered in e-charts	Regulation on maintenance of electronic personal health record
Dental documentation must be accurate, detailed, and dated, covering patient's status and treatment	Law on dental medicine
Documentation in electronic form must be protected from changes, unauthorised use, and early destruction	Law on dental medicine
Dental documentation consists of dental record with status chart, medical/dental history, radiographs, and photographs	Law on dental medicine
Obligation to allow patient to access documentation	Law on dental medicine
Obligation of record retention for 10 years	Law on dental medicine
Patient's right to informed consent Content of informed consent form/refusal form	Law on patients' rights Law on informed consent/refusal form

Dental status changes are entered in status charts by 31% of dentists, with 28% of them doing so twice a year, which may correspond to the term "each visit", as regular dental checkups are usually performed every six months. Therefore, almost 60% of dentists regularly update dental charts. Although the proportion of dentists who do not record a detailed status at the first patient visit is small (13%), noting that approximately 40% do not update such statuses regularly, these data are somewhat worrying. In terms of children's oral health care, regularly recording changes in dentition is important, and was performed by 55% of dentists in our study. In forensic analysis, developmental changes in dentition enable estimation of dental age. As for children, there can be only a small number of restorations, if any, and dental age estimation may be crucial for individual identification. An example of such a case is the plane crash over Vrbovec (Croatia), which happened in 1976, where dental age estimation provided supportive evidence for the identification of eight child victims of the accident [10].

Dental anomalies are also important for dental identification because they are relatively rare and provide a unique characteristic to dentition without caries and dental procedures. As the incidence of caries decreases in highly developed countries, the importance of anomalies for dental identification will increase even more. This study shows that dentists rarely recorded dental anomalies except for tooth number anomalies, which were recorded by 60% of respondents (Table 2). Also, only 35% of respondents recorded non-carious dental lesions such as erosion, attrition, and abrasion.

After performing a restorative procedure, data on materials and methods should be entered in the progress notes in the patient record. The majority of surveyed dentists, about 70%, use abbreviations or codes for recording treatment, while only 30% keep old lists of abbreviations after changes. This is a worrying fact because analysis of premortem dental data requires legible, clear, and easily accessible information [1,15]. Statistical analysis has shown that keeping old codes was more often done by dentists who practice in health centers. The reason for this is the fact that dentists in health centers use codes for the purpose of charging of fees to the CHIF, while in private practices payments are made by patients.

For tooth notation, 72% of dentists most often use the FDI tooth numbering system, while the Palmer–Zsigmondy system is more commonly used by respondents who graduated from the University of Split.

The most common choice of radiological image for a routine check-up was an orthopantomogram (95%). Five respondents (3%) answered that they do not routinely take X-rays. Although this is small in number, it is a warning which indicates insufficient education on the importance of X-rays in diagnosing various conditions otherwise undetectable in clinical examinations, as well as in planning therapy and monitoring development in children.

Though not obligatory except in orthodontics and oral rehabilitation, intraoral and extraoral photographs are an excellent complementary record for dental documentation and have great importance in forensics. According to the survey results, photographs were used by 61% of respondents. We consider this a good result, given that it is optional in dental documentation. In modern private practices, dental photography is increasingly used in documenting the initial status of patients and therapy planning.

Most of the respondents (93%) keep documentation in digital form, with 73% using storage on additional media as protection against alteration, premature destruction, or unauthorized use, as required by law [9]. The duration of archiving X-rays was most often 5 to 10 years (37%), with a further 40% of respondents archiving X-rays for even longer. Comparing antemortem and postmortem radiographs may be crucial for dental identification. Even old radiographs can be used to compare tooth morphology and surrounding bone structures.

More than 94% of respondents keep dental casts and temporary replacements in dental documentation. Serial numbers of implants are recorded by 61% of respondents. Statistical analysis showed that dentists working in private practices keep implant serial numbers for significantly longer than dentists in health centers. The reason may be that most implants are used in private surgeries since the CHIF does not cover the costs of implant treatment. Another explanation may be the high cost of implants and possible complaints.

In our study, when asked about barriers to better record keeping, 76% of respondents said it was a lack of time, while 30% indicated a lack of education.

The obligation to keep dental records in Croatia is regulated by the Dental Medicine Act [9]. Only 57 respondents (39%) answered that they know about the period that the law prescribes for archiving documentation, and only 47 (32%) gave the correct answer of 10 years. Most respondents acquired training in forensic dentistry in their undergraduate studies (72%), with more than a fifth of respondents stating that they have no knowledge about forensic odontology and its purpose. Statistical analysis shows that most dentists lacking knowledge of forensic odontology studied outside Croatia (abroad).

Australian dentists record basic personal data of patients in 82% of cases, with only 29% taking additional personal details, which is less often than Croatian dentists [1]. The study by Thampan et al. on a sample of 543 dentists from southern India showed that almost all respondents (97%) record basic patient data; however, the recording of additional data was not investigated [16]. Survey results of American dentists showed similar results to their Croatian counterparts regarding updating information in dental documentation [17]. Most dentists agree on the importance of updating information and cite time constraints as a major obstacle.

Two Indian studies have shown that 89% of dentists in India record dental anomalies and anatomical variations such as the torus mandibularis [16,18], significantly more so than in Croatia. Our results are similar to those in a survey on Australian dentists [1], who keep good records of personal patient data and details of restorative procedures, but somewhat less so when it comes to dental anomalies.

In terms of using abbreviations for recording treatment, our results are comparable to those from Indian dentists, with 67% of dentists using abbreviations or codes [18]. Abbreviations are kept by as much as 64% of Indian dentists as opposed to 30% of Croatian dentists.

In a paper on dental investigation in an air disaster, Ligthelm emphasized the need for international standardization of abbreviations and the maintenance of dental records [10]. This problem is particularly significant in accident investigations involving victims from other countries, as was the case in Thailand after the 2004 tsunami [19]. This is increasingly the case due to the current increasing trend of international migration. In 2019, it was estimated that there are 272 million people living in countries other than their country of birth, which is 3.5% of the world's population [20]. With approx. 82 million migrants, Europe ranks second place, after Asia which has 84 million migrants. Thousands of migrants die while trying to reach Europe, becoming "missing migrants". The Mediterranean Sea is where the highest number of known deaths during migration occur, i.e., 17,919 deaths over a span of five years (2014–2018). These trends are increasing the demand for forensic odontology expertise in human identification and age estimation for the purposes of preventing human rights violations [21]. Croatia, an EU member state, is a transit country for migrants that illegally cross EU borders while heading to Western Europe, and at the same time a country of origin for economic migrants who settle in Western European countries. Thus, legible dental documentation of Croatian citizens may be requested by dentists and forensic odontologists in other European countries, while Croatian forensic odontology experts may encounter challenges in obtaining dental records of migrants from Africa and Asia.

Poor record keeping can be expected in less developed countries [16,18,22–24], but research shows such insufficiencies even in highly developed countries such as the United Kingdom, where as many as 44% inaccurate dental records were found [25]. Research in Sudan has shown that dental students keep dental records more accurately than dentists in private clinics [23].

The situation is similar with archiving dental records, which is regulated by law in developed countries. It may come as a surprise that the legal obligation to maintain such documentation was introduced in Belgium as late as in 2004, and prior to that, it was only deontological and ethical codes that imposed the obligation on dentists to do so [12]. Dentists in India often do not keep records of treatments performed (22%), and if they keep X-rays, it is only for a few months up to a maximum of three years [18]. In Australia and New Zealand, as many as 85% of dentists keep X-rays taken by other dentists, and 63% retain even faulty X-rays [1]. Both Australian and Indian dentists are exceptionally consistent in recording implant serial numbers (70%) [1,18] and, to a lesser extent, Croatian dentists in our research (61%).

American dentists recognize the importance of adequate record keeping and archiving but, due to the lack of guidelines for updating patient records, they spend more time in other aspects of dental practice [17]. Perceived barriers to making accurate and complete dental records by Australian dentists are increased workloads in practice, time constraints, insufficient space for archives, lack of record quality check personnel, as well as lack of experience and education [1]. In our research, only a third of the dentists were familiar with the legal requirement of retaining documentation, and a fifth of the dentists had no knowledge of forensic dentistry and the possible use of dental documentation in forensic procedures.

In Croatia, forensic odontology was introduced as a mandatory course in undergraduate programs in 1997, with the establishment of the Chair of Forensic Dentistry at the School of Dental Medicine, University of Zagreb. It was later introduced in postgraduate programs and professional continuing education. Throughout the course, participants are introduced to the legal obligations of record keeping (informed consent, diagnosis, treatment plan, recording treatment) and the importance and application of documentation in dental identification and use in forensic expertise and litigation related to negligence, malpractice, and the qualification of orofacial injury. Since 2015, the harmonization of the study curriculum with recommendations of the Association for Dental Education in Europe has led to forensic odontology becoming an elective course in undergraduate programs. This has resulted in only some students enrolling onto the course, which is certainly a step backwards.

The International Organization for Forensic Odonto-Stomatology (IOFOS) investigated undergraduate education in forensic odontology and found that a specific teaching course in forensic odontology is neither mandatory nor elective in most undergraduate programs [26]. At the same time, the profile and competences for the graduating European dentist include the Professionalism domain, composed of ethics, regulation, and professional behavior [27], which are covered in a basic forensic odontology course.

5. Conclusions

The results of this research show that Croatian dentists keep and store detailed dental documentation to a great extent; however, there are some insufficiencies in recording dental anomalies and non-carious lesions, as well as omissions in taking and updating dental status, omissions in the use of codes, and inconsistencies in recording fillings, as well as insufficient knowledge of legally required conditions for archiving records. The proper maintenance of dental documentation is become increasingly important due to the development of dental tourism, bringing a large influx of patients from foreign countries. Migration is also causing an increasing demand for forensic odontology expertise, requiring assessments of dental documentation from foreign countries, if available. There is evidently a need for additional education and raising awareness on the importance of properly maintaining dental records. This new direction is necessary not only to facilitate identification of unidentified bodies or bitemark perpetrators, but also to protect dentists from possible lawsuits and litigation. Our research data also indicate the need to adopt a national and international standard for keeping detailed and legible documentation that meets contemporary trends in health care and the requirements of forensic procedures.

Including forensic odontology in compulsory undergraduate courses as well as post-graduate and continuing professional education would equip dentists with knowledge and awareness of the importance and possible application of dental documentation. At the same time, it would allow dentists to achieve and maintain competences in the domain of professionalism. We expect the IOFOS to take further steps in advising authorities to include a basic course of forensic odontology in the undergraduate dental curriculum to meet these goals. Also, dental chambers should be advised to impose a continuing education course on the legal requirements for dental practice as a prerequisite for renewal of the license.

Author Contributions: Conceptualization, I.S.P.; methodology, I.S.P., A.J. and I.M.; investigation, I.S.P., A.J. and I.M.; formal analysis, I.S.P. and J.D.; writing—original draft preparation, A.J., I.M., J.D. and A.Z.Ç.; writing—review and editing, I.S.P. and J.D.; visualization, A.J. and I.M.; supervision, I.S.P. All authors have read and agreed to the published version of the manuscript.

Funding: This research received no external funding.

Institutional Review Board Statement: The study was approved by the Ethics Committee of the School of Dental Medicine, University of Zagreb, on 18 February 2019 (approval number: 05-PA-30-IV-2/2019).

Informed Consent Statement: This research was conducted using an online questionnaire (Google Form). An invitation letter with a link to a questionnaire was sent to email addresses, available publicly or through social media. Only subjects willing to participate accessed and filled in the offered questionnaire anonymously.

Conflicts of Interest: The authors declare no conflict of interest.

References

1. Al-Azri, A.R.; Harford, J.; James, H. Awareness of forensic odontology among dentists in Australia: Are they keeping forensically valuable dental records? *Aust. Dent. J.* **2015**, *61*, 102–108. [CrossRef] [PubMed]
2. Brkić, H.; Lessig, R.; da Silva, R.H.A.; Pinchi, V.; Thevissen, P. (Eds.) *Textbook of Forensic Odonto-Stomatology by IOFOS*; Naklada Slap: Jastrebarsko, Croatia, 2021; 412p.
3. Bernardi, S.; Bianchi, S.; Continenza, M.A.; Pinchi, V.; Macchiarelli, G. Morphological study of the labial grooves' pattern in an Italian population. *Aust. J. Forensic Sci.* **2018**, *52*, 490–499. [CrossRef]
4. Chowdhry, A.; Kapoor, P. Cheiloscopy and Rugoscopy. In *Textbook of Forensic Odonto-Stomatology by IOFOS*; Brkić, H., Lessig, R., da Silva, R.H.A., Pinchi, V., Thevissen, P., Eds.; Naklada Slap: Jastrebarsko, Croatia, 2021; pp. 235–248.
5. Blažić-Potočki, Z.; Brkić, H.; Jerolimov, V.; Macan, D.; Valentić-Peruzović, M.; Varga, S.; Vojvodić, D. *Vještačenje u Stomatologiji*; Stomatološki Fakultet Sveučilišta u Zagrebu i Akademija Medicinskih Znanosti Hrvatske: Zagreb, Croatia, 2005; 107p.

6. Hinchliffe, J. Forensic odontology, part 2. Major disasters. *Br. Dent. J.* **2011**, *210*, 269–274. [CrossRef] [PubMed]
7. Brkić, H.; Petrovečki, V.; Gusić, S. Dental Identification of the Carbonized Body: Case Review. *Acta Stomatol. Croat.* **2002**, *36*, 119–125.
8. Agrawal, N.K.; Dahal, S.; Wasti, H.; Soon, A. Application of Ultraviolet Light in Dental Identification of Avalanche Vic-tims. *J. Nepal. Health Res. Counc.* **2017**, *15*, 193–196. [CrossRef] [PubMed]
9. Zakon o Dentalnoj Medicini. Zakon.hr. Available online: https://www.zakon.hr/z/406/Zakon-o-dentalnoj-medicini (accessed on 2 May 2019).
10. Dumančić, J.; Kaić, Z.; Njemirovskij, V.; Brkić, H.; Zečević, D. Dental Identification after Two Mass Disasters in Croatia. *Croat. Med. J.* **2001**, *42*, 657–662. [PubMed]
11. Croatian Dental Chamber. Strategija Razvoja Dentalne Medicine 2017–2025. 2018. Available online: http://www.hkdm.hr/pic_news/files/pdf/2019/strategija-dent-medicine-2017-2025.pdf (accessed on 2 May 2019).
12. Dierickx, A.; Seyler, M.; De Valck, E.; Wijffels, J.; Willems, G. Dental records: A Belgium study. *J. Forensic Odonto Stomatol.* **2006**, *24*, 22–31.
13. Gambhir, R.S.; Singh, G.; Talwar, P.S.; Gambhir, J.; Munjal, V. Knowledge and awareness of forensic odontology among dentists in India: A systematic review. *J. Forensic Dent. Sci.* **2016**, *8*, 2–6. [CrossRef] [PubMed]
14. Karahasanović, V. Dental Tourism Marketing in Istrian County. Graduation Thesis, Juraj Dobrila University of Pula, Pula, Croatia, 25 September 2017. Available online: https://urn.nsk.hr/urn:nbn:hr:137:185351 (accessed on 1 May 2019).
15. Charangowda, B. Dental records: An overview. *J. Forensic Dent. Sci.* **2010**, *2*, 5–10. [CrossRef] [PubMed]
16. Thampan, N.; Janani, R.; Ramya, R.; Bharanidharan, R.; Kumar, A.; Rajkumar, K. Antemortem dental records versus individual identification. *J. Forensic. Dent. Sci.* **2018**, *10*, 158–163. [CrossRef] [PubMed]
17. Tokede, O.; Ramoni, R.B.; Patton, M.; Da Silva, J.D.; Kalenderian, E. Clinical documentation of dental care in an era of electronic health record use. *J. Evid. Based Dent. Pract.* **2016**, *16*, 154–160. [CrossRef] [PubMed]
18. Sarode, G.S.; Sarode, S.C.; Choudhary, S.; Patil, S.; Anand, R.; Vyas, H. Dental records of forensic odontological importance: Maintenance pattern among dental practitioners of Pune city. *J. Forensic Dent. Sci.* **2017**, *9*, 48. [PubMed]
19. Schuller-Götzburg, P. Dental Identification of Tsunami Victims in Phuket, Thailand. *Acta Stomatol. Croat.* **2007**, *41*, 295–305.
20. International Organisation of Migration. World Migration Report. 2020. Available online: https://publications.iom.int/system/files/pdf/wmr_2020.pdf (accessed on 10 January 2021).
21. Nuzzolese, E. Missing people, migrants, identification and human rights. *J. Forensic Odonto Stomatol.* **2012**, *30*, 47–59.
22. Wadhwani, S.; Shetty, P.; Sreelatha, S. Maintenance of antemortem dental records in private dental clinics: Knowledge, attitude, and practice among the practitioners of Mangalore and surrounding areas. *J. Forensic Dent. Sci.* **2017**, *9*, 78–82. [CrossRef] [PubMed]
23. Waleed, P.; Baba, F.; Alsulami, S.; Tarakji, B. Importance of Dental Records in Forensic Dental Identification. *Acta Inform. Med.* **2015**, *23*, 49–52. [CrossRef] [PubMed]
24. Preethi, S.; Einstein, A.; Sivapathasundharam, B. Awareness of forensic odontology among dental practitioners in Chennai: A knowledge, attitude, practice study. *J. Forensic Dent. Sci.* **2011**, *3*, 63–66. [CrossRef] [PubMed]
25. Brown, N.L.; El Jephcote, V.; Morrison, J.N.; Sutton, J.E. Inaccurate dental charting in an audit of 1128 general dental practice records. *Dent. Updat.* **2017**, *44*, 254–260. [CrossRef] [PubMed]
26. Pinchi, V. Education and Qualification in Forensic Odontology. In *Textbook of Forensic Odonto-Stomatology by IOFOS*; Brkić, H., Lessig, R., da Silva, R.H.A., Pinchi, V., Thevissen, P., Eds.; Naklada Slap: Jastrebarsko, Croatia, 2021; pp. 387–406.
27. Field, J.C.; Cowpe, J.G.; Walmsley, A.D. The Graduating European Dentist: A New Undergraduate Curriculum Frame-work. *Eur. J. Dent. Educ.* **2017**, *21* (Suppl. 1), 2–10. [CrossRef]

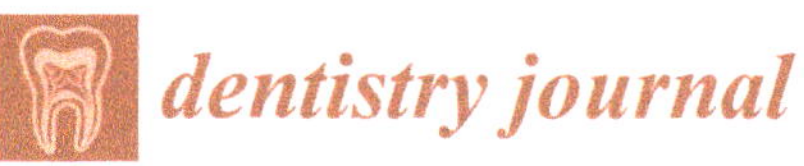

MDPI

Article

Identifying Risk Factors Affecting the Usage of Digital and Social Media: A Preliminary Qualitative Study in the Dental Profession and Dental Education

Rayan Sharka [1,2,*], Jonathan P. San Diego [1,*], Melanie Nasseripour [1] and Avijit Banerjee [3]

1 Centre for Dental Education, Faculty of Dentistry, Oral & Craniofacial Sciences, King's College London, London SE1 9RT, UK; melanie.nasseripour@kcl.ac.uk

2 Oral and Maxillofacial Department and Diagnostic Sciences, Faculty of Dentistry, Umm Al-Qura University, Makkah 24381, Saudi Arabia

3 Centre of Oral Clinical Translational Sciences, Faculty of Dentistry, Oral & Craniofacial Sciences, King's College London/Guy's & St. Thomas' NHS Hospitals Trust, London SE1 9RT, UK; avijit.banerjee@kcl.ac.uk

* Correspondence: rayan.sharka@kcl.ac.uk (R.S.); jonathan.p.san_diego@kcl.ac.uk (J.P.S.D.)

Abstract: Aims: This study aimed to identify the risk factors of using DSM to provide an insight into the inherent implications this has on dental professionals in practice and trainee professionals' education. Materials and methods: Twenty-one participants (10 dental professionals and 11 undergraduate and postgraduate dental students) participated in this qualitative study using semi-structured interviews in a dental school in the UK. The interviews were analysed and categorised into themes, some of which were identified from previous literature (e.g., privacy and psychological risks) and others emerged from the data (e.g., deceptive and misleading information). Results: The thematic analysis of interview transcripts identified nine perceived risk themes. Three themes were associated with the use of DSM in the general context, and six themes were related to the use of DSM in professional and education context. Conclusions: This study provided evidence to understand the risk factors of using DSM in dental education and the profession, but the magnitude of these risks on the uptake and usefulness of DSM needs to be assessed.

Keywords: undergraduate dental education; postgraduate dental education; continuing education; professionalism in dentistry; online education; digital media; social media; perceived risks

Citation: Sharka, R.; San Diego, J.P.; Nasseripour, M.; Banerjee, A. Identifying Risk Factors Affecting the Usage of Digital and Social Media: A Preliminary Qualitative Study in the Dental Profession and Dental Education. *Dent. J.* **2021**, *9*, 53. https://doi.org/10.3390/dj9050053

Academic Editors: Jelena Dumancic and Božana Lončar Brzak

Received: 23 February 2021
Accepted: 3 May 2021
Published: 8 May 2021

1. Introduction

The digital and social media (DSM) are defined in this study as internet-based applications that allow the creation and exchange of user-generated content and the associated digital technologies used in this creation and exchange [1]. Prominent examples of DSM include a range of communication modes across social media platforms (e.g., Twitter, Facebook, and Instagram), instant messaging apps (e.g., WhatsApp, WeChat), and video conferencing platforms (e.g., Zoom, MS Teams) through users' smartphone or computer devices. The current 3.8 billion global DSM users suggest there is an increasing impact of DSM in the private and working lives of the general population [2]. This has extended to dental students and dental professionals, with up to 98% of dental students and 75% of dental professionals reporting that they used DSM for professional and personal use [3,4], for example, for communication (with friends and family), professional education (teaching and learning dentistry), or dental practice advertisement (promoting oral health care and marketing dental services) [5–7]. The literature suggests that both user groups have highlighted perceived risks associated with the use of DSM [8,9]. Perceived risks can be defined as a possible loss, harm, or uncertainty of using DSM services [10]. Previous studies in the general online services context have applied this definition to understand and address the risk associated with the use of information technology and social media to advance the uptake of its services in the general population [10,11]. In this paper, these are referred to risks associated with the use of DSM in the general context.

Dental professionals in academic and practice settings have a professional reputation as well as regulatory requirements to uphold and be sensitive to since they have a professional standing that elicits society's trust [12]. Concerns about breaching patients' confidentiality and compliance with regulations and professional standards could also hinder the uptake of DSM in the professional context [13]. In this paper, these are referred to risks associated with the use of DSM in the professional and education context.

Despite the ongoing debate of the usefulness of DSM in dentistry [13], there have been few attempts to identify the risks of using DSM between the contexts in terms of general usage and how usage specific to dental education and profession affects the uptake of using DSM. Additionally, although this body of knowledge about dental students and professionals' compliance is crucial [14,15], there are several other general and professional risks that need to be explored and discussed. Moreover, without a doubt, the COVID-19 pandemic has brought immense challenges to dental education worldwide, which has caused a sudden transition to implement online technologies, including DSM [16]. Therefore, identifying risk perceptions associated with the implementation of such technologies seems to be justified and rational. This study aimed to identify the risk factors of using DSM to provide an insight into the inherent implications this has on dental professionals in practice and the education of trainee professionals. Dental students and professionals' risk perceptions appeared to differ from the public risk perceptions of using DSM. The research questions were:

RQ1: What are the perceived risks that can be identified associated with dental students and professionals using DSM in dental education and practice?

RQ2: Do the identified risks associate specifically with dental education and professional context and/or general usage context?

2. Materials and Methods

2.1. Participants and the Setting

Ethical approval was granted by King's College London Ethics Committee (LRS-18/19-8867). The study participants included dental students (undergraduate/postgraduate students) and dental professionals (clinical teachers providing dental care and teaching) and were recruited by email and invitation posters using purposive sampling to give participants a chance to participate in this study voluntarily [17,18]. The interviews were conducted until the interview responses reached saturation, that is when the responses did not provide new perceived risk themes during interview analysis [19]. Using these procedures, a total of 21 participants, 11 dental students, and 10 dental professionals participated in this study, of which, 12 were male, and nine were female. The median age of the dental students was 22 years (range 18–35), and for the dental professionals, the median age was 33 years (range 30–51).

2.2. Interview Procedure

A semi-structured interview guide, including open-ended questions followed by prompting questions to probe into details, was followed during interviews to elicit responses about perceived risks. The main aspects discussed in the interviews included the anticipated perceived risks and factors that influence their current use and activities of DSM and any particular challenges that could be hindering dental students and professionals' use of DSM in general and professional contexts. The interview guide was piloted with two dental students to ensure that the questions were appropriate and understandable [20]. The interviews were conducted face-to-face in a quiet office over five months between 2019 and 2020 and lasted between 15–30 min. They were audio-recorded and transcribed verbatim. An incentive Amazon voucher worth £10 was offered to each participant at the end of the interview in appreciation of their time.

2.3. Thematic Analysis Process and Coding

The initial code descriptions were developed and informed by previous studies [3–11]. Following the transcription of each interview, the main researcher read the transcripts to highlight and note the risks identified in the process of familiarisation. To ensure systematic coding and reflexivity, phrases were first coded into perceived risks and other non-risks, the risk phrases were then scrutinised to produce preliminary codes of perceived risks, which were peer-validated with a second researcher (J.S.D.) to ensure the rigour and validation of the codes. Coding descriptions not identified previously in the literature which emerged from the data were added to the coding scheme [21]. This process formed a working coding scheme which was subject to several iterations of refinement to review and refine each risk code (Table 1). To ensure the reliability of a coding scheme, the assessment of the inter-coder reliability (ICR) and the level of consistency was established following the methodology of MacPhail et al. (the overall Kappa score = 0.70) [22]. A consensus agreement was achieved through the feedback from the two coders, with any discrepancies between the two coders reconciled.

All transcripts were then imported into Nvivo12 software (QSR International Pty Ltd., Melbourne, Australia) for thematic analysis, and each code of the coding scheme was entered as a node. The illustrative phrases of perceived risks from all interview transcripts were assigned into each code. The researchers then examined the coded data for further validation. The process of coding and developing risk codes is summarised in Figure 1.

Table 1. The coding scheme developed based on literature review and interviews to code the interview transcripts.

Codes	Description	Example
• Negative effect on self-esteem and self-image	The possibility of an adverse effect on the users' peace of mind or self-esteem from using DSM.	"I believe that DSM does affect self-esteem due to exposing users to a vast number of photos, such as ideal body image, that would affect self-esteem or self-image".
• Scrutiny and negative comments concerns	The possibility of receiving negative comments and criticism from using DSM.	"I will receive negative remarks from others if I use DSM"
• Disclosure of personal data without the user's knowledge	The potential loss of control over personal information leads to the information being used without the user's knowledge or permission.	"Someone else can take the photo that I posted on my profile and use it without my consent".
• Intrusion into personal space	The state when personal/private life is observed or disturbed by others.	"Using DSM would allow others to observe my private life".
• Fear of hacking and identity fraud	The potential loss of control over the DSM profile and account due to hacking and criminal attacks.	"Internet hackers (criminals) might take control of my checking account if I used a DSM".
• Spending excessive time	The possibility of losing time when using DSM by wasting time searching and browsing different activities on DSM.	"There is a possible time loss due to engaging in different activities on DSM".
• Keeping away from doing pertinent tasks	The possibility of losing the time for doing important tasks (e.g., studying, exercising, etc.)	"If I had begun to use DSM, there are chances that I will lose time doing other essential tasks".
• Social loss	The potential loss of status in one's social group due to adopting DSM.	"My signing up for and using DSM would lead to a social loss for me because my friends and relatives would think less highly of me".
• Financial loss	The potential loss of money due to adopting DSM.	"There are the chances that you stand to lose money if you use DSM".
• Performance issues	The possibility of the DSM not performing as it was designed and advertised.	"DSM might not perform well and create problems".

Table 1. *Cont.*

Codes	Description	Example
• Lack of validity and reliability of the information	The possibility of using/sharing unreliable and invalid information on DSM.	"The information posted on DSM is poorly referenced and unreliable".
• Not evidence-based information	The possibility of using/sharing not evidence-based information on DSM.	"On YouTube and Google, you have to be careful in terms of what you are taking as evidence-based or not".
• Information has a lack of quality assurance	The possibility that the information shared on DSM is not critically appraised to ensure its quality.	"The information posted on DSM has a lack of quality assurance."
• Facing disciplinary action from regulatory bodies	The possibility of facing disciplinary action from using DSM.	"You must be aware and not make a mistake when using DSM to avoid disciplinary action".
• Legal and ethical issues	The possibility of exposure to legal penalties from using DSM.	"There is a risk of legal and ethical issues associated with DSM usage".
• Damage the professional image and reputation	The state of damage the professional image when using DSM inappropriately.	"I think using DSM is risky because anything you put could stay forever and affect your professional image".
• Not following governing bodies guidelines	The possibility of violating guidelines when using DSM.	"It is crucial to make sure that all the regulations are followed when using DSM".
• Breaching patient confidentiality	The possibility of violating and breaching patients' confidentiality when using DSM.	"I believe that using DSM is good as long as they do not expose patient privacy".
• Obtaining explicit consent	The possibility of sharing patients' information on DSM without explicit consent.	"There is a risk of sharing patients' photos on DSM without explicit consent".
• False and misleading information	The state of sharing misleading information when using DSM.	"There is lots of misleading and false information shared on DSM".
• Being deceptive in dental promotions	The state of sharing deceptive dental promotions on DSM.	"Someone can easily photoshop and play with the quality of clinical work and enhance how the treatment looks".

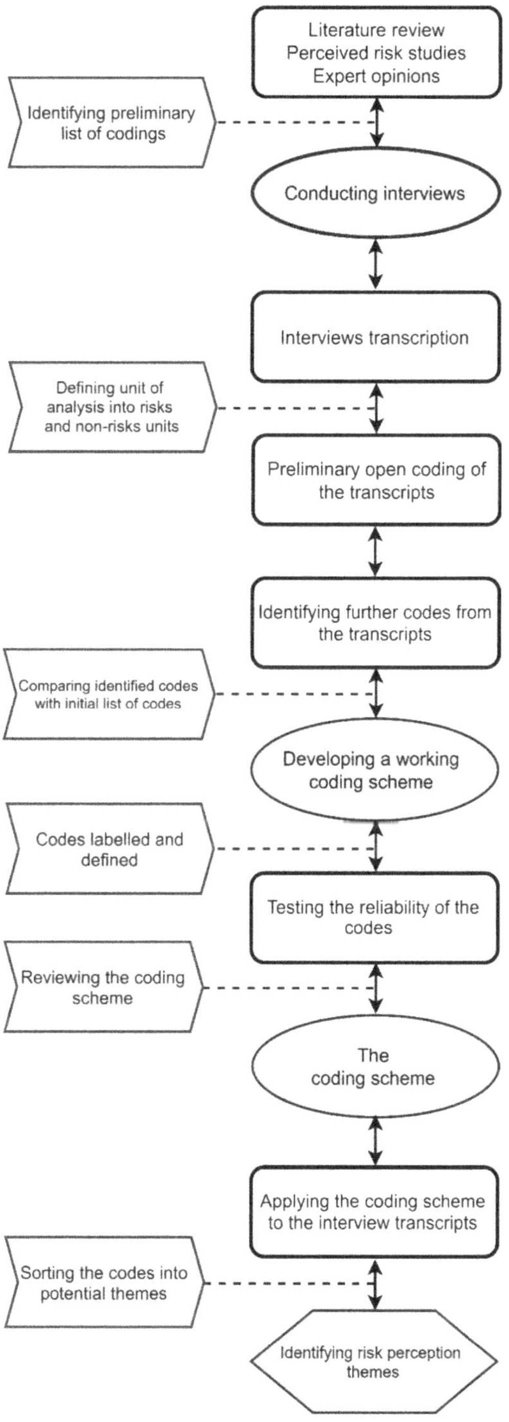

Figure 1. Process of analysis and developing themes.

3. Results

From the thematic analysis of the 21 interviews, a total of 302 phrases were identified and coded (140 risk codes and 162 non-risk codes). The 140 risk codes were assigned to 21 sub-themes, then clustered to identify nine main risk themes (Figure 2), three of which were associated with using DSM in the general context, and six themes which were associated with using DSM in professional and education context. In the following Sections 3.1 and 3.2, each perceived risk theme is defined and presented with illustrated exemplar quotes. Table 2 presents the distribution of themes by the number of participants and the frequency of occurrence.

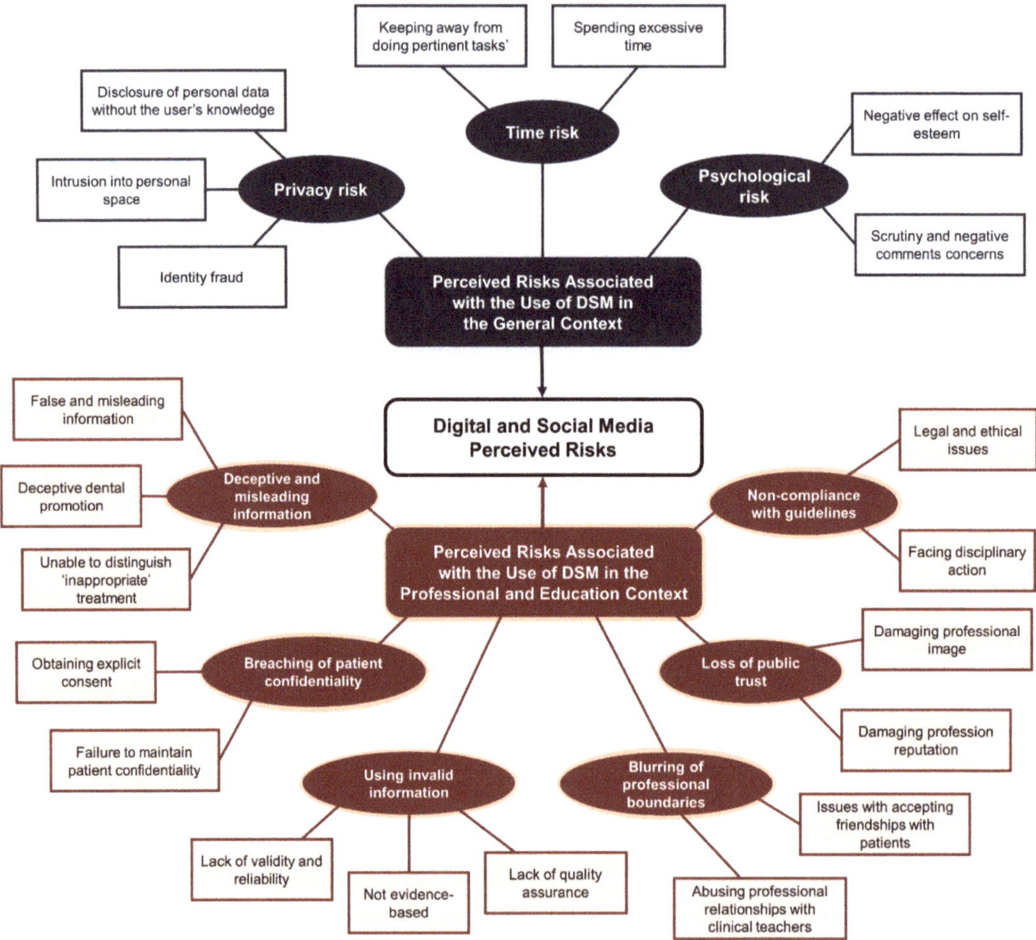

Figure 2. Thematic map showing the 21 sub-themes (rectangular shape) and nine main themes (oval shape).

Table 2. Distribution of themes, by number of total participants (n = 21) and number of total occurrences (n = 140).

Perceived Risk Themes Associated with the Use of DSM in the General Context	Number of Participants	Number of Occurrences
1. Privacy risks	14	25
2. Psychological risks	14	18
3. Time risks	11	13
Perceived Risk Themes Associated with the Use of DSM in the Professional and Education Context	**Number of Participants**	**Number of Occurrences**
4. Using invalid information	14	20
5. Non-compliance with guidelines	10	17
6. Breaches of patients' confidentiality	10	15
7. Deceptive and misleading information	9	12
8. Blurring of professional boundaries	8	10
9. Loss of public trust	7	10

3.1. Perceived Risk Themes Associated with the Use of DSM in the General Context

3.1.1. Theme (1): Privacy Risk

This theme showed highest occurrence (25 codes) across interviews, with seven out of 11 dental students having concerns about revealing personal information, such as posting and sharing private photos and specific personal life areas to the public on DSM. They preferred to use DSM within a narrow circle of people, such as families and friends, without intrusion from stranger users. For example, one dental student mentioned that "My personal accounts are private, and only my friends and family members follow me" (DS.9).

Furthermore, seven dental professionals considered that the wide availability and easy accessibility of personal information on DSM could lead to identity fraud and ID theft. For example, one dental professional described how DSM allows scammers to steal users' identity and personal information, leading to damage to a person's credit or reputation. He explained, "someone can create a fake account and post stuff as yourself, especially if you are a well-known person; you definitely have friends and enemies, and they can use your information on DSM and write untrue information about you" (DP.6).

3.1.2. Theme (2): Psychological Risk

Seven out of 11 dental students reported that DSM is an open space for users to share and post contents. This kind of usage is not protected from scrutiny and negative comments, which adversely affect feelings and self-esteem. For example, one dental student described this situation by saying that "some people posting their work, they think it is good but everyone else making fun of their work saying that your work is bad, it is too invasive; there are always risks like humiliation, and personally I do not like that" (DS.9). Similarly, seven dental professionals mentioned that they decreased their interaction with people through DSM due to the possibility of receiving negative remarks from others. One dental professional commented "I do not like to use DSM to avoid any unnecessary negative comments that make me inconvenient" (DP.5).

3.1.3. Theme (3): Time Risk

A concern of spending excessive time on DSM was discussed during interviews. Eleven out of 21 of dental students and professionals had concerns of spending too much time on DSM. One dental student noted that DSM platforms use a variety of means that encourage users to engage and spend time. He explained that "you can spend ages browsing and achieving nothing in your work, especially if you have a deadline" (DS. 11).

Also, five dental professionals described the same issue, supporting this opinion, and reported that using DSM in browsing and socialising with others wastes time and hinders them from doing pertinent tasks. "With regards to personal use, it is very time-consuming; it keeps you away from daily physical activities just by staying on it and browsing" (DP. 8).

3.2. *Perceived Risk Themes Associated with the Use of DSM in the Professional and Education Context*

3.2.1. Theme (4): Using Invalid Information

This theme presented the second highest occurrence across interviews (20 codes), with seven dental students perceiving uncertainty about using information shared on DSM because the quality of the information was different from that taught in the authentic academic environment. One dental student noted that "there is much information out there so that you do not know what is evidence-based and what is not" (DS.4). Another student supported this claim by saying that "sometimes it is questionable, and sometimes the stuff we learnt is different from what they are doing" (DS.6).

Similarly, seven dental professionals acknowledged that the main drawback of using DSM for learning is a lack of assurance of the quality of the information; "there is no filtering feature that helps the user to distinguish between the right and wrong information" (DP.9), explained one dental professional.

3.2.2. Theme (5): Non-Compliance with Guidelines

Dental students and professionals were aware of DSM guidelines issued by professional governing bodies and subsequent disciplinary actions. Six dental students reported their cautious use of DSM to avoid violation of these guidelines. For example, one student noted that "if you are a dental student, you have to be aware and do not make a mistake" (DS.11). Additionally, four dental professionals mentioned the importance of complying with authority guidelines. One dental professional noted, "it is good to make sure that all the regulations are followed" (DP.3).

3.2.3. Theme (6): Breaches of Patients' Confidentiality

Five dental students stated that, even with patient consent, using DSM to post or share patient's information still presents issues as "all photos are on the internet technically forever so any person can download and share it. There is a sticky situation in doing that" (DS.9) one dental student explained. Likewise, five dental professionals disagreed with using DSM to share dental cases. One dental professional said, "I kind of see it like a breach of patient confidentiality, even with the obtained consent form" (DP.6).

3.2.4. Theme (7): Deceptive and Misleading Information

Five dental students mentioned that DSM could be used to share information which misled or showed inaccurate dental treatments or promotions. "The public, unfortunately, gets a lot of wrong information; I think people are promoting information to get benefit from it such as [Snap-On Smile]" (DS.3), explained one dental student. Additionally, one student gave an example of such deceptive dental promotion on DSM. He stated that "You see cases posted on DSM such as [3 to 3 crowns or veneers]; did the patients need that? I think that's where the danger is, when you go online, and people think this is the normal treatment" (DS.7).

Similarly, four dental professionals discussed other aspects of misinformation such as the dental contents shared on DSM for the public not being created by specialised health care. One professional explained that "you can easily get fake information or untrue information because not all the posts are created or written by dental professionals" (DP. 6).

3.2.5. Theme (8): Blurring of Professional Boundaries

Thirty-eight percent of students and professionals interviewed felt that the line between personal and professional blurred when interacting on DSM. Six dental students described the type of interaction with dental professionals as inappropriate. One dental student said, "if I tag him on a Facebook post and say hi mate, this would be less professional" (DS.1). Similarly, dental professionals believed that their position as educators placed them in a conflicting position when interacting with their dental students on DSM. Therefore, they favoured maintaining a clear boundary between professional and personal lives. One dental professional noted, "I think it is good to have a boundary between professional life and personal life, and I think sometimes that barrier can be quite abused" (DP.3).

3.2.6. Theme (9): Loss of Public Trust

Dental students reported that using DSM could reflect negatively on their reputation and affiliated institutions if they share unprofessional content. "I would not post anything which someone could question about me as a dental professional" (DS.8), explained one dental student. Similarly, two dental professionals stated the same perception. For example, one dental professional said, "if you set up your professional profile, you cannot be perceived like a normal user! You cannot be a person who is having a party on Sunday or the weekend and posting it on DSM. You have to be a professional person" (DP. 2).

4. Discussion

This study attempted to identify the risk perceptions specific to dental students and dental professionals' usage of DSM and discuss how their perceptions are different from the public users. Interestingly, some perceived risks were consistent with the use of DSM in the general context identified in previous studies [10,11], including psychological, privacy, and time risks, and others were associated with the use of DSM in the professional and education context, such as non-compliance with guidelines, breaching patient's confidentiality, and using invalid information [8,9,14,15].

The identified risk themes indicated that DSM impacted both the professional and personal life of dental students and professionals. When they used DSM in their personal life, they perceived similar risks as users perceived in a general e-services context [10,11]. However, the significant theme was privacy risks because the nature of DSM usage is to connect and interact with colleagues or friends by revealing information, such as sharing thoughts, photos, movements, facial expressions, and interests with others. This type of activity is neither guarded against strangers nor effectively able to be protected. Such concern has been found to be an essential factor affecting the unwillingness and dissatisfaction to use DSM [11,23]. A comparable outcome was reached previously among a sample of dental students and dental educators, when 60% of them stated that privacy concerns were the major reason for not using DSM [4,15]. Nevertheless, in this study, dental students and professionals extended their perceptions to include other aspects of privacy issues, such as a high incidence of hacking and personal data breaches, making them speculate the security of their personal information on DSM.

Interestingly, psychological issues emerged from the interviews, which is in line with a growing number of studies that suggest a possible association between using DSM and a potential negative influence on self-esteem, depression, and emotions [24,25]. In this study, this could be explained by the fact that most DSM interactions were unprotected from negative remarks that may affect dental students and professionals' self-esteem, causing feelings of distress. Similarly, Davila et al. observed that depressive symptoms, including sadness and feelings of worthlessness, were associated with the quality of online communications and interactions they received while using DSM [26]. Another explanation could be due to the excessive time that dental students and professionals spend on DSM. According to a study by Iwamoto and Chun, significant positive correlations were found between the hours spent on DSM and stress, anxiety, and depression in a sample of undergraduate students [25].

Approximately half of the interviewees admitted that they were spending up to two hours per day on DSM, which could negatively impact students' academic progress and professionals' daily work. This theme indicated that DSM platforms provide various means that genuinely encourage users to allocate considerable time, ranging from connecting with friends to browsing the latest news and exploring other posts, making it time-consuming.

These findings are supported by a previous study among dental students who believed that using DSM was time-consuming and distracted them from their studies [27].

With regards to risks associated with the use of DSM in professional and education context, the interviewees shed light on a crucial risk, that is, invalid information. They noted that DSM has become an open-learning resource, providing educational materials through a user-generated content feature; however, much information shared is neither checked for its validity nor based on a reliable source. This important finding has been discussed in the literature and could have serious implications for dental education [8]; hence, dental students and professionals need additional training and education to search for evidence-based information effectively. In a recent study, Khatoon et al. demonstrated that dental students might not be competent in the skills and experience required to scrutinise the information shared online [28]. With the current dramatic move to online education and the imminent surge in the adoption of digital technologies to disseminate educational contents due to the COVID-19 pandemic, such crucial training has become a necessity [29]. Furthermore, nearly half of the dental students and professionals stated that they could be in breach of patient confidentiality if they shared their work, including clinical cases, on DSM. Additionally, some of them reported that posting patients' photos was entirely unacceptable, even if consent was obtained. The governing dental body, such as the General Dental Council (GDC) in the UK, declared that posting unidentifiable patients' photos on social media was prohibited without explicit consent from patients [30]. Patients should manifest an understanding of this reality before consenting. Several studies showed differences in the perceptions of dental students relating to this argument, suggesting the importance of introducing e-professionalism education to the curriculum of undergraduate and postgraduate students to help them avoid these pitfalls when using DSM [3,14]. Furthermore, a point worth consideration is that dental students and professionals must be familiar with the dental school and hospital guidelines governing DSM use and strictly comply to them as the laws in different countries about posting patient images on DSM could differ.

Even though this study aimed to understand the risk perceptions that concern dental students and professionals themselves as health care providers, they reported a risk that affects public users, including their patients. DSM creates uncontrolled online spaces, housing communication and dental advertising that might contain a potential threat of misinformation, which could affect the delivery of treatment care or management of patient expectations of dental practice. Some dental professionals warned of such information [31], especially for patients among young groups who are very sensitive to the perception of their dental, facial, and body appearance [32]. Shuttleworth and Smith stated that the rising incidence of cases that are influenced by the misinformation posted on DSM could open up new challenges for stakeholders in the dental health system, with the increased sharing of commercially-directed advertisements on such uncontrolled platforms [33].

It is noteworthy to mention that the impact of the ample challenges brought by COVID-19 on the perceptions of dental students and professionals have not been investigated in this study [16]. Future studies to analyse the impact of COVID-19 on the use of DSM in the professional development and training of dental students are required.

Furthermore, it is imperative to utilise quantitative methodology, e.g., a questionnaire instrument with a larger number of participants, to generalise the identified risks and assess differences between groups and their magnitude on the uptake of DSM in dental education.

5. Conclusions

This study presented the critical risks of DSM that influence dental students and professionals' usage of DSM that have not been previously explored in such a comprehensive approach. Furthermore, the combination of perceived risks in the developed framework as presented in Figure 2 is novel and provides a unique contribution to dental schools' policymakers to widen their lens about risks that affect dental students and professionals, which are different from those previously identified among public users. Dental educators can benefit from the findings of this study, which could be adopted as an introductory guideline to advance the usage of DSM among dental students and professionals with the guidance of existing governing bodies regarding social media.

Finally, dental students and professionals need to be more vigilant in using DSM so as not to damage the image of the profession and lose public trust. They need training and reassurance on how to overcome these risks and acquire a clear sense of how they might open up new avenues for knowledge dissemination, promotion ideas, and connection with the public, including their patients.

Author Contributions: R.S. conceptualised and designed the study, collected and analysed the data, interpreted the results, and wrote the original draft; J.P.S.D. conceptualised and designed the study, critically revised the manuscript, and supervised the project; M.N. conceptualised and designed the study, critically revised the manuscript, and supervised the project; A.B. conceptualised and designed the study, critically reviewed the manuscript, and supervised the project. All authors have read and agreed to the published version of the manuscript.

Funding: This study was funded by the Ministry of Education of Saudi Arabia (Umm Al-Qura University) as a part of the first author's research studies at the Faculty of Dentistry Oral & Craniofacial Sciences, King's College London. The funder had no role in study design, data collection and analysis, decision to publish, or preparation of the manuscript.

Institutional Review Board Statement: The study was approved by the Institutional Review Board of King's College London Ethics Committee (LRS-18/19-8867) on 23 April 2019.

Informed Consent Statement: Informed consent was obtained from all participants involved in the study.

Data Availability Statement: The data presented in this study are stored in a digital secured place of King's College London and available upon reasonable request.

Acknowledgments: The authors wish to thank all participants involved in the study for their effort and time.

Conflicts of Interest: The authors declare no conflict of interest.

References

1. Kaplan, A.M.; Haenlein, M. Users of the world, unite! The challenges and opportunities of Social Media. *Bus. Horiz.* **2010**, *53*, 59–68. [CrossRef]
2. Digital in 2020: Global Internet Use Accelerates. 2020. Available online: https://wearesocial.com/digital-2020 (accessed on 27 November 2020).
3. Dobson, E.; Patel, P.; Neville, P. Perceptions of e-professionalism among dental students: A UK dental school study. *Br. Dent. J.* **2019**, *226*, 73–78. [CrossRef]
4. Arnett, M.R.; Loewen, J.M.; Romito, L.M. Use of social media by dental educators. *J. Dent. Educ.* **2013**, *77*, 1402–1412. [CrossRef]
5. Gonzalez, S.; Gadbury-Amyot, C. Using Twitter for Teaching and Learning in an Oral and Maxillofacial Radiology Course. *J. Dent. Educ.* **2016**, *80*, 149–155. [CrossRef] [PubMed]
6. O'Brien, S.; Duane, B. Delivery of information to orthodontic patients using social media. *Evid. Based Dent.* **2017**, *18*, 59–60. [CrossRef] [PubMed]
7. Parmar, N.; Dong, L.; Eisingerich, A.B. Connecting with Your Dentist on Facebook: Patients' and Dentists' Attitudes Towards Social Media Usage in Dentistry. *J. Med. Internet Res.* **2018**, *20*, 101–109. [CrossRef]
8. Bhola, S.; Hellyer, P. The risks and benefits of social media in dental foundation training. *Br. Dent. J.* **2016**, *221*, 609–613. [CrossRef] [PubMed]
9. Greer, A.C.; Stokes, C.W.; Zijlstra-Shaw, S.; Sandars, J.E. Conflicting demands that dentists and dental care professionals experience when using social media: A scoping review. *Br. Dent. J.* **2019**, *227*, 893–899. [CrossRef]
10. Featherman, M.S.; Pavlou, P.A. Predicting e-services adoption: A perceived risk facets perspective. *Int. J. Hum. Comput.* **2003**, *59*, 451–474. [CrossRef]
11. Khan, G.F.; Swar, B.; Lee, S.K. Social Media Risks and Benefits: A Public Sector Perspective. *Soc. Sci. Comput. Rev.* **2014**, *32*, 606–627. [CrossRef]
12. Holden, A.C.L. Paradise Lost; the reputation of the dental profession and regulatory scope. *Br. Dent. J.* **2017**, *222*, 239–241. [CrossRef]
13. De Peralta, T.L.; Farrior, O.F.; Flake, N.M.; Gallagher, D.; Susin, C.; Valenza, J. The Use of Social Media by Dental Students for Communication and Learning: Two Viewpoints. *J. Dent. Educ.* **2019**, *83*, 663–668. [CrossRef] [PubMed]

14. Kenny, P.; Johnson, I.G. Social media use, attitudes, behaviours and perceptions of online professionalism amongst dental students. *Br. Dent. J.* **2016**, *221*, 651–655. [CrossRef] [PubMed]
15. Arnett, M.R.; Christensen, H.L.; Nelson, B.A. A school-wide assessment of social media usage by students in a US dental school. *Br. Dent. J.* **2014**, *217*, 531–535. [CrossRef]
16. Bennardo, F.; Buffone, C.; Fortunato, L.; Giudice, A. COVID-19 is a challenge for dental education—A commentary. *Eur. J. Dent. Educ.* **2020**, *24*, 822–824. [CrossRef]
17. Ritchie, J.; Lewis, J.; Nicholls, C.M.; Ormston, R. *Qualitative Research Practice: A Guide for Social Science Students and Researchers*, 1st ed.; SAGE Publications Ltd.: London, UK, 2003; pp. 78–79.
18. Bryman, A. *Social Research Methods*, 4th ed.; Oxford University Press: New York, NY, USA, 2016; pp. 418–419.
19. Saunders, B.; Sim, J.; Kingstone, T.; Baker, S.; Waterfield, J.; Bartlam, B.; Burroughs, H.; Jinks, C. Saturation in qualitative research: Exploring its conceptualization and operationalization. *Qual. Quant.* **2018**, *52*, 1893–1907. [CrossRef]
20. Abdul Majid, M.; Othman, M.; Mohamad, S.; Lim, S.A.H.; Yusof, A. Piloting for Interviews in Qualitative Research: Operationalization and Lessons Learnt. *Int. J. Acad. Res. Bus. Soc. Sci.* **2017**, *31*, 1073–1080.
21. DeCuir-Gunby, J.T.; Marshall, P.L.; McCulloch, A.W. Developing and using a codebook for the analysis of interview data: An example from a professional development research project. *Field Methods* **2011**, *23*, 136–155. [CrossRef]
22. MacPhail, C.; Khoza, N.; Abler, L.; Ranganathan, M. Process guidelines for establishing intercoder reliability in qualitative studies. *Qual. Res.* **2016**, *16*, 198–212. [CrossRef]
23. Huang, H.Y.; Chen, P.L.; Kuo, Y.C. Understanding the facilitators and inhibitors of individuals' social network site usage. *Online Inf. Rev.* **2017**, *41*, 85–101. [CrossRef]
24. Keles, B.; McCrae, N.; Grealish, A. A systematic review: The influence of social media on depression, anxiety and psychological distress in adolescents. *Int. J. Adolesc. Youth* **2020**, *25*, 79–93. [CrossRef]
25. Iwamoto, D.; Chun, H. The Emotional Impact of Social Media in Higher Education. *Int. J. High Educ.* **2020**, *9*, 239–247. [CrossRef]
26. Davila, J.; Hershenberg, R.; Feinstein, B.A.; Gorman, K.; Bhatia, V.; Starr, L.R. Frequency and Quality of Social Networking Among Young Adults: Associations with Depressive Symptoms, Rumination, and Corumination. *Psychol. Pop. Media Cult.* **2012**, *1*, 72–78. [CrossRef] [PubMed]
27. Rajeh, M.; Sembawa, S.; Nassar, A.; Al Hebshi, S.A.; Aboalshamat, K.T.; Badri, M.K. Social media as a learning tool: Dental students' perspectives. *J. Dent. Educ.* **2020**, 1–8. [CrossRef]
28. Khatoon, B.; Hill, K.; Walmsley, A.D. Mobile learning in dentistry: Challenges and opportunities. *Br. Dent. J.* **2019**, *227*, 298–304. [CrossRef] [PubMed]
29. Sharka, R.; Abed, H.; Dziedzic, A. Can Undergraduate Dental Education be Online and Virtual During the COVID-19 Era? Clinical Training as a Crucial Element of Practical Competencies. *Med. Ed. Publish.* **2020**, *30*, 215. [CrossRef]
30. General Dental Council. Guidance on Using Social Media. 2016. Available online: https://www.gdcuk.org/api/files/Guidance%20on%20using%20social%20media.pdf (accessed on 7 October 2020).
31. Tatullo, M. Science is not a Social Opinion. *Dent. J.* **2019**, *7*, 34. [CrossRef] [PubMed]
32. Rana, S.; Kelleher, M. The Dangers of Social Media and Young Dental Patients' Body Image. *Dent. Update* **2018**, *45*, 902–910. [CrossRef]
33. Shuttleworth, J.; Smith, W. NHS dentistry: The social media challenge. *Br. Dent. J.* **2016**, *220*, 153. [CrossRef]

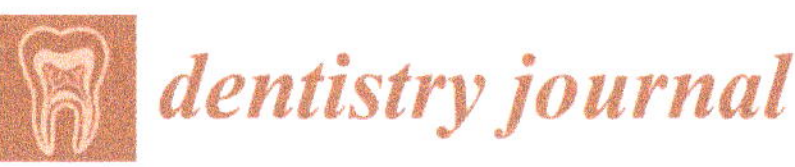 MDPI

Article

Peer Mentoring as a Tool for Developing Soft Skills in Clinical Practice: A 3-Year Study

Antonio M. Lluch [1], Clàudia Lluch [2], María Arregui [3,*], Esther Jiménez [4] and Luis Giner-Tarrida [3]

1 Integrated Dentistry Department, Faculty of Dentistry, Universitat Internacional de Catalunya, 08195 Sant Cugat del Vallés, Spain; alluch-alumni@uic.es
2 Pediatric Dentistry Department, Faculty of Dentistry, Universitat Internacional de Catalunya, 08195 Sant Cugat del Vallés, Spain; claudialluch@uic.es
3 Dentistry Department, Faculty of Dentistry, Universitat Internacional de Catalunya, 08195 Sant Cugat del Vallés, Spain; lginer@uic.es
4 Faculty of Education, Universitat Internacional de Catalunya, 08195 Sant Cugat del Vallés, Spain; ejimenez@uic.es
* Correspondence: mariaarregui@uic.es

Abstract: Education currently focuses on improving academic knowledge and clinical skills, but it is also important for students to develop personal and interpersonal skills from the start of their clinical practice. The aim was to evaluate the effect of peer mentoring in third-year students and to gauge the evolution of non-technical skills (NTS) acquisition up to the fifth year. The study groups were selected between September 2015 and May 2018, based on the NTS training they had or had not received: (1) fifth-year students with no training (G1); (2) third-year students mentored in NTS (G2a); and (3) a small group of fifth-year students who became mentors (G2b). A total of 276 students who took part in this study were assessed using a 114-item self-evaluation questionnaire. Data were collected from seven surveys conducted between September 2015 and May 2018, and statistical analysis was performed using one-way ANOVA and Fisher's post-hoc test. G2a improved their non-technical skill acquisition over three years of clinical training up to their fifth year. This group and G2b showed statistically significant differences compared to non-mentored students (G1). Peer mentoring at the beginning of clinical practice is a valid option for training students in non-technical skills.

Keywords: dental education; mentoring; non-technical skills training

Citation: Lluch, A.M.; Lluch, C.; Arregui, M.; Jiménez, E.; Giner-Tarrida, L. Peer Mentoring as a Tool for Developing Soft Skills in Clinical Practice: A 3-Year Study. *Dent. J.* **2021**, *9*, 57. https://doi.org/10.3390/dj9050057

Academic Editors: Jelena Dumancic and Božana Lončar Brzak

Received: 24 March 2021
Accepted: 11 May 2021
Published: 17 May 2021

1. Introduction

In the last decade, one of the most controversial and widely discussed topics in higher education is the development of soft or non-technical skill education [1]. In the case of health science education, the current focus is on improving academic knowledge and clinical skills improvement [2]. Both in dentistry and other health science disciplines, the dentist–patient relationship is not only technical but also based on emotional interactions [3]. This second skill is known as a non-technical skill.

Non-technical skills (NTS) can be defined as a set of social skills, including soft skills, that are perfectly compatible with technical skills, that help health professionals adapt to their environment, and that allow them to perform their work efficiently [4,5]. In medicine, dentistry has also been introduced in recent years to create a model of education that is more holistic and integrated [5]. NTS have been found to improve technical skills in professions like aviation that have been applied for many years, which include situational awareness, decision making, teamwork, leadership, and stress and fatigue management [4]. In terms of effective dental practice, both technical and non-technical skills are essential [2,6].

NTS include soft skills (i.e., social skills), which were first defined in the early 90s. Salovey and Mayer [7] defined emotional intelligence as a form of social intelligence used to control one's own emotions and those of others to discriminate between them and to harness this information to guide one's thoughts and actions. Furthermore, soft skills help people adapt to their professional and personal life to overcome new challenges [1]. Over the years, studies on emotional intelligence in health care professionals have grown exponentially [8].

The transition between preclinical and clinical practice is one of the most critical moments in dental studies [9]. The first experience in the clinical environment entails new responsibilities, as well as clinical and legal protocols that students must acquire to manage their work, interact with patients, and work as a team. Verbal and nonverbal communication is an essential element of the patient–dentist relationship [10]. An important part of this involves developing verbal communication [11] and listening skills, which help patients understand their oral health condition and needs [6]. The students' empathy and assertiveness are essential to this end [12], as are identifying and managing both their emotions and those of others [8]. Additional relevant basic skills for clinical practice include reasoning, problem-solving, decision-making, using and assessing information, and showing self-confidence. Unlike technical skills, non-technical skills in self-management, work management, and interrelationship skills enable students to think critically and are the key learning outcomes that further contribute to success or failure [13]. These skills are closely tied to safe and effective clinical practice centered on the patient and the clinical team. Indeed, providing appropriate and responsive care and listening to patients and respecting their choice, privacy, and dignity [14,15] is no less important than heading a clinical team to perform the best clinical practice [16].

Several studies have associated high levels of emotional intelligence and non-technical skills not only with strong academic performance and more satisfactory clinical results [8,17–19] but also with team work management and good rapport between students and their colleagues and staff members [6]. Despite the increasing importance of these skills, as described in the Profile and Competencies for the European Dentists (approved in 2009 by the General Assembly of the Association for Dental Education in Europe), they continue to receive inadequate attention in the curricula [20].

Nowadays, the term mentor is synonymous with a counsellor, guide, or even a coach [21]. Among the different definitions of mentoring in the literature, the most widespread is "a voluntary and reciprocal interpersonal relationship in which a person's acknowledged expertise shares their experience and learning with a less experienced person, the mentee" [21–23]. Depending on the program and the university, a mentor could be a faculty member or a senior student [24–26].

The importance and benefits of peer mentoring obtained in clinical training are well documented. These benefits are reaped by mentee and mentor alike [21,25,27–29], and they can be an effective pedagogical strategy to promote non-technical skills among students [30]. This experience helps to reduce anxiety, improve confidence, and create a more positive and productive learning experience [31]. However, some authors have identified drawbacks, including opposing perspectives of mentees and mentors and personality clashes that might lead to envy [23]; another example is an unequal distribution in the number of mentors and mentees, or that some mentors might focus on one non-technical skill only, which could leave mentees at a disadvantage compared to peers who develop all these skills [22].

Some authors have highlighted the need to train students as potential university staff [22,24,32]; student mentor training in non-technical skills could be a good step in this direction. Indeed, some studies have underlined the importance of such programs to complement the training of junior faculty staff in addition to leadership programs [23,26,27].

This study analyzed the level of NTS acquired by students between September 2015 and May 2018, based on data collected from third-year students starting clinical practice under the mentorship of fifth-year students trained in NTS. Subsequently, data were obtained from the same students' NTS training at the end of each academic year from 2016 to 2018.

The aim of this study was to evaluate the outcome of peer mentoring in third-year students and their uptake of NTS across three years, as well as compare the NTS acquisition in fifth-year students, some of whom were mentored in their third year, some of whom received no mentoring, and some of whom became mentors. The research hypothesis was to evaluate whether third-year peer mentoring during clinical practice is a valid tool for students to develop these skills.

2. Materials and Methods

The study was approved by the University's Research Ethics Committee. The head of the mentor program, in collaboration with the university's Training, Counselling, and Coaching Department, drew up a strategic soft skills framework based on three different models [2,3,6] that are used to promote NTS in the integrated clinical department. Table 1 describes the five groups of NTS studied, according to their different characteristics.

Table 1. Strategic non-technical skills framework.

Non-Technical Skills	Characteristics
Cognitive self-management	Data collection Analysis Synthetic thinking Logical judgment Reliability
Emotional self-management	Autonomy Mental resistance Self-confidence Perseverance
Connection relationship	Empathy Assertiveness Active listening
Impact relationship	Conflict management Credibility Communication
Work management	Problem solving Precision Planning and organizing Orientation in the objectives

With a view to recruiting fourth-year students who would become mentors in their fifth year, an information session was held in which the objectives of the mentor program were explained. For the selection criteria, the interested students were asked to submit a motivation letter and to pass a personal interview. The exclusion criteria were students with pending subjects or those spending part of the academic year on an exchange program. The students were selected at a ratio of 1 per 4 pairs of third-year students, which was proportionally equal to the clinical faculty.

The program was divided into three parts in which the mentors worked either together or individually depending on the training; as such, by the end of the course they had worked for about 170 h (Figure 1). At the beginning of the academic year, the students underwent 16 h of intensive training comprising communication skills with patient simulation activities, work management, relationship skills, and a group-coaching session to strengthen the importance of teamwork. During this intensive training, students also took a psychometric test to assess their self-knowledge development and to provide a starting point for individual coaching sessions to develop their self-management skills. This initial training and newly acquired knowledge taught mentors how to help third-year students develop and improve their non-technical skills for 4 h a week in a clinical environment, helping them to optimize their time and work in clinical situations like learning how to take radiographs or write up a clinical history using templates. The mentors also showed mentees how to communicate with patients in a clear and comprehensive manner. The last part of the program involved monthly group meetings, in which the mentors discussed their experiences and solved problems together with the help and supervision of faculty members who attended the meetings.

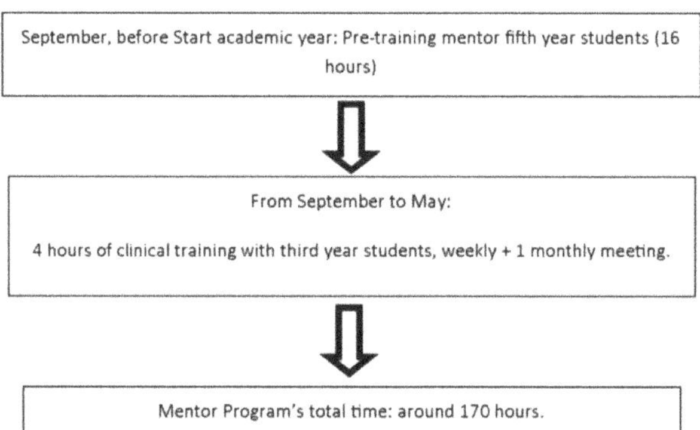

Figure 1. Mentor program framework.

The students were recruited between September 2015 and May 2018 and divided into two groups according to the NTS training they had received or not. Group 1 (G1) comprised students who did not receive NTS training; Group 2 (G2) consisted of students trained in NTS, who were subdivided into two different groups (Figure 2): G2a were third-year mentees trained in NTS, and G2b were third-year mentees who received additional NTS training in their fifth year in order to mentor third-year students.

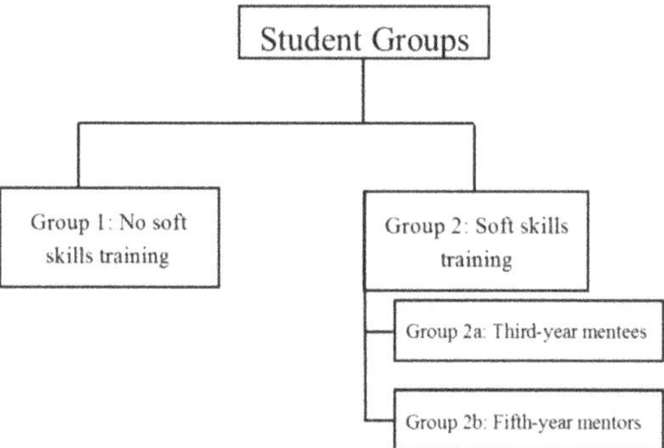

Figure 2. Student distribution.

All the students were informed of the purpose of the study, data protection, and possible risks and benefits. The students were then asked to take an online survey at the faculty. More than 90% of the students and 100% of the mentors completed the survey in person. Data collection was carried out electronically between September 2015 and May 2018 (Figure 3). The survey was composed on 114 self-assessment questions divided into the strategic NTS framework described in Table 1. The students scored the questions on a scale of 1 to 10.

Data for G1 was collected at the end of the 2015–2016 and 2016–2017 academic years. G2a students filled in the survey on four different dates: in the 2015–2016 academic year, in September (before clinical practice) and in May, and at the end of the 2016–2017 and 2017–2018 academic years. G2b took the survey only once, upon concluding their studies in May 2018.

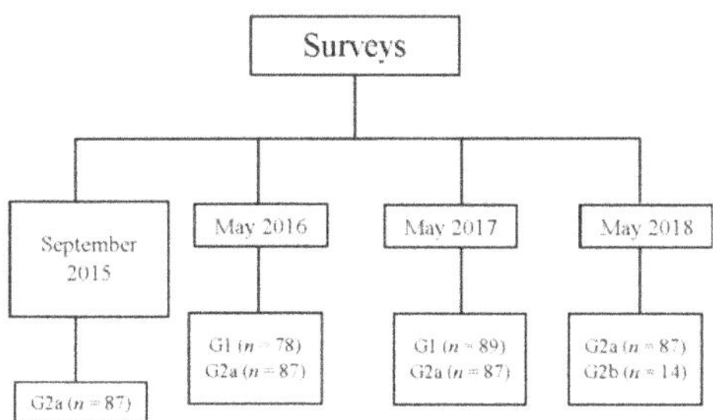

Figure 3. Data survey collection process.

All the data was collected in Excel files (Microsoft, Redmond, WA, USA), and statistical analysis was performed using the StatGraphics Centurion XV software (StatPoint Technologies, Inc., Warrenton, VA, USA). The data were analyzed with one-way ANOVA, and differences across groups were identified using the Fisher post-hoc test. The level of statistical significance was set at $p < 0.05$, with a 95% confidence interval.

3. Results

Two hundred and seventy-six students took part in the study and were divided in the following groups: G1 (n = 175) subdivided in May 2016 (n = 78) and May 2017 (n = 89), and G2 (n = 101) subdivided in G2a (n = 87) and G2b (n = 14); the last group was the mentors. The survey was filled in different moments, as shown in Figure 3. The students mentored in their first clinical training year showed an evolution in their acquisition of NTS from when they started training under mentor supervision in 2015 until they finished in 2018. One-way ANOVA showed statistically significant differences ($p < 0.05$) in the whole comparisons, but when the data were analyzed with the Fisher post-hoc test, the highest significant differences were between the students starting their clinical training in 2015 and finishing the whole clinical program three years later in May of 2018 (Table 2).

Table 2. Mean and standard deviation (SD) of mentored students (G2a).

Survey Time	Mean (SD)
September 2015	67.17 (4.23) [a]
May 2016	76.38 (3.14) [b]
May 2017	78.57 (2.51) [bc]
May 2018	81.20 (1.40) [c]

Superscript letter in the same column showed significant statistical differences ($p < 0.05$).

The highest change observed in soft-skills acquisition was in cognitive self-management, and the lowest in the connection relationship. Table 3 shows the scores of the different skills measured by year.

Table 3. Mentee acquired skills.

Non-Technical Skills	September 2015	May 2016	May 2017	May 2018
Cognitive self-management	60.91	72.02	75.36	79.13
Emotional self-management	67.62	76.57	76.83	81.09
Connection relationship	72.14	80.09	81.78	83.07
Impact relationship	69.49	78.4	79.48	81.41
Work management	65.71	74.82	79.38	81.28
Total	67.17	76.38	78.57	81.20

According to one-way ANOVA, group analysis upon completion of clinical training showed statistically significant differences ($p = 0.02$), but the Fisher post-hoc test indicated that G2a and G2b obtained similar scores, showing no statistically significant differences between them (Table 4). It should be noted that these two groups were mentored in their first clinical year. In this context, the statistical differences were between students who never were mentored (G1) and those who were mentored during their first year of clinical training (G2). It should be noted that, even though in the G2 group there was no statistical differences between being a mentor or not in fifth-year, the group of mentors were those who obtained the highest scores.

Table 4. Mean and standard deviation (SD) in 5th year students.

Group	Mean (SD)
G1	76.99 (3.51) [a]
G2a	81.20 (1.40) [b]
G2b	83.86 (1.47) [b]

Superscript letters denote statistically significant differences ($p < 0.05$).

Analysis of the non-technical skills acquired by the different groups showed that the mentors obtained the highest scores in all the skills when compared with the skills obtained by the other two groups, particularly G1 (non-mentored students). While the three groups obtained the lowest scores in cognitive self-management, the highest score differed depending on the group: the non-mentored students and the mentees scored the highest for connection relationship, while the mentors scored the highest for work management (Table 5).

Table 5. Comparison of non-technical skills acquired by students in this study.

Non-Technical Skills	G1 2016–2017	G2a May 2018	G2b May 2018
Cognitive self-management	72.01	79.13	81.89
Emotional self-management	76.86	81.09	84.37
Connection relationship	81.01	83.07	83.78
Impact relationship	79.49	81.41	83.32
Work management	75.56	81.28	85.92
Total	76.99	81.20	83.86

4. Discussion

The peer mentoring program was designed to facilitate the incorporation of third-year students in NTS acquisition during their clinical practice through mentoring by fifth-year students. The idea for implementing this program and introducing NTS training during clinical practice arose from the need to train dental students in these skills and ensure that the curriculum that is more focused on technical skills. The results of the present study showed that both mentors and mentees improved their NTS in clinical management, particularly in terms of relationships and self-management. Mentor's expertise is developed throughout their clinical training and reinforced by NTS training during the program.

In order to reduce students' stress and to increase their self-confidence, several universities that run training programs centered on NTS acquisition have stressed the importance of conducting this training alongside clinical practice [10,25,30,33]. However, some of these studies focused on one specific NTS, the most common being communication [10,11,30], followed by teamwork [30]. In the belief that all non-technical skills have equal relevance in clinical training, the authors of the present study analyzed all of them. The results showed an improvement in mentors and mentees when compared with non-mentored students, above all in self-management, relationship, and teamwork, in accordance with other studies [30,34].

To improve their skills, the mentors prepared and developed some clinical aids (videos, pictures, or templates) to show mentees how to organize working time, fill in clinical records, prepare the work area, conduct X-ray management, and fill in the periodontal card. They also improved their communication skills explaining all these procedures to mentees, and other abilities such as solving problems or making decisions when they counselled third-year students in patient management, and showed them strategies to speak with patients. This system is more centered on an in situ clinical scenario than other systems described in the literature that combined portfolio development with clinical recommendation and supervision by a mentor faculty member [33]. In the present study, when comparing the evolution of three years of mentees, the authors showed an improvement in their non-technical skills. It is important to highlight that they only received a mentor's support in their first year of clinical training, but the acquired knowledge was well assimilated. This outcome could be related to the view of Alzahem et al. [9], who stated that supervision at this critical juncture reduces stress levels and enhances technical and non-technical skills. In addition, it was observed that by the time they reached the final year of clinical practice (i.e., based on results from May 2018), although the mentors received extra training, there was not much difference between them and the rest of their peers who were not trained in this type of skill. However, in contrast, the systematic review by Nicolaides et al. [5] highlights the need for regular training of non-technical skills because it has been found that these skills diminish over time. Therefore, it is important to introduce these types of skills into the curriculum in combination with clinical skills for the benefit of all students. The professional development of students' clinical skills and knowledge should not be underestimated.

While some universities used faculty staff as mentors [23,26,28,33], the facilitators of the mentor program opted to use a group of fifth-year students, with whom third-year mentees felt more at ease when discussing their doubts. Hence, mentors must undergo specific training before starting the program. The decision to assign 16 h of mentor training conforms to the average training time of between 2 and 35 h, as described in the systematic review conducted by Carey et al. [10]. The training observed in the present study was supplemented by monthly meetings in which the mentors consolidated their training and expressed any problems or doubts concerning their mentees. These meetings also served to encourage teamwork and to avoid the problems of calibration described in some studies [9,33]. Furthermore, these meetings allowed the facilitators to mentor the students in a similar way to how the literature described mentoring and leadership programs to train new staff members [23,26]. While coaching sessions for mentor students in dentistry have not been reported in the literature, the facilitators considered it important to use a professional coach from outside the dentistry profession to reinforce and empower mentors as future clinicians and as people. The results of this study showed that student mentors obtained the highest scores in NTS, especially in emotional self-management and work management, a finding that could relate to the additional training. These results are in accordance with the description of Nicolaides et al. [5], as they stated that NTS could be a catalyst at an individual improvement level, which would allow for better organization of multidisciplinary teamwork.

Since its inception, the program has seen an increase in the number of students applying to become mentors, in accordance with the findings of Stenfors-Hayes et al. [35]. This kind of program shows that mentors are suitably trained for inclusion in the faculty staff [24,32,35] or used to complement junior staff training courses [23,26]. At present, some of the mentors who took part in the program under this study joined the clinical faculty.

The limitations of the present study are related to the study plans and the schedules of mentors. It was challenging to find suitable times for monthly meetings that avoided class times or were compatible with clinical trainings, which is consistent with findings in other studies [30]. In addition, given the facilitators' need to adapt their own schedules to those of the students, they need to consider the cost benefits of the program (as discussed in Romanelli et al. [19] and Stewart et al. [31]). Future perspectives could involve the study of new faculty staff's NTS, with or without prior preparation in this field, as well as whether third-year students improve their development of NTS with or without mentor assistance. Patients' views on the non-technical skills of students' post-treatment should also be investigated in future research.

As a consequence of the health situation caused by COVID-19, we will have to consider whether part of the NTS training should be done online for the mentor group, as it is important to keep the training of the 3rd year students in the clinical environment. If this is not possible, online strategies should be explored to help students learn these skills outside the clinical scenario by solving clinical cases and role-playing sessions online, as other universities have done during the duration of the pandemic situation [36–38].

5. Conclusions

Due to the clinical faculty's difficulties in simultaneously training third-year students in technical and NTS, peer mentoring among students is a valid option for NTS training. The results showed that mentees improved their confidence and development of the acquired NTS without specific mentoring. Furthermore, mentors increased their NTS training in clinical practice, which could be a factor in their incorporation into clinical faculty.

Author Contributions: Conceptualization, A.M.L. and L.G.-T.; methodology, A.M.L. and M.A.; investigation, A.M.L. and M.A.; writing—original draft preparation, A.M.L., C.L. and M.A.; writing—review and editing, L.G.-T. and E.J.; supervision, A.M.L., L.G.-T. and E.J. All authors have read and agreed to the published version of the manuscript.

Funding: This research received no external funding.

Institutional Review Board Statement: The study was conducted in accordance to the guidelines of the Declaration of Helsinki, and approved by the Ethics Committee in Research of Universitat Internacional de Catalunya (REC-ENC-2017-01) on 7 February 2017.

Informed Consent Statement: Informed consent was obtained from all the subjects involved in the study.

Data Availability Statement: Not applicable.

Acknowledgments: The authors are grateful to Blanca Paniagua for her efforts in the first stage of this research. We also acknowledge the coaching skills of Evaristo Aguado, Edith Castellarnau, and Artur Lázaro, as well as of Victor Gil, Carlos Areales, and Ana María Silva, for their support in this study. We also thank Mark Lodge for language support. The mentor program received a grant from the ADEE Scholarship program in 2017.

Conflicts of Interest: The authors declare no conflict of interest.

References

1. Succi, C.; Canovi, M. Soft skills to enhance graduate employability: Comparing students and employers' Perceptions. *Stud. High. Educ.* **2020**, *45*, 1834–1847. [CrossRef]
2. Dalaya, M.; Ishaquddin, S.; Ghadage, M.; Hatte, G. An interesting review on soft skills and dental practice. *J. Clin. Diagn. Res.* **2015**, *9*, ZE19–ZE21. [CrossRef]
3. Bisquerra Alzina, R.; Pérez Escoda, N. Emotional competences. *Educ. XX1* **2007**, *10*, 61–82.
4. Flin, R.; Patey, R.; Glavin, R.; Maran, N. Anaesthetists' non-technical skills. *Br. J. Anaesth.* **2010**, *105*, 38–44. [CrossRef]
5. Nicolaides, M.; Cardillo, L.; Theodoulou, I.; Hanrahan, J.; Tsoulfas, G.; Athanasiou, T.; Papalois, A.; Sideris, M. Developing a novel framework for non-technical skills learning strategies for undergraduates: A systematic review. *Ann. Med. Surg.* **2018**, *36*, 29–40. [CrossRef]
6. Gonzalez, M.A.; Abu Kasim, N.H.; Naimie, Z. Soft skills and dental education. *Eur. J. Dent. Educ.* **2013**, *17*, 73–82. [CrossRef] [PubMed]
7. Salovey, P.; Mayer, J.D. Emotional intelligence. *Imagin. Cogn. Personal.* **1990**, *9*, 185–211. [CrossRef]
8. Victoroff, K.Z.; Boyatzis, R.E. What is the relationship between emotional intelligence and dental student clinical performance? *J. Dent. Educ.* **2013**, *77*, 416–426. [CrossRef] [PubMed]
9. Alzahem, A.M.; van der Molen, H.T.; Alaujan, A.H.; Schmidt, H.G.; Zamakhshary, M.H. Stress amongst dental students: A systematic review. *Eur. J. Dent. Educ.* **2011**, *15*, 8–18. [CrossRef] [PubMed]
10. Carey, J.A.; Madill, A.; Manogue, M. Communications skills in dental education: A systematic research review. *Eur. J. Dent. Educ.* **2010**, *14*, 69–78. [CrossRef] [PubMed]

11. Hannah, A.; Lim, B.T.; Ayers, K.M. Emotional intelligence and clinical interview performance of dental students. *J. Dent. Educ.* **2009**, *73*, 1107–1117. [CrossRef] [PubMed]
12. Neumann, M.; Edelhäuser, F.; Tauschel, D.; Fischer, M.R.; Wirtz, M.; Woopen, C.; Haramati, A.; Scheffer, C. Empathy decline and its reasons: A systematic review of studies with medical students and residents. *Acad. Med.* **2011**, *86*, 996–1009. [CrossRef]
13. Quieng, M.C.; Lim, P.P.; Lucas, M.R.D. 21st century-based Soft Skills: Spotlight on non-cognitive skills in a cognitive-laden dentistry Program. *Eur. J. Contemp. Educ.* **2015**, *11*, 72–81. [CrossRef]
14. Field, J.C.; Kavadella, A.; Szep, S.; Davies, J.R.; DeLap, E.; Manzanares Cespedes, M.C. The graduating European dentist-domain III: Patient-centred care. *Eur. J. Dent. Educ.* **2017**, *21*, 18–24. [CrossRef] [PubMed]
15. McLoughlin, J.; Zijlstra-Shaw, S.; Davies, J.R.; Field, J.C. The graduating European dentist-domain I: Professionalism. *Eur. J. Dent. Educ.* **2017**, *21*, 11–13. [CrossRef]
16. Field, J.C.; DeLap, E.; Manzanares Cespedes, M.C. The graduating European dentist-domain II: Safe and effective clinical practice. *Eur. J. Dent. Educ.* **2017**, *21*, 14–17. [CrossRef] [PubMed]
17. Azimi, S.; AsgharNejad Farid, A.A.; Kharazi Fard, M.J.; Khoei, N. Emotional intelligence of dental students and patient satisfaction. *Eur. J. Dent. Educ.* **2010**, *14*, 129–132. [CrossRef]
18. Lam, L.T.; Kirby, S.L. Is emotional intelligence an advantage? An exploration of the impact of emotional and general intelligence on individual performance. *J. Soc. Psychol.* **2002**, *142*, 133–143. [CrossRef]
19. Romanelli, F.; Cain, J.; Smith, K.M. Emotional intelligence as a predictor of academic and/or professional success. *Am. J. Pharm. Educ.* **2006**, *70*, 69. [CrossRef]
20. Cowpe, J.; Plasschaert, A.; Harzer, W.; Vinkka-Puhakka, H.; Walmsley, A.D. Profile and competences for the graduating European dentist—Update 2009. *Eur. J. Dent. Educ* **2010**, *14*, 193–202. [CrossRef]
21. Friedman, P.K.; Arena, C.; Atchison, K.; Beemsterboer, P.L.; Farsai, P.; Giusti, J.B.; Haden, N.K.; Martin, M.E.; Sanders, C.F., Jr.; Sudzina, M.R.; et al. Report of the ADEA President's Commission on Mentoring. *J. Dent. Educ.* **2004**, *68*, 390–396. [CrossRef]
22. Gironda, M.W.; Bibb, C.A.; Lefever, K.; Law, C.; Messadi, D. A program to recruit and mentor future academic dentists: Successes and challenges. *J. Dent. Educ.* **2013**, *77*, 292–299. [CrossRef]
23. Wilson, N.H.F.; Verma, M.; Nanda, A. Leadership in recruiting and retaining talent in academic dentistry. *J. Dent.* **2019**, *87*, 32–35. [CrossRef]
24. Bagramian, R.A.; Taichman, R.S.; McCauley, L.; Green, T.G.; Inglehart, M.R. Mentoring of dental and dental hygiene faculty: A case study. *J. Dent. Educ.* **2011**, *75*, 291–299. [CrossRef]
25. Lopez, N.; Johnson, S.; Black, N. Does peer mentoring work? Dental students assess its benefits as an adaptive coping strategy. *J. Dent. Educ.* **2010**, *74*, 1197–1205. [CrossRef]
26. Sinkford, J.C.; Valachovic, R.W. Growing our own: Mentoring in the dental academic pipeline. *J. Dent. Educ.* **2019**, *83*, 981–987. [CrossRef]
27. John, V.; Papageorge, M.; Jahangiri, L.; Wheater, M.; Cappelli, D.; Frazer, R.; Sohn, W. Recruitment, development, and retention of dental faculty in a changing environment. *J. Dent. Educ.* **2011**, *75*, 82–89. [CrossRef]
28. Schrubbe, K.F. Mentorship: A critical component for professional growth and academic success. *J. Dent. Educ.* **2004**, *68*, 324–328. [CrossRef]
29. Zerzan, J.T.; Hess, R.; Schur, E.; Phillips, R.S.; Rigotti, N. Making the most of mentors: A guide for mentees. *Acad. Med.* **2009**, *84*, 140–144. [CrossRef]
30. Abu Kasim, N.H.; Abu Kassim, N.L.; Razak, A.A.A.; Abdullah, H.; Bindal, P.; Che' Abdul Aziz, Z.A.; Sulaiman, E.; Farook, M.S.; Gonzalez, M.A.; Thong, Y.L.; et al. Pairing as an instructional strategy to promote soft skills amongst clinical dental students. *Eur. J. Dent. Educ.* **2014**, *18*, 51–57. [CrossRef] [PubMed]
31. Stewart, R.A.; Hauge, L.S.; Stewart, R.D.; Rosen, R.L.; Charnot-Katsikas, A.; Prinz, R.A.; Association for Surgical Education. A CRASH course in procedural skills improves medical students' self-assessment of proficiency, confidence, and anxiety. *Am. J. Surg.* **2007**, *193*, 771–773. [CrossRef]
32. Bibb, C.A.; Lefever, K.H. Mentoring future dental educators through an apprentice teaching experience. *J. Dent. Educ.* **2002**, *66*, 703–709. [CrossRef]
33. Schwartz, B.; Saad, M.N.; Goldberg, D. Evaluating the students' perspectives of a clinic mentoring programme. *Eur. J. Dent. Educ.* **2014**, *18*, 115–120. [CrossRef]
34. Haist, S.A.; Wilson, J.F.; Fosson, S.E.; Brigham, N.L. Are fourth-year medical students effective teachers of the physical examination to first-year medical students? *J. Gen. Intern. Med.* **1997**, *12*, 177–181. [CrossRef]
35. Stenfors-Hayes, T.; Lindgren, L.E.; Tranaeus, S. Perspectives on being a mentor for undergraduate dental students. *Eur. J. Dent. Educ.* **2011**, *15*, 153–158. [CrossRef] [PubMed]
36. Bianchi, S.; Gatto, R.; Fabiani, L. Effects of the SARS-COV-2 pandemic of medical education in Italy: Considerations and tips. *Eur. Biomed. J.* **2020**, *15*, 100–101.
37. Stoopler, E.T.; Tanaka, T.I.; Sollecito, T.P. Hospital-based dental externship during COVID-19 pandemic: Think virtual! *Spec. Care Dent.* **2020**, *40*, 393–394. [CrossRef]
38. Varvara, G.; Bernardi, S.; Bianchi, S.; Sinjari, B.; Piatelli, M. Dental education challenges during the COVID-19 pandemic period in Italy: Undergraduate student feedback, future perspectives, and the needs of teaching strategies for professional development. *Healthcare* **2021**, *9*, 454. [CrossRef] [PubMed]

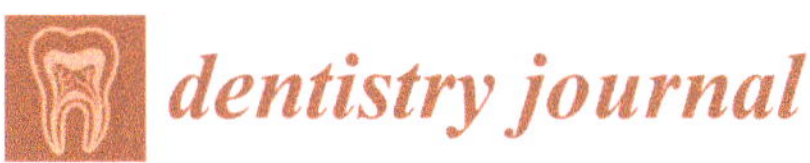 MDPI

Article

The Best Dentistry Professional Visual Acuity Measured under Simulated Clinical Conditions Provides Keplerian Magnification Loupe: A Cross-Sectional Study

Iris Urlic [1,*], Josip Pavan [1], Zeljko Verzak [2], Zoran Karlovic [3] and Dubravka Negovetic Vranic [2]

[1] Department of Ophthalmology, Clinical Hospital Dubrava, Av.GojkaŠuška6, 10000 Zagreb, Croatia; josip.pavan@kbd.hr

[2] Department of Pediatric and Preventive Dentistry, School of Dental Medicine, University of Zagreb, Gundulićeva 5, 10000 Zagreb, Croatia; verzak@sfzg.hr (Z.V.); dnegovetic@sfzg.hr (D.N.V.)

[3] Department of Endodontics and Restorative Dentistry, School of Dental Medicine, University of Zagreb, Gundulićeva 5, 10000 Zagreb, Croatia; karlovic@sfzg.hr

* Correspondence: iris.urlic@gmail.com; Tel.: +385-91-4874-700

Abstract: Visual acuity plays an important role in dentists' vision in their daily clinical routine. This study aimed to determine dental students' visual acuity without optical aids and when using magnification devices in simulated clinical conditions. The participants were forty-six students at the School of Dental Medicine with a visual acuity of 1.0 in decimal values or 100% in percentage. The central visual acuity was tested using a miniature Snellen eye chart placed in the molar cavity of a dental phantom, in simulated clinical conditions under five different settings (natural visual acuity, by applying head magnifying glasses x1,5 and binocular magnifying devices using Galileo's x2,5/350 mm, Keplerx3,3/450 mm and Keplerx4,5/350 mm optical system). The Wilcoxon Signed Rank test shows that the distribution of measurements of the visual acuity undertaken by the application of magnifying devices (VNL, VGA2,5, VKP3,3, VKP4,5) contained higher values of visual acuity than those received by the use of natural vision (VSC) ($p < 0.001$ for the comparison to the VNL, VGA2,5, VKP3,3 and VKP4,5 groups). The highest and statistically most significant increase in visual acuity is achieved using the Keplerian telescope x4.5/350 mm. The application of magnifying devices provided dentistry professionals with better visual acuity, improving detail detection in an oral cavity during dental procedures by magnifying the oral structure. The use of magnification devices means much more precise work, decreases the operating time, improves posture and reduces muscle pain in the shoulder during dental treatment.

Keywords: visual acuity; miniaturized Snellen optotype; Galilean and Keplerian telescope optical system in dentistry

Citation: Urlic, I.; Pavan, J.; Verzak, Z.; Karlovic, Z.; Negovetic Vranic, D. The Best Dentistry Professional Visual Acuity Measured under Simulated Clinical Conditions Provides Keplerian Magnification Loupe: A Cross-Sectional Study. *Dent. J.* **2021**, *9*, 69. https://doi.org/10.3390/dj9060069

Academic Editor: Changxiang Wang

Received: 19 April 2021
Accepted: 7 June 2021
Published: 11 June 2021

Publisher's Note: MDPI stays neutral with regard to jurisdictional claims in published maps and institutional affiliations.

1. Introduction

By using magnifying aids, a dentist achieves ergonomic, musculoskeletal and optical benefits, and the magnification compensates for the weakening of eye accommodation, which occurs after the age of forty (presbyopia). The use of telescope magnification devices proved to improve the diagnosis and treatments in dental medicine [1,2]. Magnification in dentistry upgrades soft and hard tissue evaluation, calculus and periodontal pocket detection, restorative evaluation and radiological interpretation [3,4].

Highly demanding eye-hand coordination and tactile perception require the highest visual function, three-dimensional image creation, stereo vision and object depth perception as well as other psychological and neurological qualities [3].

Magnification is achieved by a system of lenses used in the Galileo and Kepler optical systems. The Galilean telescope has a diverging and the Keplerian telescope a converging lens eyepiece [5]. The loupe's ergonomic factors are the declination angle, working distance and frame size [6].

A study that is examining the visual acuity of dentists with age proved a wide variability in near visual acuity and a significant improvement in visual acuity within the dental workspace by 100–379% when using Galileo's x2,5 and Kepler's x4,3 magnifying glass, regardless of age [7]. Kepler's magnifier x4,3 achieved the highest visual acuity in the clinical work of dentists due to the highest magnification, but also due to the absence of chromatic and optical aberrations [8]. Dentists under the age of 40 statistically have significantly greater visual acuity than older dentists. Dentists under the age of 40 can significantly improve their visual acuity by reducing the eye–object distance or by using magnifying glasses [9]. The use of magnification aids does not weaken the eye. After wearing loupes for a period, the user becomes accustomed to seeing more detail than is apparent with natural vision [10].

The most commonly used proximity visual test of the British Faculty of Ophthalmology [11] is not sensitive enough to examine visual acuity in the dentist's workplace, and a standardized, generally accepted proximity visual acuity test in dentistry with magnifications, which would meet optical parameters, is not yet available [8].

The miniaturization of Snellen's optotype that was carried out for this research enabled the study to examine how properly fitted magnification loupes improve visual acuity at close range, therefore producing higher-quality dentistry.

2. Materials and Methods

2.1. Participants

The study was carried out in the Dentistry Pre-clinic of the School of Dental Medicine, University in Zagreb from September to December 2015. The participants were students at the School of Dental Medicine, University of Zagreb (N = 46) who voluntarily agreed to participate in the study. The participants were of both genders, aged between 20 and 25 years. Before being included in the study, their eye status was examined by an ophthalmologist in an ophthalmology practice. The inclusion criteria for participants were a central visual acuity of 1.0 in decimal values examined using a Snellen visual chart, a near visual acuity of 1.0 examined using Jäger tables, regular ocular movement and convergence, regular pupil reaction and an oval or round shaped optic nerve head.

2.2. Miniature Snellen Visual Test

The visual acuity was examined by means of a miniature visual test invented for this study in cooperation with the Croatian State Archives, Central Photo Laboratory. A sample of an A4 Snellen optotype was created in high resolution, printed and copied onto a 35-millimeter B/W microfilm. A microfilm camera, Zeutscheu Documator, was used to reduce the high-resolution A4 Snellen chart to the highest possible reduction of 28,5x compared to the initial size of the optotype. The size of the miniaturized Snellen chart for the near visual acuity examination of dentists was 5.2 × 2.8 mm and the optotype dimensions ranged from 0.05 mm to a maximum of 0.6 mm (Figure 1).

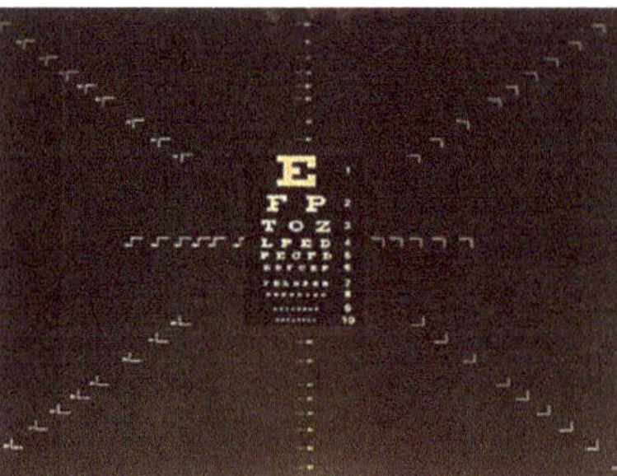

Figure 1. Miniaturized visual Snellen optotype (under magnification ×4) by courtesy of the Croatian State Archive.

2.3. Dentistry Professional Visual Acuity with Magnification Telescopes

The participants were examined in a working zone lit by a 60 W surgery lamp parallel to the participants' visual axis, sitting in a dental chair with a maximum head deflection of 25° forward in an upright position. Their feet were fully placed on the floor, their knees were placed below and their elbows level with the dental phantom. The examination room was illuminated by sunlight and artificial light ranging from 250 to 500 lux, measured using a luxmeter. The miniature visual chart was fixed in the dental phantom's molar cavity (Figure 2). The visual acuity was registered by decimal graduation between 0.1 to 1.0 as the smallest optotype of the miniaturized Snellen optotype that an examinee managed to read at a working distance without correction (VSC), by application of x1.5 head magnifying glasses (VNL), using Galileo's x2,5/350 mm binocular magnifying devices (VGA2,5), Kepler x3,3/450 mm optical magnification system (VKP3,3) and a x4,5/350 mm optical system (VKP4,5) (Figure 3). The study was approved under No. 05-PA-26-6/2015 by the Ethics Committees of the School of Dental Medicine, University of Zagreb.

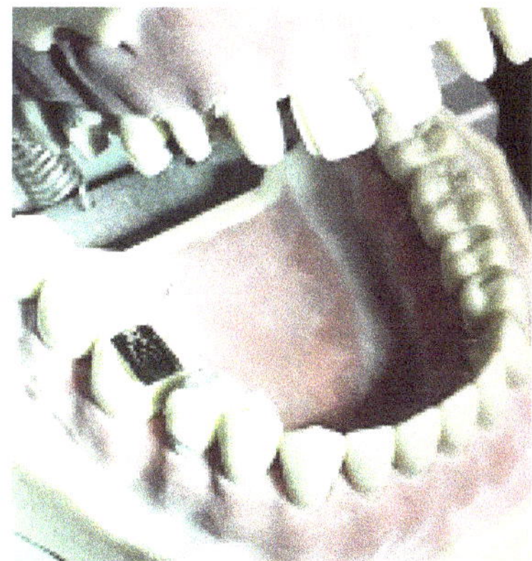

Figure 2. Miniaturized visual Snellen chart placed in the tooth cavity of a dental phantom.

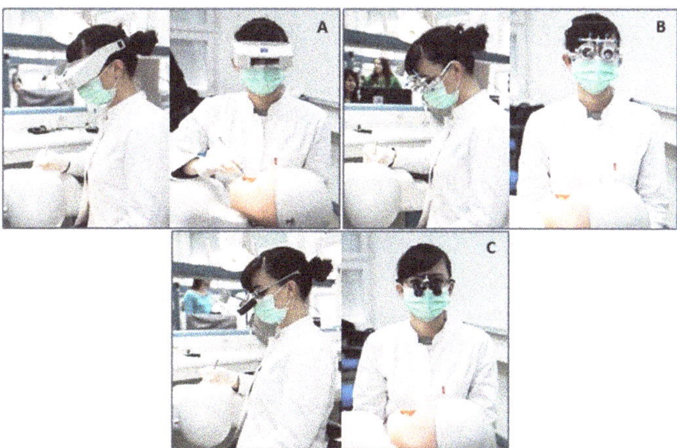

Figure 3. Examining the dentistry visual acuity under simulated clinical conditions by applying (**A**) head magnifying glasses, (**B**) a Galilean telescope, (**C**) and a Keplerian telescope.

2.4. Statistical Analysis

Prior to performing the differential analysis, the normality of the data's distribution was tested. The Shapiro–Wilk test rejected the null hypothesis of the data's normality

($p < 0.05$). As the data were not normally distributed, nonparametric statistical tests were used for their analysis.

Data on visual acuity during the use of five different optical systems were collected from the same subjects and analyzed using the following non-parametric tests for repeated measurements: the Friedman test and the Wilcoxon Signed Rank test. The Friedman test examined whether there was a statistically significant difference in visual acuity between the different optical systems. In order to find out between which pairs of systems significant deviations in visual acuity were recorded, the Wilcoxon's Signed Rank test was performed after the Friedman test. The analysis was performed using the SAS System software package (SAS Institute Inc., Cary, NC, USA).

3. Results

3.1. *Standard Deviation of Dentistry Professional Visual Acuity*

Statistical analysis included 46 subjects, 25 females and 21 males, with an average age of 21.8 years. Visual acuity was examined at close range within each individual group and the following were compared: the control group with each individual group corrected by a magnifying aid; visual acuity in the vicinity of the Kepler/Galileo systems; visual acuity in the vicinity of the Keplerian optical systems.

The mean value (standard deviation) of visual acuity using natural vision without magnifying aids at a distance of 300 to 400 mm (VSC) was 0.411 (0.074); using head magnification glasses x1,5 (VNL), 0.504 (0.076); using a Galilean magnifying telescope x2,5 at a distance of 350 mm (VGA2,5), 0.517 (0.077); using a Kepler optical system x3,3 at a distance of 450 mm (VKP3,3), 0.541 (0.086); and when using Kepler x4.5 at a distance of 350 mm (VKP4,5) the average value (standard deviation) of the recorded visual acuity measurements was 0.646 (0.081) (Table 1).

Table 1. Descriptive indicators of visual acuity distribution *.

Optical System	N	Mean	Std Dev	CV (%)	Median	Q1	Q3	Min	Max
VSC	46	0.411	0.074	17.9	0.4	0.4	0.5	0.3	0.6
VNL	46	0.504	0.076	15.0	0.5	0.5	0.6	0.4	0.7
VGA 2,5	46	0.517	0.077	14.9	0.5	0.5	0.6	0.4	0.7
VKP 3,3	46	0.541	0.086	15.9	0.6	0.5	0.6	0.4	0.7
VKP4,5	46	0.646	0.081	12.5	0.6	0.6	0.7	0.5	0.8

* N, sample size; Mean, arithmetic mean; Std Dev, standard deviation; CV, variation coefficient; Q1, 1st quartile; Q3, 3rd quartile; Min, minimum; Max, maximum.

3.2. *The Friedman Test*

Consistent with the results of the descriptive analysis, the Friedman test indicated the existence of statistically significant differences in the distribution of the visual acuity measurements between the different optical systems ($p < 0.001$).

3.3. *The Wilcoxon Signed Rank Test*

A comparison of a VNL with a VGA 2,5, VKP 3,3 and VKP4,5 indicated a statistically significant difference in the distribution of the visual acuity measurements in relation to Kepler's magnifying glass x3,3 (VKP 3,3; $p = 0.014$) and Kepler's magnifying glass x4.,5 (VKP4,5; $p < 0.001$), but not in relation to the Galilean magnifying glass x2,5 (VGA 2,5; $p = 0.288$). When using Kepler's magnifiers, higher values of visual acuity were generally recorded. The Wilcoxon Signed rank test indicated a statistically significant difference between the distributions of visual acuity (VGA 2,5) in relation to Kepler's magnifying glass x4,5 (VKP4,5; $p < 0.001$), but not in relation to Kepler's magnifying glass x3,3 (VKP 3,3; $p = 0.064$). Compared to the Galilean magnifying glass x2.5 (VGA 2,5), Kepler's magnifying glass x4,5 (VKP4,5) generally recorded higher values of visual acuity. A comparison of Kepler's magnifiers indicated that the distribution of the measured visual acuity values after using the Kepler magnifying glass x4,5 (VKP4,5) generally contained higher visual acuity values compared to the distribution of measured values after using the Kepler magnifying glass x3,3 (VKP 3,3) (Wilcoxon Signed Rank test; $p < 0.001$). The results of the Wilcoxon Signed Rank test concluded that the distributions of visual acuity measurements when using magnifying aids (groups VNL, VGA 2,5, VKP 3,3 and VKP4,5) generally contained higher values of measured visual acuity compared to the use of natural vision without magnifying aids (VSC) ($p < 0.001$ for comparison with VNL, VGA 2,5, VKP 3,3 and VKP4,5 groups) (Table 2).

Table 2. Wilcoxon Signed Rank test results to compare visual acuity recorded when using different optical systems *.

Optical System Comparison	Test Statistics W	*p*-Value
VNL vs. VSC	390,0	<0.001
VGA 2,5 vs. VSC	403,5	<0.001
VKP 3,3 vs. VSC	423,0	<0.001
VKP4,5 vs. VSC	517,5	<0.001
VGA 2,5 vs. VNL	22,5	0.288
VKP 3,3 vs. VNL	103,5	0.014
VKP4,5 vs. VNL	473,0	<0.001
VKP 3,3 vs. VGA 2,5	55,0	0.064
VKP4,5 vs. VGA 2,5	480,5	<0.001
VKP4,5 vs. VKP 3,3	430,5	<0.001

* VSC, visual acuity without correction; VNL, visual acuity with the application of x1.5 head magnifying glasses; VGA2,5, visual acuity with the Galileo x2.5/350 mm magnifying device; VKP3,3, visual acuity with the Kepler x3,3/450 mm optical system; VKP4,5, visual acuity with the Kepler x4,5/350 mm optical system.

4. Discussion

The range of visual acuities close to the normal eye status of subjects who do not use optical aids for eye correction is from 0.3 to 0.6 in decimal values. Statistically significant near visual acuity compensation relative to visual acuity without optical aids is achieved using a head magnifier x1,5, a Galileo telescope x2,5 and a Kepler system x3,3, and the range of near visual acuity is from 0.4 to 0.7. There was no statistically significant difference between the visual acuity of head magnifier x1,5, Galileo x2,5 and Kepler x3,3. This study shows that it is justified to start using the Galileo optical systems x2,5 at a working distance of 350 mm for dental students, dental technicians and dentists who are beginning to adapt to magnification [12]. A study examining the use of magnifications at the New Zealand School of Dentistry found that out of 285 first-year students, 23% used a magnification of up to 48% in their final year of study. In addition, 72% of professors use magnifiers, with the most common magnification of x2.5, and half of them use magnifiers with an added light bulb [13]. Eichenberger et al. evaluated the self-assessed near visual acuity of sixty-nine dentists in a private practice in Switzerland as well as their experience with magnification devices. The study showed that many dentists were not aware of their individual or age-related visual deficiencies that can be compensated with telescope systems and should be used early enough to compensate for those vision irregularities [14].

With the Keplerian telescope x4,5, a minimum value of visual acuity of 0.5 is achieved and a maximum of 0.8. A statistically significant increase in visual acuity is achieved by increasing the magnification, changing the Galileo x2,5 to Kepler's optical system x4,5 and by increasing the magnification within the Kepler x3,3 to x4,5.

Kepler's x4.5/350 mm magnifier achieves a maximum visual acuity that is not achieved with any other magnifier used in this study. A study conducted by Wajngarten examined dental students' visual acuity and forward head posture when using telescope systems in the operating field. The Galilean and Keplerian magnification systems provided the best visual acuity and the lowest angulation of the operator's neck in comparison to the naked eye, simple loupe and operating microscope [15]. The visual threshold was reached with the Keplerian telescope by dentists under the age of 40, both with and without coaxial light, and dentists under the age of 40 identified a 0.05 mm structure within the root canal [16].

It was observed that 100% visual acuity or 1.0 by the Snellen optotype was not achieved even with the best correction, despite the fact that the study was performed in simulated conditions with young subjects, without refraction error or presbyopia. The use of turbine and the effect of aerosol on blurred vision were not taken into consideration.

This study includes emetropic (normovision) students without refractive anomalies (myopia, hyperopia). By involving dental students, we excluded dentists over the age of forty, presbyopic participants. A future step for this study is to examine the visual acuity of myopic, hyperopic and presbyopic dentists with and without optical aids.

5. Conclusions

The major optical goal for central visual acuity by using telescopes is to magnify the image in the dental visible path. Visual performance increases with the application of head magnifying glasses and binocular magnifying devices. The highest increase in visual acuity is achieved using the Keplerian telescope x4.5/350 mm. The Galilean telescope is small and lightweight but the Keplerian telescope, in comparison with Galileo's, allows for a higher magnification, greater depth of field, wider field of view and greater focal length.

Author Contributions: Conceptualization, I.U., J.P. and D.N.V.; methodology, I.U., J.P. and D.N.V.; software, I.U. and D.N.V.; validation, I.U. and D.N.V.; formal analysis, I.U. and D.N.V.; investigation, I.U.; resources, I.U.; Z.V., Z.K.; data curation, I.U. and D.N.V.; writing—original draft preparation, I.U.; writing—review and editing, I.U. and D.N.V.; visualization, J.P. and D.N.V.; supervision, J.P. and D.N.V.; project administration, I.U.; funding acquisition, I.U. All authors have read and agreed to the published version of the manuscript.

Funding: This research received no external funding.

Institutional Review Board Statement: The study was approved by the Ethics committee of the Dental School, University of Zagreb (05-PA-26-6/2015, 16-03-2015).

Informed Consent Statement: Informed consent was obtained from all subjects involved in the study.

Data Availability Statement: The data presented in this study are available on request from corresponding author.

Conflicts of Interest: The authors declare no conflict of interest.

References

1. Strassler, H.E.; Syme, S.E.; Serio, F.; Kaim, J.M. Enhanced visualization during dental practise using magnification system. *Compend. Contin. Educ. Dent.* **1998**, *9*, 595–598.
2. Sunell, S.; Rucker, L. Surgical magnification in dental hygiene practice. *Int. J. Dent. Hyg.* **2004**, *2*, 25–26. [CrossRef] [PubMed]
3. Syrimi, M.; Ali, N. The role of stereopsis (three-dimensional vision) in dentistry: Review of current literature. *Br. Dent. J.* **2015**, *218*, 597–598. [CrossRef] [PubMed]
4. Syme, S.E.; Fried, J.L.; Strassler, H.E. Enhanced visualization using magnification. *J. Dent. Hyg.* **1997**, *71*, 202–206. [PubMed]
5. Telescopes and Microscopes. Available online: http://electron9.phys.utk.edu/optics421/modules/m3/telescopes.htm (accessed on 1 May 2009).
6. Valachi, B. Magnification in dentistry: How ergonomic features impact your health. *Dent. Today* **2009**, *28*, 133.
7. Eichenberger, M.; Perrin, P.; Neuhaus, W.K.; Bringolf, U.; Lussi, A. Visual acuity of dentists under simulated clinical conditions. *Clin. Oral Investig.* **2013**, *17*, 725–729. [CrossRef] [PubMed]
8. Eichenberge, M.; Perrin, P.; Neuhaus, W.K.; Bringolf, U.; Lussi, A. Influence of loupes and age on the near visual acuity of practicing dentists. *J. Biomed. Opt.* **2011**, *16*, 035003. [CrossRef]
9. Perrin, P.; Ramseyer, S.T.; Eichenberger, M.; Lussi, A. Visual acuity of dentists in their respective clinical condition. *Clin. Oral Investig.* **2014**, *18*, 2055–2058. [CrossRef] [PubMed]
10. Christensen, G.J. Magnification in dentistry: Useful tool or another gimmick? *J. Am. Dent. Assoc.* **2003**, *134*, 1647–1650. [CrossRef]
11. Mahmoud, A.L.S. Arabic reading types. *BMJ* **1986**, *70*, 314–316.
12. Urlic, I.; Verzak, Z.; Negovetić, V.D. Measuring the influence of Galilean loupe system on near visual acuity under simulated clinical conditions. *Acta Stomatol. Croat.* **2016**, *3*, 235–241. [CrossRef] [PubMed]
13. Murray, C.M.; Chandler, N.P. Magnification: Magnifying the point. *BDJ* **2015**, *218*, 369. [CrossRef] [PubMed]

14. Eichenberger, M.; Perrin, P.; Ramseyer, S.T.; Lussi, A. Visual acuity and experience with magnification devices in Swiss dental practices. *Oper. Dent.* **2015**, *40*, E142–E149. [CrossRef] [PubMed]
15. Wajngarten, D.; Garcia, P.P.N.S. Effect of magnification devices on dental students' visual acuity. *PLoS ONE* **2019**, *14*, e0212793. [CrossRef] [PubMed]
16. Perrin, P.; Neuhaus, K.W.; Lussi, A. The impact of loupes and microscopes on vision in endodontics. *Int. Endod. J.* **2014**, *47*, 425–429. [CrossRef]

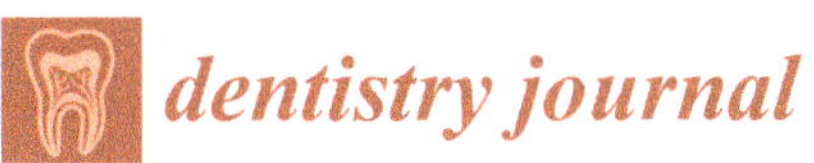

MDPI

Article

The Effect of Extra Educational Elements on the Confidence of Undergraduate Dental Students Learning to Administer Local Anaesthesia

Mats Sjöström [1] and Malin Brundin [2,*]

1 Department of Oral and Maxillofacial Surgery, Umeå University, 90187 Umeå, Sweden; mats.sjostrom@umu.se
2 Department of Endodontics, Umeå University, 90187 Umeå, Sweden
* Correspondence: malin.brundin@umu.se

Abstract: Local anaesthesia is taught early in the practical part of dental programs. However, dental students express uncertainty and concern before their practical training in local anaesthesia. The aim of this study was to evaluate how extra educational elements in the teaching of local anaesthesia affect students' confidence using local anaesthesia. The students were divided into three groups (A, B and C). Group A received the same education that was used the previous year (i.e., four hours of theoretical lectures followed by four hours of practical exercises performed on a fellow student). Group B did their practical training on fellow students in groups of three, with each student taking turns performing, receiving and observing the procedure. Group C received training using an anatomically correct model before their practical training on a fellow student. After each training step, the students completed a questionnaire about their confidence administering local anaesthesia. The students experienced a significant increase in confidence after each educational step. Combining theory and practical instruction, including the use of anatomically correct models and peer instruction, improved students' confidence in administering local anaesthesia. The greatest increase in confidence was in the students placed in groups of three where each student performed, received and observed the procedure.

Keywords: undergraduate dental education; clinical skills teaching; teaching methodology; local anesthesia

Citation: Sjöström, M.; Brundin, M. The Effect of Extra Educational Elements on the Confidence of Undergraduate Dental Students Learning to Administer Local Anaesthesia. *Dent. J.* **2021**, *9*, 77. https://doi.org/10.3390/dj9070077

Academic Editors: Jelena Dumancic and Božana Lončar Brzak

Received: 20 May 2021
Accepted: 28 June 2021
Published: 1 July 2021

1. Introduction

Dental education involves clinical training on patients. This implies a need for student teaching of local anesthesia for patient comfort. A recently published review of teaching local anaesthesia in dental schools in the USA identified three main pedagogical approaches: didactic instruction via books and lectures; practical exercises conducted in peer groups; and practice using anatomically correct models. However, due to the heterogeneity of the studies, the authors were unable to analyse the pedagogical effects of the three teaching methods and the students' confidence administering local anaesthesia. The authors concluded that the lack of evidence makes it difficult to determine an optimal way to teach local anaesthesia [1].

Dental professionals can feel anxious about local anaesthesia, resulting in stress and anxiety before administering local anaesthesia to a patient. The amount of practice affects stress and anxiety levels, where less practice or experience increases stress and anxiety. Stress and reasons for stress have been evaluated in previous studies. For example, Wong et al. studied dental hygiene students' experiences of anxiety related to their confidence performing local anaesthesia. An increased degree of confidence reduced students' stress associated with administering local anaesthesia [2]. In a paediatric anaesthesia study, a higher degree of stress was found in dental students compared with experienced specialist colleagues [3]. Methods other than direct clinical training have been found to be effective and improve students' confidence administering local anaesthesia. For example, Kenny et al. found that students trained in administering local anaesthesia to children using videos showed significantly increased confidence immediately after the training as well as at follow-up [4]. The use of anatomically correct models designed to verify whether local anaesthesia is correctly administered is a teaching method that can eventually become a complement to the use of peers for practice. Moreover, training with these models provides an opportunity to train an unlimited number of times and without continuous supervision. Previous evaluations of preclinical model training have concluded that students who practiced on a model before their clinical training were significantly better prepared and more confident administering local anaesthesia to a peer [5]. In addition, training on a model has been associated with increased confidence and better motor control [6]. However, model training does not automatically increase a dental student's ability to safely administer local anaesthesia to a patient [7]. Accessibility to reflection is an important part of the learning process according to Kolb's learning cycle [8]. The time and opportunities for this should be included in practical training elements. This can be done by ensuring that there is time for students to observe clinical situations without them being the one performing the procedure.

Dental students in Umeå are taught local anaesthesia as one of the first clinical topics, early in the fifth semester. The teaching curriculum includes literature studies, lectures, demonstrations, focus groups and treatment of patients. The practical training of local anaesthesia is carried out on a fellow student after demonstration followed by personal clinical training under the supervision of an oral surgeon. As a final element of the course, the student administers local anaesthesia under supervision to a patient prior to tooth extraction. The stepwise education of local anaesthesia, with clinical observations during instruction and demonstrations of how to administer local anaesthesia performed by the oral surgeon, followed by personal training under supervision, can be compared to a master teaching a novice or a novice studying under a master. Solid knowledge grounded in theory is important to achieve excellence in the students' practice. Active learning by using instructional activities and involvement with the students who are being trained in local anaestheisia gives the students space to reflect on the clinical situation and their own performance. This reflective thought and an internal processing links the experience with previous learning [9]. The student evaluations collected after each completed course report that the students express a need for more clinical training to increase their confidence when administering local anaesthesia to patients.

This study aimed to evaluate three different teaching models, including one that utilized anatomical models in addition to clinical observations, during training of dental students in local anaesthesia at Umeå University. Hopefully, the results can improve the teaching of local anaesthesia to dental students in Umeå University and increase the students' confidence during application of local anaesthesia.

2. Materials and Methods

In 2020, all undergraduate dental students at Umeå University in their fifth semester (n = 72, 50 women/22 men, mean age: 25, range 21–39) were invited to a study evaluating whether extra educational elements can improve student confidence for local anaesthesia. The students were informed orally and in writing about the study and that their participation was voluntary. After acceptance, all students were given a survey consisting of a statement to be answered with a classification for confidence on a visual analogue scale ranging between zero and ten (0 = I feel absolutely unconfident in independently administering anaesthesia to patients and 10 = I feel completely confident in independently administering anaesthesia to patients) [10,11] (Appendix A).

The students were divided into three groups (A, B and C) during their dental program. One group received the traditional education while two groups received modified education. All groups received training in accordance with the syllabus. A randomization between the groups was performed, resulting in group A (n = 24, 14 women/10 men, mean age: 25, range 21–31) receiving the traditional education of practical training in local anaesthesia—i.e., in groups of two, with a four-hour theory lecture followed by four hours of practical training on a fellow student. Group B (n = 25, 19 women/6 men, mean age: 25, range 22–39) received a four-hour theory lecture followed by four hours of practical training in groups of three—i.e., each member of the group performed, received and observed the procedure. Group C (n = 23, 17 women/6 men, mean age: 25, range 22–36) received a four-hour theory lecture followed by four hours of practical training on an anatomically correct model (Frasaco, AG-3 IB) (Figure 1).

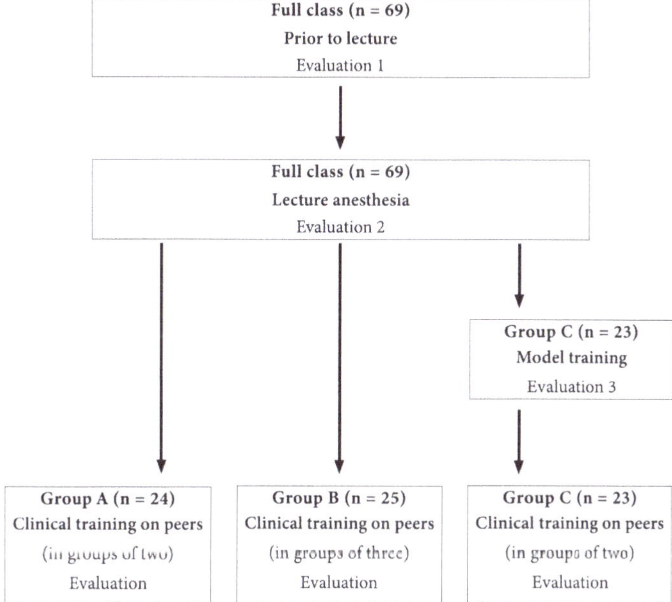

Figure 1. Study design for evaluation of students' self confidence in using local anesthesia during the course "Oral surgery 1", fifth semester. Three students were not present at the theoretical lecture, which is why their answers are missing in evaluations 1 and 2. At the clinical training, all 72 students participated.

The model has four contact points (mental foramen, mandibular foramen, incisive foramen and greater palatine foramen) covered by rubber simulating covering mucosa. The students simulated injections with dry injection needles and the right positioning of the needle tip was indicated with acoustic signals (Figure 2).

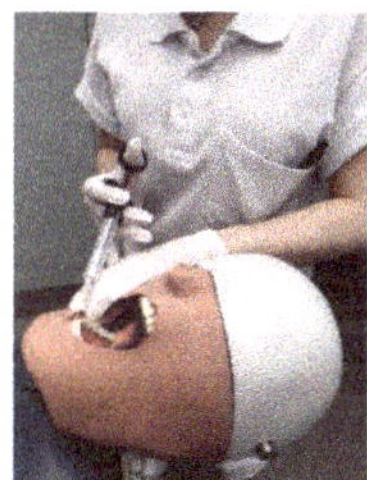

Figure 2. Dental student during model training.

After model training, group C had four hours of practical training on a fellow student (i.e., a group of two). As group C was uneven, one sub-group consisted of three students instead of two. All students (groups A, B and C) were taught the inferior alveolar block technique using the direct standard technique. During all the local anaesthesia attempts, four oral surgeons supervised the groups. After each training step, the students completed the survey described above. The responses were compiled on two occasions and the mean of the two measured values was used in the statistical calculations.

Parts of the course (the clinical training) were performed during the COVID-19 pandemic. At the end of March, all teaching at universities in Sweden was conducted digitally. Exceptions were made, however, for education where clinical elements were included. Clinical training was allowed to be performed under special restrictions, including full protective equipment and adaptation of training facilities. The clinical education at the School of Dentistry in Umeå thus continued during the pandemic. The introductory lecture in this case could be held on the university's premises in the traditional way, as this preceded in time the transition to digital education.

Statistics

The non-parametric Mann–Whitney U-test was used to compare the students' self-evaluated measures of perceived safety between the three groups. For all tests, the p-value was set to ≤ 0.05. The responses to the survey are presented as mean values and the corresponding standard error of the mean for each occasion (Figure 3). All statistical tests were performed using IBM SPSS Statistics for Windows, Version 26.0 (IBM Corp: Armonk, NY, USA).

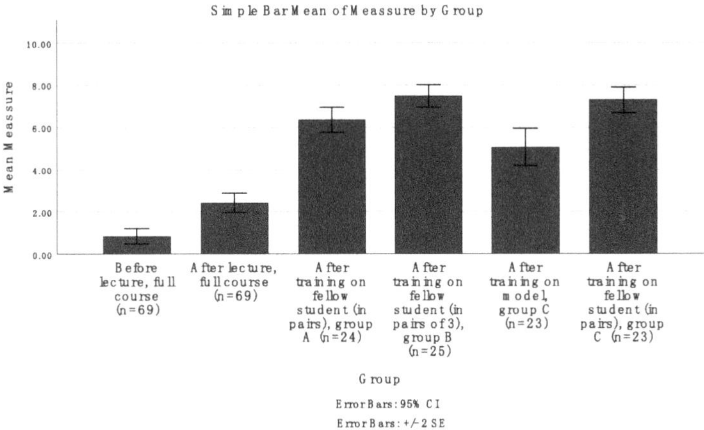

Figure 3. Students' self-evaluation about self-confidence in independently administering anesthesia to patients before the theoretical lecture, after the theoretical lecture, after training on a model and after training on a fellow student. Each question was answered based on self-assessment on a 10-point graded scale (0 = absolutely not confident in independently administering anesthesia to patients, 10 = completely confident in independently administering anesthesia to patients).

3. Results

The results of the students' self-evaluation for confidence after each educational step are presented in Figure 3. Three students were not present at the theoretical lecture, which is why their answers are missing in evaluations 1 and 2. At the clinical training all 72 students participated.

Table 1 describes the statistical analysis of differences between the educational steps as expressed in students' confidence administering local anaesthesia. A significant increase in confidence administering local anaesthesia was seen after the theoretical lecture (p-value < 0.01). Significant differences in confidence administering local anaesthesia were also seen between the theoretical lecture and the students training on each other (i.e., peer training under supervision of an oral surgeon) (p-value < 0.01). A non-significant difference was seen between group C (training with the model followed by peer training in pairs) and group B (peer training in groups of three; p-value 0.69).

Table 1. Statistical comparison between each education step using the Mann–Whitney U-test.

Comparacy between Each Education Steps	p-Value
Before lecture (full course, n = 69) vs. After lecture (full course, n = 69)	<0.01
After lecture (full course, n = 69) vs. After training in pair (Group A, n = 24)	<0.01
After training in pair (Group A, n = 24) vs. After training on model (Group C, n = 23)	0.01
After training in pair (Group A, n = 24) vs. After training 3 and 3 (Group B, n = 25)	0.03
After training in pair (Group A, n = 24) vs. After training on model and then in pair (Group C, n = 23)	0.02
After training 3 and 3 (Group B, n = 25) vs. After training on model and then in pair (Group C, n = 23)	0.69

4. Discussion

The results from this study, on the effects of extra educational elements on the confidence of undergraduate dental students learning to administer local anaesthesia, indicate a stepwise increase of confidence during the course. It is evident that students did not feel completely confident in independently administering anaesthesia to patients after the clinical training irrespective of the teaching method. Surprisingly, some students reported self-confidence prior to the first theoretical lecture. This was probably the consequence of previous professional experience working as dental hygienists or dental nurses.

The largest increase in perceived confidence was seen after the clinical exercise with students training on each other (i.e., peer training under supervision of an oral surgeon). Training with models increased the students' confidence administering anaesthesia, but peer training in groups of three, where each student performed, received and observed the procedure, produced similar results as training on models in combination with peer training in pairs. In a full teaching schedule, it is necessary to analyse which training effort is most effective for the students. Students who were trained using anatomical models (group C) resulted in increased confidence. Training using anatomical models significantly increased students' confidence compared to instruction using only theory. When combined with theory instruction, training on a peer increased students' confidence even more. A survey study of 267 dental schools in Europe and Israel found that most students experienced uncertainty associated with injecting patients and desired an introduction involving anatomical models and more instruction [12]. Students positively responded to training on an anatomical model before injecting real patients.

However, studies that have investigated training primarily relying on models of jaws found no difference in the students' ability to successfully administer local anaesthesia to a peer [5]. These findings support the idea that several teaching methods should be used in clinical training. Using models to train students in how to administer local anaesthesia does not necessarily mean that a student's knowledge base increases [7], but such training can increase a student's confidence and make them more comfortable for the next learning step. Wong et al. studied dental hygiene students' experiences of anxiety related to their confidence performing local anaesthesia. An increased degree of confidence reduced students' stress associated with administering local anaesthesia [2]. Methods other than direct clinical training have been found to be effective and improve students' confidence administering local anaesthesia. For example, Kenny et al. found that students trained in administering local anaesthesia to children by using videos showed significantly increased confidence immediately after the training as well as at follow-up [4].

All students in the present study trained on fellow students under supervision. In group B, three students worked together—i.e., the students took turns performing, receiving and observing the procedure. In groups A and C, the students worked in pairs and administrated local anaesthesia on each other. Compared to groups A and C, group B showed significantly better results regarding student confidence administering local anaesthesia. In addition, group C, where the students practiced the procedure on one another after training on an anatomical model, showed higher confidence administering local anaesthesia than group A, where the students did not practice on an anatomical model before practicing on one another (group A). Training on a model increases students' confidence, but training on a partner, with whom one can communicate and observe reactions, gives a better possibility of increasing self-confidence during training in local anaesthesia.

Instruction and demonstration, performed by an oral surgeon, of how to administer local anaesthesia can be compared to a master teaching a novice or a novice studying under a master. Traditionally, this has been the main pedagogical method used to train young people [13]. In medical education, much of the practical learning takes place with younger colleagues learning from older, more experienced colleagues. According to Nielsen and Kvale, observation and imitation are legitimate pedagogical methods [13]. Practical training of administering local anaesthesia can be seen as an example of legitimate peripheral participation. In the context of this study, the student observes via lectures and demonstration before administering anaesthesia on a fellow student under the supervision of a teacher. Only after practicing on a peer is the student allowed to administer local anaesthesia to a patient, also under the supervision of a teacher. According to Kary et al., the combination of these three pedagogical methods prepares students to confidently inject a patient independently of a teacher [1].

During the clinical training with local anaesthesia, students practice on each other. This arrangement, of course, raises some ethical issues. In a study on ethical issues related to the teaching of local anaesthesia at dental schools in the USA, the authors showed that the majority of training is done without oral or written consent [14]. In a survey of three dental schools in the USA, Hossaini found that many students raised ethical questions about administering anaesthesia to their peers for the sole purpose of training [15]. Furthermore, Hossaini's generalization of the results revealed that this type of training is unethical [15]. In a survey from eleven Turkish dental colleges on how students are trained in local anaesthesia, the authors found that the clinical teaching started in the fifth semester but that the theory education started earlier [16]. The first injection was performed on peers supervised by oral surgeons. None of the schools stated that they required permission from a medical ethics committee to inject fellow students. Other dental education institutions in Sweden have similar arrangements as in Umeå, and two of the four dental schools have their students train on anatomical models before practicing local anaesthesia on a fellow student (personal communication MS). In Umeå, discussions about undergraduate training using local anaesthesia on a fellow student have been taking place, but Umeå students also expressed that they find the exercise valuable as it gives them experience with the effect of local anaesthesia. From an ethical perspective, one can ask whether receiving anesthesia in any way adds something to a student's educational project [14]. Depending on their oral health, many young people in Sweden have never received local anesthesia during their lifetime. Gaining experience of this is important knowledge, as this experience helps students understand what their future patients will experience. The syllabus in Oral Surgery is anchored in the program council. Today, students do not give their informative consent to receive local anesthesia during the clinical training, which of course is something that should be considered in the future. However, no student is forced to receive local anesthesia if there is a contraindication, such as medical reasons or severe anxiety.

The literature describes different strategies for teaching local anaesthesia. The choice of strategies varies based on tradition, teacher availability, materials and premises and patient access. As a result of the different conditions, the literature must be evaluated based on the conclusions of each article. The readers can then apply the findings to their own institution. From the literature, we can conclude that several dental programs are working to improve the way local anaesthesia is taught. From course evaluations we know that dental students in Umeå have asked about more clinical training. Although offering more clinical training is a reasonable request, it must be incorporated into an already full training schedule. Therefore, future teaching will be conducted as before but in groups of three, with each student taking turns performing, receiving and observing the procedure. After each member of the group has performed the procedure, the clinical supervisor will guide the students in a discussion and reflection on the experience. Providing time to observe a clinical moment gives space for reflection [17]. In the situation where the student is the one administrating the anaesthetics, the focus is on the technicality of the procedure, which very likely requires the student's full attention. The opportunity to take part in the procedure, i.e., observe the technical aspects of the injection and at the same time have the opportunity to observe the patient's reaction, provides a greater opportunity for reflection on the overall clinical situation. This study indicates that training in groups of three improves student confidence in administering local anaesthesia compared to training only on an anatomical model.

The number of included students was limited to students who were enrolled in the course at the start of the study in spring 2020. A larger number of informants would of cause have given more strength to the study. Additionally, the students were not randomized in the different groups. At the start of the dental program, students are divided into three groups by the study administration due to technical schedule issues. All groups receive the same course content and the same amount of clinical training as previous years' students. This means that no student is disadvantaged compared to earlier dental students.

We performed a randomization when the three groups (A, B and C) were randomized for the three test methods. The groups were not compensated for gender and age, which could have affected the results of the study, as differences in male and female dentists' self-assessment of their clinical competence, favoring male dentists, have been reported [18]. On the other hand, the number of participants ranged between 23 and 25 and all groups had the same mean age and female dominance, although the proportion varied. In this study, we used a visual analogue scale ranging between 0–10 for evaluation of confidence. This range for the scale is often used to measure pain, but it is also used for measuring other subjective experiences, such as confidence [10,11,19]. The selected scaling method is easy to administer and easy for the students to use, and it also has good reliability and validity [20]. Additionally, the instrument has been used in other studies [10,11,21,22], which allows comparisons. A shortcoming of this measuring instrument is that the students' self-esteem with regard to their confidence cannot always be translated into ability. The fact that the students feel safe before administrating does not mean that they have mastered it. However, it has been shown that good self-confidence and a feeling of control have a positive effect on learning [23,24].

5. Conclusions

The results from this study indicate that, with extra training using anatomical models before peer training in pairs, students experience a higher level of confidence when it comes to administering local anaesthesia. It was also shown that the same effect was achieved by letting students work in groups of three in the clinical situation, where each student was given the opportunity to observe and reflect on the injection procedure.

Author Contributions: Conceptualization, M.S. and M.B.; methodology, M.S. and M.B.; investigation, M.S.; resources, M.S. and M.B.; data curation, M.S.; writing–original draft preparation, M.S. and M.B.; writing–review and editing, M.S. and M.B.; project administration, M.S. and M.B. Both authors have read and agreed to the published version of the manuscript. Both authors have read and agreed to the published version of the manuscript.

Funding: The present research was funded by the Faculty of Medicine of Umeå University.

Institutional Review Board Statement: The study was carried out at the Department of Dentistry, Faculty of Medicine, Umeå University. As this was not medical research, the protocol was not reviewed by the Ethics Committee; it was, however, approved by the advisory committee for the odontology programs, Faculty of Medicine, Umeå University.

Informed Consent Statement: Informed consent was obtained from all subjects involved in the study. Participation in the study was voluntary. No student received education that deviated from the curriculum for the course "Oral and Maxillofacial Surgery 1, 3 hp". The study was performed in accordance with the principles of the Helsinki Declaration regarding anonymity and integrity.

Data Availability Statement: The data presented in this study are available on request from the corresponding author.

Acknowledgments: We would like to express our thanks to all the dental students who participated in this study. Their participation made this study possible. We also would like to express our gratitude to Björn Tavelin for his statistical advice during the preparation of this paper.

Conflicts of Interest: The authors declare no conflict of interest.

Appendix A

Questionnaire

Each question should be answered based on self-assessment on a scale where 0 = I feel absolutely not confident to independently place anesthesia on the patient. 10 = feel completely confident to independently apply anesthesia to the patient.

Before the education in oral anesthesia started: How confident did you feel to independently place local anesthesia on a patient (Group A, B and C)

0____10

After the theoretical lecture over anesthesia techniques: How cconfident did you feel to, independently place local anesthesia on a patient (Group A, B and C)

0____10

After the practical exercise with anesthesia on model: How confident did you feel to, independently place local anesthesia on a patient (group C only).

0____10

After the practical exercise with anesthesia on peer student: How confident did you feel to, independently place local anesthesia on a patient (Group A, B and C).

0____10

Figure A1. Questionnaire.

References

1. Kary, A.L.; Gomez, J.; Raffaelli, S.D.; Levine, M.H. Preclinical Local Anesthesia Education in Dental Schools: A Systematic Review. *J. Dent. Educ.* **2018**, *82*, 1059–1064. [CrossRef]
2. Wong, G.; Apthorpe, H.C.; Ruiz, K.; Nanayakkara, S. Student-to-Student Dental Local Anesthetic Preclinical Training: Impact on Students' Confidence and Anxiety in Clinical Practice. *J. Dent. Educ.* **2019**, *83*, 56–63. [CrossRef] [PubMed]
3. Farokh-Gisour, E.; Hatamvand, M. Investigation of Stress Level Among Dentistry Students, General Dentists, and Pediatric Dental Specialists During Performing Pediatric Dentistry in Kerman, Iran, in 2017. *Open Dent. J.* **2018**, *12*, 631–637. [CrossRef] [PubMed]
4. Kenny, K.P.; Alkazme, A.M.; Day, P.F. The effect of viewing video clips of paediatric local anaesthetic administration on the confidence of undergraduate dental students. *Eur. J. Dent. Educ.* **2018**, *22*, e57–e62. [CrossRef]
5. Lee, J.S.; Graham, R.; Bassiur, J.P.; Lichtenthal, R.M. Evaluation of a Local Anesthesia Simulation Model with Dental Students as Novice Clinicians. *J. Dent. Educ.* **2015**, *79*, 1411–1417. [CrossRef]
6. Lopez-Cabrera, C.; Hernandez-Rivas, E.J.; Komabayashi, T.; Galindo-Reyes, E.L.; Tallabs-Lopez, D.; Cerda-Cristerna, B.I. Positive influence of a dental anaesthesia simulation model on the perception of learning by Mexican dental students. *Eur. J. Dent. Educ.* **2017**, *21*, e142–e147. [CrossRef] [PubMed]
7. Knipfer, C.; Rohde, M.; Oetter, N.; Muench, T.; Kesting, M.R.; Stelzle, F. Local anaesthesia training for undergraduate students—How big is the step from model to man? *BMC Med Educ* **2018**, *18*, 308. [CrossRef]
8. Kolb, D.A. *Experiential Learning: Experience as the Source of Learning and Development*; Prentice-Hall: Englewood Cliffs, NJ, USA, 1984; Volume 1.
9. Wrenn, J.; Wrenn, B. Enhancing Learning by Integrating Theory and Practice. *Int. J. Teach. Learn. High. Educ.* **2009**, *21*, 248–265.
10. Rodd, H.D.; Farman, M.; Albadri, S.; Mackie, I.C. Undergraduate experience and self-assessed confidence in paediatric dentistry: Comparison of three UK dental schools. *Br. Dent. J.* **2010**, *208*, 221–225. [CrossRef]
11. Wong, S.; Wong, X.; Vaithilingam, R.; Rajan, S. Dental undergraduates' self-assessed confidence in paediatric dentistry. *Ann. Dent.* **2015**, *22*, 22–30.
12. Brand, H.S.; Tan, L.L.; van der Spek, S.J.; Baart, J.A. European dental students' opinions on their local anaesthesia education. *Eur. J. Dent. Educ.* **2011**, *15*, 47–52. [CrossRef]
13. Nielsen, K.; Kvale, S. *Mästarlära—Lärande som Social Praxis*; Studentlitteratur: Lund, Sweden, 2000.
14. Rosenberg, M.; Orr, D.L., 2nd; Starley, E.D.; Jensen, D.R. Student-to-student local anesthesia injections in dental education: Moral, ethical, and legal issues. *J. Dent. Educ.* **2009**, *73*, 127–132. [CrossRef] [PubMed]
15. Hossaini, M. Teaching local anesthesia in dental schools: Opinions about the student-to-student administration model. *J. Dent. Educ.* **2011**, *75*, 1263–1269. [CrossRef] [PubMed]
16. Tomruk, C.O.; Oktay, I.; Sencift, K. A survey of local anesthesia education in Turkish dental schools. *J. Dent. Educ.* **2013**, *77*, 348–350. [CrossRef] [PubMed]
17. Abelsson, A.; Bisholt, B. Nurse students learning acute care by simulation—Focus on observation and debriefing. *Nurse Educ. Pract.* **2017**, *24*, 6–13. [CrossRef] [PubMed]
18. Karaharju-Suvanto, T.; Napankangas, R.; Koivumaki, J.; Pyorala, E.; Vinkka-Puhakka, H. Gender differences in self-assessed clinical competence–a survey of young dentists in Finland. *Eur. J. Dent. Educ.* **2014**, *18*, 234–240. [CrossRef]
19. Finch, E.; Fleming, J.; Brown, K.; Lethlean, J.; Cameron, A.; McPhail, S.M. The confidence of speech-language pathology students regarding communicating with people with aphasia. *BMC Med. Educ.* **2013**, *13*, 92. [CrossRef]
20. McCormack, H.; Horne, D.; Sheather, S. Clinical applications of visual analogue scales: A critical review. *Psychol Med.* **1988**, *18*, 1007–1019. [CrossRef]
21. Sonbol, H.N.; Abu-Ghazaleh, S.B.; Al-Bitar, Z.B. Undergraduate experience and self-assessed confidence in paediatric dentistry at the University of Jordan Dental School. *Eur. J. Dent. Educ.* **2017**, *21*, e126–e130. [CrossRef] [PubMed]
22. Rajan, S.; Chen, H.Y.; Chen, J.J.; Chin-You, S.; Chee, S.; Chrun, R.; Byun, J.; Abuzar, M. Final year dental students' self-assessed confidence in general dentistry. *Eur. J. Dent. Educ.* **2020**, *24*, 233–242. [CrossRef]
23. Akbari, O.; Sahibzada, J. Students' Self-Confidence and Its Impacts on Their Learning Process. *Am. Int. J. Soc. Sci. Res.* **2020**, *5*, 1–15. [CrossRef]
24. Fine, P.; Leung, A.; Bentall, C.; Louca, C. The impact of confidence on clinical dental practice. *Eur. J. Dent. Educ.* **2019**, *23*, 159–167. [CrossRef] [PubMed]

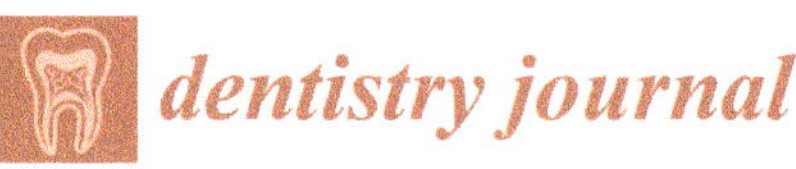

MDPI

Article

Early Clinical Experience and Mentoring of Young Dental Students—A Qualitative Study

Rod Moore *, Simone Molsing, Nicola Meyer and Matilde Schepler

Institute of Dentistry and Oral Health Sciences, Aarhus University, 8000 Aarhus C, Denmark; simonemolsing@hotmail.com (S.M.); nicola_meyer@hotmail.com (N.M.); matildeschepler@hotmail.com (M.S.)
* Correspondence: rod.moore@dent.au.dk

Abstract: The literature reports that student transition between preclinical and clinical dental education can be traumatic and stressful for many reasons. Early clinical experience has been reported to provide some relief. In this qualitative study, twelve final year dental students were interviewed about their perceptions and experiences with a mentee/mentor (FOAL) program in Aarhus, Denmark, to see if it (1) counteracted stress perceptions from preclinical education to the clinic, (2) inspired professionalism and a sense of study relevance, (3) helped in learning to reflect on competencies and attitudes, (4) helped with clinical social perspectives (communication/contact), (5) helped with motivation to learn and (6) helped to reaffirm one's professional study choice. Using qualitative description methods with purposeful sampling, data from interviews were collected, transcribed, analyzed and validated with a short questionnaire. The FOAL program, today, has several benefits for mentees, including partially helping in the preclinic to clinic transition and the increased insight into mentors' clinical tasks and communication with patients. Informants described that FOAL also contributed positively to both mentee and mentor students' learning motivation, collaborative skills and professional attitudes. Challenges were lack of organization/planning, not enough clinical hours, lack of clinical knowledge and persistent stress levels at the clinical transition. These issues are already being considered in the curriculum reform currently in progress and are also relevant to other dental curricula internationally.

Keywords: clinical education; early clinical experience; dental students; motivation; stress perceptions; self-determination theory; self-efficacy; social learning theory

Citation: Moore, R.; Molsing, S.; Meyer, N.; Schepler, M. Early Clinical Experience and Mentoring of Young Dental Students—A Qualitative Study. *Dent. J.* **2021**, *9*, 91. https://doi.org/10.3390/dj9080091

Academic Editors: Jelena Dumancic, Božana Lončar Brzak and Patrick R. Schmidlin

Received: 19 June 2021
Accepted: 29 July 2021
Published: 6 August 2021

1. Introduction

The literature [1–4] shows that the preclinic to clinic transition in dental education can be emotionally traumatic and stressful, which can lead to poor learning experiences [2], decreased motivation for learning [4] and, in the worst case, signs of anxiety and depression [1]. Building and maintaining motivation seems to be essential to averting poor outcomes [5–7]. Motivation for clinical learning has been applicably described in self-determination theory (SDT) [8–11], where degrees of motivation are divided into three main categories: amotivation, external motivation and internal motivation. SDT also clarifies that the quality of learning is based on the quality of motivation. Amotivation describes students with low or no motivation. In external motivation, students are affected by various external parameters that span several phases of development towards higher-quality motivation. The first and least autonomous phase is *externally regulated motivation*, where students study, for example, mainly because teachers or instructors have expectations of them and not because they themselves are optimally interested or engaged in learning or see its relevance or relatedness to becoming a professional. The next two phases of learning motivation are gradual transitions in a student's improving self-motivation levels. The fourth phase of external motivation is *integrated regulation*, where students transition to becoming self-motivated. Finally, internal motivation is the most autonomy-building motivation due to engagement by students' own volition, their needs for growth in self-awareness and social awareness and their sense of relatedness to the profession that they have chosen [9,10]. This means that in this phase, students are highly self-motivated to learn, wanting to show they have fully understood the relevance of the curriculum. As suggested above, SDT posits that these phases of motivation often progress from external to internal, depending on the student's experiences during the study period [9,10]. Mentorship support is thought to specifically direct mentees towards creating an understanding of the value of their chosen profession and towards a gradual internalization of this value [11,12], which is a topic of interest in this paper.

Knowledge of early clinical experience as a teaching strategy and the theory of the benefits of these strategies are plentiful in the health literature [13–17]. As alluded to above, SDT proposes that different qualities of motivation affect different outcomes. There appears to be a link between early clinical experience and less stress [15,16] as well as the idea that students feel more confident about their future professional role at the clinic after these early experiences [14,17,18]. Dental students with early clinical experience have also been reported to have greater internal motivation for learning [5–7]. Since internal motivation favors optimal learning, the need for early clinical experiences for dental students seems to be supported by SDT [6,7]. As reasons for engaging in activities become more self-determined, positive outcomes are expected such as deeper learning, less superficial information processing, better performance, less intention to drop out, greater creativity and improved well-being or adjustment [11,16,19]. Mentorship support during the early years of medical education also appears to stimulate feelings of volition and needs for professional autonomy and relatedness, which are the tenants of SDT's concept of internal motivation [11]. However, this is still a hypothesis in relation to dental education [6,7].

The present study aims to contribute to the international dental education literature and to inform educational policy considerations about early clinical experience and mentorship. It specifically evaluates student perceptions and experiences with a program at Fællesklinikken (FK), a comprehensive care clinic at the dental school in Aarhus, Denmark. To achieve this, specific aims were formulated. These took the form of the following research questions about early clinical experience as mentors and mentees and their implicit hypotheses:

Hypothesis 1 (H1). *Does early clinical experience help reduce stress/anxiety during the transition from preclinical education to the clinic?*

Hypothesis 2 (H2). *Is it inspiring to see older students treat patients (enhanced relevance to profession, according to SDT)?*

Hypothesis 3 (H3). *Did you learn to reflect on your own competencies and attitudes (enhanced self-awareness, according to SDT)?*

Hypothesis 4 (H4). *Did you learn about social perspectives (communication/contact) in the clinic (enhanced social awareness, according to SDT)?*

Hypothesis 5 (H5). *Did early clinical experiences increase your motivation for study activity and general learning within the education?*

Hypothesis 6 (H6). *Did you ever think of dropping out of dentistry? Did early clinical experience help you reaffirm your choice?*

2. Materials and Methods

2.1. Setting

The so-called "FOAL program" was first introduced, quite intuitively, to FK at the Aarhus Dental School. Here, first and second year students could acquire some experience at the clinic as respite from their heavy theoretical teaching load in the basic sciences. The program was formally introduced in 2012 in the form that it is now in in 2021, but there was also a program from 1979 to 2011, which was on a voluntary basis. That voluntary program was established at the time in an attempt to reduce first year drop-out rates, i.e., intended as a source of professional inspiration and motivation. Currently, dental students are required to be mentees 12 h per semester during the 1st–4th semesters.

The current mandatory FOAL program still occurs in the 1st–4th semesters, and FOAL students (mentees) act as assistants mainly for 7th–10th semester students (mentors) who have their own patients, since 5th–6th semester students work mostly in dyad pairs. Otherwise, in the first 4 semesters, students only have preclinical dental skill instruction in simulation clinics. Student contact with patients can only occur within the FOAL program. The clinical leader gives a lecture to 1st semester students as a short introduction to the teaching clinic and the role of foals. Mentee tasks under the program include suction assistance, entering measurement results in electronic journals and help in fetching materials, and, in some cases, a foal (mentee) may be allowed to polish off some work after depuration, or to carry out some other easier treatment tasks. Therefore, mentees get an introductory insight into the daily function of the teaching clinic before they themselves become clinicians. In addition, they also obtain opportunities to gain some social skills during the treatments, as in many cases, while sitting alone with patients, they have the chance to make independent contact.

2.2. Interviews

Twelve female final year Danish dental students aged 23–28 volunteered to be informants about their perceptions and experiences in the FOAL program using semi-structured interviews in Danish. Students were recruited in October–November 2020. Female dental students at the Aarhus School of Dentistry usually make up about 80% of the students, which is why only female participants were chosen in these interviews [20]. In this sample, 12 out of 46 possible female students were recruited. This was part of a purposeful sampling strategy [21] in which the women were recruited equally from each of the two clinical floors and with different clinical days of the week to cover any possible differences between student groupings and teacher influences. As they were in their final year, these informants had experience as both mentees and mentors, which was purposeful, since they could then reflect on both situations. Each interview was conducted, transcribed and validated among three female dental student co-authors. For anonymity, the subjects were code numbered from 1 to 12. These students were from the same class as subjects chosen for the study and were aware of many of the learning phenomena to be studied. They were given several hours of training in qualitative methods, interview techniques and transcription as instructed by the first author, who is both a clinical teacher and a senior researcher formally trained in qualitative methods. The questions are shown in Table 1.

To encourage more detail and greater in-depth answers, there were follow-up questions such as "Can you tell me more about that?" Thus, standard interview techniques were used that embraced qualitative description methods [22,23] such as confirmations and follow-ups, in order to check and supplement initial statements until each subject's knowledge about topics appeared to be exhausted and the informant and interviewer agreed to stop. A quantitative validation method [24,25], in the form of a brief questionnaire, was also used in a follow-up re-visitation of the same informants. It consisted of sixteen true/false items based on group identification and the main findings of the students' interview data. All 12 students subsequently completed the validation survey. The questions are listed in a table in the Results section.

Table 1. Interview questionnaire items.

(1) What is your overall assessment of the FOAL program?
(2) What are the benefits of the FOAL program at the clinic as a mentee? ... mentor?
(3) What challenges have arisen in connection with the FOAL program as a mentee?
(4) Have you had a feeling that you were inspired by your time as a mentee, i.e., as a foal?
(5) Are there (other) things you became aware of about yourself as a mentee? ... mentor?
(6) Have you ever been in doubt about whether you wanted to become a dentist?
Has the FOAL program had an influence on it?
(7) Do you have something you would like to add in relation to the FOAL program?

The research was carried out in accordance with the Declaration of Helsinki and Aarhus Municipality's ethical committee rules, including, but not limited to, that there was no potential harm to participants, that the anonymity of participants was guaranteed and that informed verbal and written consent of the participants was obtained.

2.3. *Analyses*

The students' audio-recorded interviews were transcribed verbatim via the dictation program in Word 2016 and saved according to appropriate measures to ensure the anonymity of the subjects and their identities. The text files of the interviews were then imported into NVivo software [26] to assist with a general inductive analytic approach [27] to explore categories and compare contexts related to students' experiences of the FOAL program. NVivo aids in structuring and analyzing the files, making it easier to find supportive material with concrete text quotations when exemplifying phenomena and common themes [27] which reoccur throughout the various interviews.

A "Code Book" [26] was prepared, in which brief descriptions with illustrative quotes for each category or theme developed in the NVivo program were documented. (The Code Book topics are listed in a table in the Results section.) To ensure that there was sufficient theoretical saturation, the data analysis ended only when there was redundancy of descriptions and no new categories of phenomena or themes could be found [27,28].

All student interviews and validation questionnaires were analyzed within their social contexts and were further defined by the following scientific assumptions: (1) that informants were members of the same socio-cultural group (Danish dental students of the same class, age and gender), (2) that they answered questions independently of each other and (3) that the questions were about a specific domain (early clinical experiences in the teaching clinic) [29].

The true/false survey provided the estimated validity and consistency in informants' use of descriptions and findings from the entire sample, that is, estimates of consensus for the interviewed informants. This also made it possible to evaluate if there were sufficient numbers of informants for valid results at the 95% confidence level. Questionnaire responses were analyzed according to cultural consensus theory, which is based on a formal mathematical model [29]. This theoretical approach makes it possible to judge how accurately the informants described the relevant social phenomena in their responses, as well as the strength of agreement between informants. Unicet 6.0 software [30] was used to calculate these consensus and informant competency parameters. Unicet 6.0 provides Cronbach's alpha calculations, factor analysis and Bayesian probability estimates based on patterns of subject agreement. Standardized values for intersubject agreement and minimum sample size required for testing at the given confidence levels, which are provided in the Results section and guided assessment of students' results [31].

3. Results

The results in Table 2 below are the coded categories of student perceptions and descriptions of early clinical experience. Details of the coding descriptions and quotes in the text after the table correspond to the order of findings summarized in Table 2. As expected, students described a broad range of categories due to their "insider" role as users of early clinical experience. Results by specific aims and categories of findings are reported below, and many are accompanied by cogent quotations that illustrate each. Students' quotations are identified as S1 to S12 for anonymity.

Table 2. Categories of informants' interview answers. (See details in text sections below by corresponding section numbers).

Categories of Interview Findings re. FOAL Program	
Overall assessment of FOAL program = positive; needs improvements	(Section 3.1)
Advantages of the FOAL program	(Section 3.2)
As mentees (foals):	
To try something other than bookwork	
Learning something about communication/contact with patients	
Legitimized lack of knowledge	
Opportunity to reduce the preclinical to clinic transition crisis (5th sem.)	
Experienced students are seen as role models	
As mentors:	
An extra pair of hands helps	
Mentee's active engagement is crucial to the program	
Learning by teaching others	
No need for special preparations to have a foal	
Challenges with the FOAL program	(Section 3.3)
Fetch something for a mentor, but you do not know what it is	
Lack of knowledge about clinical dentistry	
A scary social situation	
"Lost, but cool"—feeling overwhelmed, yet exhilarated	
Lack of training of foals about the basics	
Focus of mentor's attention to the foal can disappear with pressurized situations	
As a foal, you can feel more like a hindrance than a help	
Competition for foal times at the clinic	
Becoming inspired as a foal	(Section 3.4)
"Of course the older students were cool! I want to be too."	
Foals reaffirming their choice of profession It helped to be a foal	(Section 3.5)
Considerations or suggestions for improvement	(Section 3.6)
Better distribution of times as foals	
Increase the number of mentee hours	
Not enough time for FOAL program in 2nd year; best in 1st year	
Do simple treatments early	
Have the same mentor every time	

3.1. Overall Assessment of the FOAL Program

The informants mainly thought that the FOAL program had been positive, since as a mentee or foal, a student could acquire some early clinical experience and inspiration about their chosen profession. At the same time, there were also reports of shortcomings that had affected the experience. A good example of an overall assessment of the FOAL program is as follows:

> S2: "It's a good thing that in the first semesters they come up to get some experience at the clinic and that they are allowed to see and ask about things and get some knowledge about the clinic (and the profession). But they know nothing. So, it could be nice with some more introduction."

Praise for the program in general, but also a lack of more introduction and theory, was also pointed out by another informant:

> S5: "It was good to get up to the clinic early in the study and see how it works at the clinic and what and how to expect to work as a dentist. But it was also sometimes difficult to follow any theory behind what actually happened. So yes, you had seen a little, but still a little difficult to assess what had happened."

3.2. *Advantages with the FOAL Program*

As a mentee/foal

Students got to try something other than bookwork: Informants lauded the FOAL program as an opportunity to try out their hands in the clinic rather than more basic sciences. Among other things, one informant formulated the following:

> S4: "It was good to get a little away from the books, and come up to the clinic to see what you really will be doing someday."

> S3: "Then I was allowed to polish with a prophylaxis cup once, I can remember. It was mega cool!"

Learning something about communication/contact with patients: For better or worse, informants described different situations where they could appreciate the importance of good communication. As one informant put it:

> S3: "You find out you like to have that kind of human contact, so you really have to talk with the patients. You have to make them feel comfortable and safe. I found that I actually think it is a cool way to work with people and the clinical environment up there."

Another informant reported learning from watching mentors communicate with patients:

> S6: "I actually think it was easier to see when there was not a very good communication between patient and mentor compared to when there was a good relationship and communication between them."

> Learning small talk was often part of the communication related to patient treatment, as described in the quote below:

> S2: "There is a lot of small talk at the clinic. So it's nice that you're sometimes allowed to talk to patients a little bit before you (actually) have them yourself."

"Legitimized lack of knowledge": Informants described that as a foal, students do not have much experience or knowledge, neither about patients nor treatments, which is why it is not possible to hold them responsible for ignorance about theory or practice. Thus, many stated that it is better to just relax with expectations as a foal:

> S5: "It was nice that they knew you were a foal. In this way you were allowed to ask more questions, i.e., legitimized ignorance. You didn't really know enough. It was really minimal knowledge you had."

> S11: "I became less afraid of patient contact (with time), so it became more harmless. You can just sit on the sidelines quietly and learn things one step at a time. First you suction and then you can just sit and chat, since you are not in charge. Then you build up your knowledge up from there. I think that was really very good."

Opportunity to reduce the preclinical to clinical transition crisis in the fifth semester: Theoretical learning during the first 2 years of dental education is supplemented with preclinical lab or simulation work, i.e., in the form of modules within the main clinical disciplines (restorative, periodontal, prosthetics, etc.). Learning these lab or simulation skills is part of the preparation to transition into the clinic environment. The FOAL program could also contribute to a less stressful transition according to many informants:

> S11: "If you have not been a foal and you are in the fifth semester and have never sat in front of a patient before, it would be something completely different to have to go up and do your first filling or anesthesia. The FOAL program has contributed by making students familiar with the clinic and routines. They may even become familiar with the teachers. I definitely think it helps."

Other informants stated that the FOAL program did not significantly reduce this stressful transition.

> S5: "It makes the transition a little smaller. But, it is a very big leap to go from meeting up for 3 h at a time, sitting and suctioning, not really knowing what exactly has gone on and then to having your own patients. You have to call up patients and prepare for the whole treatment, with all that it entails. So yes, a big leap, still."

Experienced students are seen as role models: Informants described that a foal records in their memory when their mentors are acting professionally, both in terms of behavior and treatment. The following quotations illustrate this.

> S1: "You see how other older students handle situations and that they can be exposed to pressured situations. Yes, you have seen them talk to the patient and seen that they can make some small mistakes and thought yes okay, and that also worked out."

> In addition to seeing how mentors act with patients and the teachers, the foals also became familiar with the clinical environment from early participation.

> S2: "There was a little everyday life at the clinic and you saw a little about what it was all about."

As a mentor

An extra pair of hands helps: Overall, the informants as mentors thought that the great advantage of having a foal was the hands-on practical help they provide.

> S4: "If you are in the middle of having trouble with something, you can ask: 'Would you be so kind to fetch my teacher, because I need to stay with this in the meantime?"

The mentee's active engagement is crucial to the program: According to the informants, the cooperation between a mentor and a foal depends on the level of interest and commitment of the foal.

> S11: "It's fun to have the younger ones up. Especially if it's someone who wants to interact a lot and inquiries into things, not just suctioning a meter away. Then I think it's fun to be a mentor."

Informants added that interested and committed foals ask more questions, which is why the mentor, in addition to the practical help, also benefits from teaching them and testing their own theoretical knowledge.

> S1: "You get to refresh your memory, because if they are curious and ask questions, you can explain what you are doing. Then you become even more confident (and say to yourself)—"Well, (I) actually know what (I am) doing!""

Learning by teaching others: As shown in the quote above, many informants explained that they learned by explaining treatments to foals, thus reaffirming their role as clinicians.

In the process, mentors test their own knowledge by formulating and refreshing previously learned knowledge.

> S3: "You do not always think about why you do this or that until there is someone sitting next to you and you have to explain it. Then you recall why you actually do things the way (you do) and more aware of your own way of operating."

Simultaneously to the above, several mentors tried to make the treatment situation exciting and learned to be more educational. This pedagogical attitude was often inspired from the time they themselves were foals.

> S2: "At least I try to make it exciting for them at the clinic, because I myself was a foal for a mentor who was not very inspiring to be with. So I teach and explain and allow (them) to get their fingers wet in the patient's mouth. Just being allowed to touch a patient makes a big difference."

As a mentor, you can also learn about your own stress reactions, and to relax during treatment, even when you have a new foal.

> S6: "You want to have a good relationship with your patient, and if you have a relatively new foal, which you also have to start up, then you must at least learn (to) be able to relax with it all one way or another. Because it can quickly get stressful if it is also a new treatment that you are trying to learn."

No need for any special preparation to have a foal: Most mentors did not prepare very much to have foal assistance. They did not think it necessary to prepare.

> S4: "Many of the things we do come automatic, so I can explain without having to review a manual ahead of it."

However, many mentors gave foals personal introductions before treatment began.

> S11: "I always ask what semester they are in and if it is something they have done before. Then I tell them about the patient, and what we are going to do, and what we did last time. If it is a slightly special patient, who may present some challenges, then I also mention that."

3.3. Challenges with the FOAL Program

Told to fetch something, but the foal does not know what it is: A significant challenge for foals at the clinic was described as their lack of knowledge about clinic organization, equipment, supplies and staff, since they were not introduced to this.

> S6: "If you were sent out to find something, did not really hear what it was that the mentor said and you did not know who to ask for help, it could all be overwhelming."

Lack of knowledge about clinical dentistry: Some informants remembered the feelings of being ignorant and unsure about how to behave as well as the requirements and expectations demanded of them.

> S12: "I was very scared (at first) to do something wrong. I think it was enormously anxiety-provoking to have to sit with that suction and have no idea: "Does it hurt to get it on your tongue? Does it hurt to suction on the cheek? You sat and were completely panicky.""

A scary social situation: Coming up to the clinic as a foal and meeting patients, older students, teachers and staff can be very overwhelming for some new students. In some cases, some students experience it almost as anxiety-provoking, as expressed in this quote:

> S7: "If you are actually a little unsure of yourself and you have to actively go in and ask 'I want to come and help you.', it can be a personal challenge for a young foal; just to take that step and sit with strangers for 3 h."

"Lost, but cool": On the other hand, informants experienced both the challenges above as a foal and, at the same time, the exhilaration of being among clinicians in their chosen profession:

> S10: "I was lost in a way because you do not really know people or the place (at first). You were just told to show up at a chair and you did. But I also felt a little buff, because we all knew that it was mega cool."

Lack of training of foals about the basics: Although the informants described that they as mentors introduced their foals to treatments, there was a lack of basic mandatory training in being a foal, for example, to learn something about materials and equipment or the use of suction equipment.

> S2: "I didn't know the difference between a laser tip and a plastic instrument. You know nothing, so you should get a better introduction, since you feel a little stupid."

Focus of mentor's attention to the foal can disappear with pressurized situations: Besides lacking some type of basic training, the foals lacked orientation about what they could expect of mentors in stressful clinical situations:

> S1: "If something is really difficult and I (as a mentor) am under pressure, then my focus of attention on the foal disappears. You have to have energy reserves in order to maintain attention to making explanations."

As a foal, you can feel more like a hindrance than a help:

> S2: "Sometimes the students you help are in pressured situations, so you feel more like a hindrance than a help. That's how it is sometimes."

Competition for foal times at the clinic: It could be urgent for either a foal or a mentor to find a partner because of periods with heavy demand. At the beginning of a semester, many foals want to help, which is why there may be competition between the foals to come up to the clinic and help. On the other hand, at the end of the semester, it is typically the mentors who find it difficult to get help, as foals have already fulfilled their foal times and are starting to study up for exams. These issues create stressful conditions for students.

3.4. Becoming Inspired as a Foal

Some informants said they were inspired by their foal experiences. Most found it inspiring that their mentors could be so proficient, and this had also motivated them to want to become proficient.

> S3: "I just think it was really cool seeing how much they could do. I really wanted to be able to do the same. By being allowed to see someone good at their job, I also wanted to be good myself."

3.5. Foals Reaffirming Their Choice of Profession

Most informants had considered and been in doubt about their educational choice to become a dentist. The most prominent reason for this was the stressful crisis that arose during the transition between their fourth and fifth semesters when starting at the teaching clinic. However, the FOAL program eased the difficult transition slightly. This is because, as a young student, you have an opportunity to gain insight into and engage in some clinical treatments, even though you are not a fully responsible clinical student yet.

> S9: "Especially the fifth semester, I think, I was almost ready to drop it all. It was not so much FK, but more things around it that made it tiring. I liked FK. Do I think that the FOAL program helped to make me be less in doubt? Yes. Because there you just want to get started by seeing what they (mentors) sat and did, which made it quite clear. So, did I reaffirm my study choice as a foal? Yes, I think so."

Another informant thought the FOAL program made little difference:

> S12: "Yes, I have been in doubt many times, after we started at the clinic ourselves. There was all the pressure of seeing patients and at the same time having to juggle theoretical subjects on top of it. There were just too many balls in the air. So I think many times I thought "Oh, am I good enough for this, since now, again, I am sitting and fiddling around with an impression. The others can figure it out, why can't I?"

This quote also indicates that self-doubt plays a prominent role in the preclinical to clinic transition crisis.

3.6. Considerations or Suggestions for Improvement

Better distribution of times as foals: The informants displayed a desire for a more structured FOAL program so that the planning schedule is optimized and there is no overlap between foal times and coursework.

> S1: "One challenge is that it can be a little difficult if everyone from 1–3 semesters has coursework and (a mentor) needs a foal. Where there is small group course-work, that's okay. But sometimes they all have a lecture that is at a really stupid time, like from 10 am to 12 noon, so you can't get help then at all. So either they could put coursework either (earliest) in the morning or after clinic hours."

> S6: "(The school needs) to come up with something where different teams of foals are assigned certain days. Then it would not be as stressful to find someone when times are just totally booked."

Increase the number of mentee hours: Many informants believed that more mentee hours will benefit clinical insight and reduce feelings of ignorance.

> S10: "I think there could have been a few more hours because it can take a long time between times when you can be there. Then you lose a bit of (the routine). So maybe if there was one day a week where there was an hour or two where you could (flexibly) manage to be there, I think it would make more sense."

Not enough time for FOAL program in second year; best in first year: Some informants pointed out that there is already a lot of pressure on students to complete theoretical courses in the second year, and that the FOAL program can be a stress factor. Thus, it would be better to complete all of the foal hours during the first year.

> S9: "There may not have been enough foal hours in the first semester as it is right now. In the third and fourth semesters there is more pressure because you had several larger (theoretical) subjects."

Do simple treatments early as foals: Several informants came up with the proposal to try small simple treatments on patients already in what is now the preclinical phase.

> S12: "There are types of treatment you could perhaps start doing earlier (than the 5th sem). I think it could be cool because a simple periodontal treatment or instruction on tooth brushing or holding a mirror and probe at the same time is not something we've really done (systematically)."

> Several informants also expressed a wish that foals would receive a "clinical mini-course" so that they were better equipped to start in the clinic.

Have the same mentor every time: Several informants as foals thought it best to have the same mentor every time they were at the clinic as it made them feel safe in the new and sometimes overwhelming setting. As mentors, they also agreed it was best to have the same mentee each time, as previously described above.

> S5: "I think it was an advantage to be associated with a (specific) mentor or a group of mentors, to feel more secure. It gave more of a sense of the routine, since there was not just a new one every time."

The results from the questionnaire responses are shown in Table 3 below. There was significantly high consensus and informant competence among the informants, suggesting, as shown in Table 4 below, that the sample size was adequate at the 0.95 confidence level, given the assumptions described in the methods.

Table 3. Questionnaire results: percentages of true vs. false answers for the 12 senior students.

Statistics: Consensus α Reliability = 0.94; Mean Competence = 0.74, SD = 0.20	T	F
(1) I am a female dental student in my 9th–10th semester.	100%	0
(2) I am between 20 between 30 years old.	100%	0
(3) I speak fluent Danish.	100%	0
(4) As a foal, there were no opportunities to see what the clinic was like, as well as what the training would lead to in the end.	33%	67%
(5) The first hours as a mentee in the clinic were overwhelming for many students for several reasons.	67%	33%
(6) As a foal, it was possible to experience that you belonged in "the clinical life", even if you were not an official clinician yet.	83%	17%
(7) It was not an advantage if a foal was given the opportunity to do a simple treatment such as toothbrushing, rubber cup polishing or applying fluorides.	17%	83%
(8) A foal got the most out of mentors who could not maintain contact with them, even during pressured clinical situations.	0	100%
(9) As a foal, you had an opportunity to take part in a completely new social network, which was important for when you yourself would start up as a clinician.	58%	42%
(10) Both as a mentor or foal, there was no benefit in having the same partner from time to time, if it went well.	0	100%
(11) The FOAL program can help the often-stressful transition from pre-clinic to clinic by knowing a little about the clinic and the people there.	75%	25%
(12) As a foal, it did not help that mentors could put themselves in your shoes (empathy).	0	100%
(13) Mentors got the most out of active, curious foals, which affected the amount of explanation and teaching.	75%	25%
(14) As a mentor, you learn from teaching, i.e., meaningful communication reinforces what you have learned as well as your professional pride.	92%	8%
(15) The current FOAL program seems a bit disorganized, as not enough time was set aside for foal orientation or mentor training.	75%	25%
(16) Changing the number of foal hours and/or better distribution of hours would be advantageous.	92%	8%

Table 4. Standardized chart for minimal number of informants needed to classify a desired percentage of questions with a specified confidence level for various levels of cultural competence (note for clarity: 0.50 is considered "good" mean intersubject agreement according to [31]).

	Proportion of Questions				
Answered "correctly"	Consensus (average level of cultural competency:)				
	0.5	0.6	0.7	0.8	0.9
At 0.95 confidence level:	(Minimal number of informants needed:)				
0.80	9	7	4	4	4
0.85	11	7	4	4	4
0.90	13	9	6	4	4
0.95	17	11	6	6	4
0.99	29	19	10	8	4
	At 0.99 confidence level:				
0.80	15	10	5	4	4
0.85	15	10	7	5	4
0.90	21	12	7	5	4
0.95	23	14	9	7	4
0.99	>30	20	13	8	6

4. Discussion

The purpose of this study was to investigate early clinical learning and evaluate the FOAL program's influence on students' perceptions at the Aarhus Dental School. Twelve last year clinical students' perceptions and experiences about the benefits of and challenges with the FOAL program, as well as suggestions for improvements to the FOAL program, were explored.

There are important caveats to keep in mind regarding the present results. (1) Although these qualitative results may be representative of Danish female dental students, who are the large majority of Danish dental students, they may not be representative of males or other student nationalities. Cultural influences on student motivations and learning environments can vary from nation to nation and by gender. (2) No specific measures of stress or self-efficacy were used for comparisons with the results in this study. Efforts were focused solely on informants describing their own experiences and perceptions about early clinical experience as mentees and in mentorship in order to gain knowledge that would contribute to variable selection in future research and informed educational policy.

Overall, informants were positive about the FOAL program but often felt there was room for improvement. They described a large number of benefits, both as mentees and mentors. They also described that it was positive early in the curriculum to experience the clinical context of the profession and not just the theoretical studies that dominate the first two years. Informants described that the FOAL program helped to allay the crisis from preclinical education to the clinic, but only in part. Therefore, Hypothesis 1 could only be partially confirmed, but the program helped according to many informants. They had an opportunity to become familiar with the clinical environment, the teachers and the activities at the clinic. On the other hand, informants expressed that there should have been more time for foal activities since foals only received a limited insight into daily life at the clinic. Additionally, they stated that foals do not acquire an overall picture of the workload expected of clinical students, as they do not experience the extra tasks that come with being a responsible clinician, such as post-clinic lab work and making patient appointments. Many foals chose to use the same mentor because they felt that the learning environment was safer. On the other hand, this precluded opportunities to see different mentors' work tasks, working methods and other ways of coping with the stresses of first year clinicians.

The present findings support a recent study by the Association for Dental Education in Europe (ADEE) about "Transition to Clinical Training in Dentistry" [4] which recognized early clinical experience as an important factor in achieving contextual learning and better integration of theory and practice [4]. These results support Hypothesis 2, that is, the FOAL program "provided professional inspiration and study relevance."

There were also benefits on the mentor side of the mentor/mentee relationship. A student or resident, placed in the position of a teacher of near-peers, experiences a different relation to them [12]. Acting as a relative expert makes a mentor feel like an expert with feelings of competence, relative autonomy and self-esteem before others, which, in turn, can motivate the peer-teacher in further professional development [12]. Not only did mentors increase their self-awareness about their competencies (Hypotheses 3) but they also exhibited professional pride and attitudes when teaching young mentees.

Another advantage mentioned by several informants was that the FOAL program contributed to learning about contact with patients and communication, which supports Hypotheses 4. The ability to communicate clearly is an essential cornerstone skill for future professionals. Some informants reasoned that had it not been for the FOAL program, meeting patients and communication would have been an additional stress factor in the fifth semester, had they not tried it as a foal. This supports another recent English study that reported that dental student informants perceived early clinical experience to be an advantage in developing interpersonal skills for communication with patients and clinical staff, by acquiring gradual familiarity with the clinical environment [13].

As foals, many informants experienced increased internal motivation to learn more about theory as well as learning clinical skills (Hypothesis 5). Some even went so far as to say that had the FOAL program not existed, then their motivation would have suffered since it would depend solely on theoretical and laboratory teaching. A medical student study showed similar results in reports of acquisition of clinical knowledge and skills, self-confidence, improved performance, validation of career plans and increased motivation to study the basic sciences [14].

For most informants, the FOAL program contributed to reaffirming their choice of dentistry as a career (Hypothesis 6), since they had the opportunity to gain insight into clinical treatment, at the beginning of the education, and this makes it easier to confirm or deny the choice of dentistry as the correct career. Early clinical experience can lead to a full sense of volition, choice and self-determination [9,10]. This means that a student pursues an activity for the satisfaction that is derived from it regardless of external pressure [6]. Kusurkar et al. [19] also found that autonomous motivation in medical students correlated positively and significantly with not dropping out. On the other hand, the current mandatory 12 foal hours per semester may not provide sufficient experience to be able to make this decision.

Informants determined that one of the advantages for mentors, among others, was that an actively engaged foal could more likely test the mentor's theoretical knowledge. This was perceived to give the mentor increased self-confidence and motivation by confirming their own mastery of clinical treatments and theory, i.e., professional identity, as described above. These findings support Hypotheses 3–5 since more actively involved foals contribute to greater learning benefits for both mentors and themselves. Thus, synergism in the mentor/mentee relationship promotes learning reflections, learning about communication and contact and learning motivation for both learners. Serrano et al. [4] described that self-motivation is regulated by satisfaction and performance. If a foal seems less involved, informants admitted that this did not contribute anything positive to a mentor's learning curve. In another study, this lack of motivation (amotivation) was also found to be negatively correlated with medical students' reflections about learning [19]. SDT concepts of controlled external motivation and amotivation are associated with negative outcomes, including low competence, poor well-being and insufficient psychological adaptation to university life [6].

The concept of self-efficacy in the context of mentee/mentor learning [32,33] also seems highly relevant to the discussion of the present results. Self-efficacy is a student's "sense of being able to do" a task and/or "feeling confident or competent" to execute learned skills or attitudes in their education [34]. Self-efficacy is based on Bandura's social learning theory [35] which posits that besides theoretical and directly conditioned learning, people also learn via (1) observation, (2) imitation and (3) modeling. Observational learning occurs constantly, and exposure to a mentor's behaviors provides new learning through the modeling process. Studies on medical students have also confirmed that mentee/mentor relationships provided learning through observation, feedback and cognitive support [12,33,36], often even more than teacher contacts in some cases [37]. The present mentees had the opportunity to observe and consult with their mentors constantly, thus providing abundant opportunities for them both to build up self-efficacy and self-confidence. Thus, social learning theory is very fundamental to self-determination theory and professional motivational development [19]. Foals experienced, first-hand, multiple levels of learning by observing mentors with their patients. These are likely the first steps young dental students make in becoming more mature, acclimatizing to professional settings and identifying with their future role [17].

The interviews also revealed a number of challenges and needs for improvement in the current FOAL program. Almost all informants pointed out a lack of clinical knowledge as being their biggest challenge. This contributes to insecurity and can be overwhelming, since there are no experiences to fall back on. As a mentor, the clinical naiveté of the foal can also be a challenge if the mentor is already in a high-pressure treatment situation. The clinically naive foal may amplify the mentor's irritation or frustration. Lack of knowledge about standards of treatment in a clinical situation can be frustrating or even a source of stress, according to Moore et al. [2]. The informants described that this problem was greatest in the first and second semesters and suggested a more structured orientation at the beginning of the FOAL program.

The current FOAL program revealed rifts about foal times as well as issues in relation to foals' academic schedule. Therefore, another suggestion was to improve the distribution of times and thus provide a more structured FOAL program. Presently, the responsibility for achieving compulsory foal hours is placed on the individual student, which can contribute to increased stress and anxiety. Besides the obvious challenge of booking their own times, it also requires that a foal must confront social barriers with which he/she may not be comfortable. Thus, to confront these challenges, the informants suggested that a foal should be able to choose to work with the same mentor for all the hours, in order to provide security and better conditions for motivation and learning.

Another suggestion was that an even earlier start of clinical treatments should be implemented in the clinical curriculum. Earlier starts would have younger clinical students start with easier treatments on patients and would presumably provide additional experience, motivation and self-confidence to try gradually more difficult treatments. However, Dyrbye et al. [14] pointed out that even if one sees positive results with early clinical experience, more insight is still needed into how these affect students' professional development. Perhaps an earlier start to clinical treatments in the third and fourth semesters, along with streamlined and clinically relevant theoretical support, as is now in the planning phase with a new curriculum reform at Aarhus, will ultimately provide an additional positive intrinsic motivation for students' professional development. The idea seems at least good, in relation to trying to break the stress curve from the fourth to fifth semesters of the preclinical to clinic transition, which still exists at present (2021). At any rate, it seems that an improved FOAL program in the first and second semesters still has a lot of relevance and would provide a more nuanced and formative professional orientation for both foals and mentors.

5. Conclusions

The informants in this study felt that there were many benefits to the FOAL mentee/mentor program. They described, as mentees, that it helped them gain insight into the clinical world and the relevance of their studies, which contributed to a less stressful transition from the preclinical to clinical semesters. The study also found that a well-functioning FOAL program required an actively involved mentee, as this positively affected the mentee/mentor relationship and improved the motivation of both for learning, acquisition of social perspectives and professional reflection. In other words, mentees and mentors got out of the program what they put into it. Teachers in similar clinical learning situations need to point this out both in introductory orientations and in daily clinical experiences.

Although there is still pronounced stress among students in their transition to the clinic, the Aarhus Dental School is currently in the process of redesigning the curriculum to include an optimized early FOAL program in the first year combined with clinical transition to treating patients with easier treatments in the third and fourth semesters. The reflection on the present results indicates that this might provide an even greater benefit for the students that could further help eliminate the current clinical transition crisis period. These results should also have some interest internationally, since the Association of Dental Education in Europe has called for more attention to this problem.

Author Contributions: Conceptualization, R.M.; methodology, R.M.; software, R.M.; validation, S.M., M.S. and N.M.; formal analysis, R.M.; investigation, R.M., S.M., M.S. and N.M.; resources, R.M.; data curation, R.M., S.M., M.S. and N.M.; writing—original draft preparation, R.M., S.M., M.S. and N.M.; writing—review and editing, R.M., S.M., M.S. and N.M.; visualization, R.M.; supervision, R.M.; project administration, R.M.; funding acquisition, not relevant. All authors have read and agreed to the published version of the manuscript.

Funding: No funding sponsors were used or involved with the choice of research project, design collection, analyses, interpretation of data, writing of the manuscript or in the decision to publish the results.

Institutional Review Board Statement: The study was conducted according to the guidelines of the Declaration of Helsinki, and approved by the Project Institutional Review Board of the Institute of Dentistry and Oral Health, Aarhus University (protocol code 331122U018, 1 March 2021).

Informed Consent Statement: Informed consent was obtained from all subjects involved in the study.

Data Availability Statement: The original data supporting the reported results are in Danish and can be requisitioned from the first author.

Conflicts of Interest: The authors declare no conflict of interest.

References

1. Moore, R.M.; Madsen, L.V.; Trans, M. Stress Sensitivity and Signs of Anxiety or Depression among First Year Clinical Dental and Medical Students. *Open J. Med. Psychol.* **2020**, *9*, 7–20. [CrossRef]
2. Moore, R. Psychosocial student functioning in comprehensive dental clinic education: A qualitative study. *Eur. J. Dent. Educ.* **2018**, *22*, e479–e487. [CrossRef] [PubMed]
3. Grandy, T.G.; Westerman, G.H.; Combs, C.E.; Turner, C.H. Perceptions of stress among third-year dental students. *J. Dent. Educ.* **1989**, *53*, 718–721. [CrossRef] [PubMed]
4. Serrano, C.M.; Botelho, M.G.; Wesselink, P.R.; Vervoorn, J.M. Challenges in the transition to clinical training in dentistry: An ADEE special interest group initial report. *Eur. J. Dent. Educ.* **2018**, *22*, e451–e457. [CrossRef]
5. Orsini, C.; Binnie, V.I.; Fuentes, F.; Ledezma, P.; Jerez, O. Implications of motivation differences in preclinical-clinical transition of dental students: A one-year follow-up study. *Educ. Med.* **2016**, *17*, 193–196. [CrossRef]
6. Orsini, C. Self-determined motivation in Dental Education: Are we supporting autonomy or controlling behaviour? *J. Oral Res.* **2015**, *4*, 86–87. [CrossRef]
7. Orsini, C.; Evans, P.; Binnie, V.; Ledezma, P.; Fuentes, F. Encouraging intrinsic motivation in the clinical setting: Teachers' perspectives from the self-determination theory. *Eur. J. Dent. Educ.* **2016**, *20*, 102–111. [CrossRef]
8. Deci, E.L.; Ryan, R.M. Self-determination theory: A macrotheory of human motivation, development, and health. *Can. Psychol.* **2008**, *49*, 182–185. [CrossRef]
9. Ng, J.Y.; Ntoumanis, N.; Thøgersen-Ntoumani, C.; Deci, E.L.; Ryan, R.M.; Duda, J.L.; Williams, G.C. Self-Determination Theory Applied to Health Contexts: A Meta-Analysis. *Persp. Psychol. Sci.* **2012**, *7*, 325–340. [CrossRef]
10. Ryan, R.M.; Deci, E.L. Self-determination theory and the facilitation of intrinsic motivation, social development, and well-being. *Am. Psychol.* **2000**, *55*, 68–78. [CrossRef]
11. Ten Cate, O.T.J.; Kusurkar, R.A.; Williams, G.C. How self-determination theory can assist our understanding of the teaching and learning processes in medical education. AMEE Guide No. 59. *Med. Teach.* **2011**, *33*, 961–973. [CrossRef]
12. Ten Cate, O.; Durning, S. Dimensions and psychology of peer teaching in medical education. *Med. Teach.* **2007**, *29*, 546–552. [CrossRef]
13. Ali, K.; Zahra, D.; McColl, E.; Salih, V.; Tredwin, C. Impact of early clinical exposure on the learning experience of undergraduate dental students. *Eur. J. Dent. Educ.* **2018**, *22*, e75–e80. [CrossRef]
14. Dyrbye, L.N.; Harris, I.; Rohren, C.H. Early Clinical Experiences from Students' Perspectives: A Qualitative Study of Narratives. *Acad. Med.* **2007**, *82*, 979–988. [CrossRef]
15. Ebrahimi, S.; Kojuri, J.; Ashkani Esfahani, S. Early clinical experience, a way for Preparing Students for clinical setting. *Galen Med. J.* **2012**, *1*, 42–47.
16. Kashbour, W.A.; Kendall, J.; Grey, N. Students' perspectives of early and gradual transitioning between simulation and clinical training in dentistry and their suggestions for future course improvements. *Eur. J. Dent. Educ.* **2019**, *23*, 471–481. [CrossRef]
17. Littlewood, S.; Ypinazar, V.; Margolis, S.A.; Scherpbier, A.; Spencer, J.; Dornan, T. Early practical experience and the social responsiveness of clinical education: Systematic review. *Br. Med. J.* **2005**, *331*, 387–391. [CrossRef]
18. Zijlstra-Shaw, S.; Robinson, P.G.; Roberts, T. Assessing professionalism within dental education; the need for a definition. *Eur. J. Dent. Educ.* **2012**, *16*, e128–e36. [CrossRef]
19. Kusurkar, R.A.; Ten Cate, T.J.; Van Asperen, M.; Croiset, G. Motivation as an independent and a dependent variable in medical education: A review of the literature. *Med. Teach.* **2011**, *33*, e242–e262. [CrossRef]
20. Moore, R.; Freitag, A.-S.; Hansen, A.D. Dental Student Perceptions of Learning in Dyad Practice—A Qualitative Study. *Arch. Dent. Oral Health* **2021**, *4*, 1–14. [CrossRef]
21. Palinkas, L.A.; Horwitz, S.M.; Green, C.A.; Wisdom, J.P.; Duan, N.; Hoagwood, K. Purposeful Sampling for Qualitative Data Collection and Analysis in Mixed Method Implementation Research. *Adm. Policy Ment. Health* **2015**, *42*, 533–544. [CrossRef] [PubMed]
22. Sandelowski, M. What's in a name? Qualitative description revisited. *Res. Nurs. Health* **2010**, *33*, 77–84. [CrossRef] [PubMed]

23. Neergaard, M.A.; Olesen, F.; Andersen, R.S.; Sondergaard, J. Qualitative description—The poor cousin of health research? *BMC Med. Res. Methodol.* **2009**, *9*, 52. [CrossRef] [PubMed]
24. Moore, R. Combining qualitative and quantitative research approaches in understanding pain. *J. Dent. Educ.* **1996**, *60*, 709–715. [CrossRef]
25. Moore, R.; Brødsgaard, I.; Miller, M.L.; Mao, T.-K.; Dworkin, S.F. Consensus analysis: Reliability, validity and informant accuracy in use of American and mandarin Chinese pain descriptors. *Ann. Behav. Med.* **1997**, *19*, 295–300. [CrossRef]
26. NVivo. *Qualitative Data Analysis Software*; QSR International Pty Ltd.: Brisbane, Australia; Los Angeles, CA, USA; London, UK, 2018.
27. Thomas, D.R. A general inductive approach for analyzing qualitative evaluation data. *Am. J. Eval.* **2006**, *27*, 237–246. [CrossRef]
28. Weller, S.C.; Vickers, B.; Bernard, H.R.; Blackburn, A.M.; Borgatti, S.; Gravlee, C.C.; Johnson, J.C. Open-ended interview questions and saturation. *PLoS ONE* **2018**, *13*, e0198606. [CrossRef]
29. Romney, A.K.; Weller, S.C.; Batchelder, W.H. Culture as consensus: A theory of cultural and informant accuracy. *Am. Anthropol.* **1986**, *88*, 313–338. [CrossRef]
30. Borgatti, S.P.; Everett, M.G.; Freeman, L.C. *Ucinet 6 for Windows: Software for Social Network Analysis*; Analytic Technologies: Harvard, MA, USA, 2002.
31. Weller, S.C.; Romney, A.K. *Systematic Data Collection*; SAGE: Newbury Park, CA, USA, 1988. [CrossRef]
32. Topping, K.J. Trends in Peer Learning. *Educ. Psychol.* **2005**, *25*, 631–645. [CrossRef]
33. Tolsgaard, M.G.; Kulasegaram, K.M.; Ringsted, C.V. Collaborative learning of clinical skills in health professions education: The why, how, when and for whom. *Med. Educ.* **2016**, *50*, 69–78. [CrossRef]
34. Bandura, A. Self-efficacy: Toward a unifying theory of behavior change. *Psychol. Rev.* **1977**, *84*, 191–215. [CrossRef]
35. Bandura, A. *Social Learning Theory*; Prentice-Hall: Upper Saddle River, NJ, USA, 2002.
36. Tolsgaard, M.G.; Rasmussen, M.B.; Bjørck, S.; Gustafsson, A.; Ringsted, C.V. Medical students' perception of dyad practice. *Perspect. Med. Educ.* **2014**, *3*, 500–507. [CrossRef]
37. Bandura, A.; Schunk, D.H. Cultivating competence, self-efficacy, and intrinsic interest through proximal self-motivation. *J. Pers. Soc. Psychol.* **1981**, *41*, 586–598. [CrossRef]

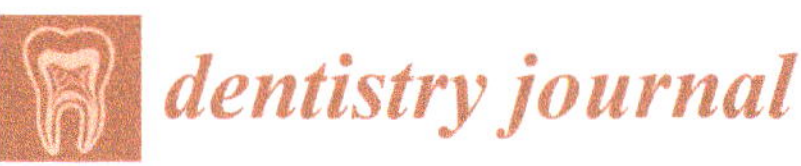 MDPI

Article

Education Regarding and Adherence to Recommended Nutrition Guidelines among Dental Students

Camille Frayna [1], Christoffer Devantier [2], Braden Harris [2], Karl Kingsley [3,*] and Joshua M. Polanski [3]

1 Pediatric Dentistry Postgraduate Program, School of Dental Medicine, University of Nevada, 1700 W. Charleston Blvd., Las Vegas, NV 89106, USA; frayna@unlv.nevada.edu
2 Department of Clinical Sciences, School of Dental Medicine, University of Nevada, 1700 W. Charleston Blvd., Las Vegas, NV 89106, USA; devantie@unlv.nevada.edu (C.D.); harrib11@unlv.nevada.edu (B.H.)
3 Department of Biomedical Sciences, School of Dental Medicine, University of Nevada, 1001 Shadow Lane, Las Vegas, NV 89106, USA; Joshua.Polanski@unlv.edu
* Correspondence: Karl.Kingsley@unlv.edu; Tel.: +1-702-774-2623; Fax: +1-702-774-2721

Abstract: The Dietary Guidelines for Americans (DGA) were developed to reduce or prevent many types of chronic illness, including cancer, heart disease and diabetes. Healthcare provider recommendations may be influenced by understanding of and adherence to the DGA, which may be incorporated into provider training, medical and dental clinical curricula—although few studies have evaluated adherence to the DGA among dental students. This approved retrospective study of voluntary student responses from a first-year dental school nutrition course included a short dietary and exercise survey administered as part of the DGA learning module. A total of N = 299 students completed the voluntary nutrition survey, yielding a response rate of 91.4%. Daily fruit and vegetable intake, dairy and whole grain servings among UNLV-SDM students were significantly lower than the DGA recommendations but higher than U.S. averages for 18–30-year-olds—although neither group met DGA recommendations. This study represents one of the first to evaluate the dietary intake of U.S. dental students for comparison with the DGA for positive health behaviors. These data demonstrate a lack of adherence to the DGA among highly educated dental students and the need for the curricular inclusion of diet and nutrition into the dental school curriculum.

Keywords: Dietary Guidelines for Americans (DGA); diet; dental student; education

Citation: Frayna, C.; Devantier, C.; Harris, B.; Kingsley, K.; Polanski, J.M. Education Regarding and Adherence to Recommended Nutrition Guidelines among Dental Students. *Dent. J.* **2021**, *9*, 93. https://doi.org/10.3390/dj9080093

Academic Editors: Jelena Dumancic, Božana Lončar Brzak and Cortino Sukotjo

Received: 6 May 2021
Accepted: 5 August 2021
Published: 9 August 2021

1. Introduction

The Dietary Guidelines for Americans (DGA) were developed by the Department of Health and Human Services (HHS) and the United States Department of Agriculture (USDA) to improve or maintain the health of the United States (U.S.) population [1,2]. Many of the recommendations emphasize the epidemiological and clinical findings of health promotion associated with the consumption of nutrient-dense foods, including fruits and vegetables [3,4]. Other important DGA recommendations include limitations on saturated and trans fats, added sugars, and sodium—mostly associated with adverse health outcomes, morbidity and premature mortality [5–7].

Healthcare providers are encouraged to promote the DGA in patient consultations to limit or prevent many chronic illnesses, such as diabetes and heart disease [8,9]. Most of the evidence regarding DGA recommendations and implementations has traditionally involved primary care physicians, which have been seen as crucial in the efforts to reduce the burden of chronic diseases associated with poor dietary intake and behaviors [10–12]. However, new models of health information incorporate the use of alternative providers and educators to deliver DGA recommendations and dietary information, including teachers and other healthcare specialist providers [13,14].

Dentists are a specific subgroup of healthcare providers that have moderate to lengthy patient interactions which may benefit from these consultations, because the etiologies of many oral diseases are based in nutritional deficiencies, poor dietary intake and chronic illness, such as diabetes [15–17]. More specifically, pediatric dentists are seen as a key group of healthcare providers that can positively and significantly influence parental and pediatric patient dietary behaviors and specific policy recommendations have been made by the American Academy of Pediatric Dentistry to improve adherence to the DGA [18–20].

Some evidence now suggests that medical provider recommendations may be influenced by the understanding of and adherence to the DGA, which may be incorporated into medical education and clinical curricula [21–23]. In fact, the Academy of Nutrition and Dietetics has indicated interprofessional education in nutrition as an essential component of healthcare provider training and is indispensable for developing providers with the competence to implement this into clinical practice [24,25]. Although some studies have focused on the importance of including nutrition education among dental and dental hygiene students, few studies have evaluated adherence to the DGA among dental students [26–28].

Based upon this paucity of information in this area and the overall importance of this topic, the goal of this project was to evaluate the diet and nutrition of dental students compared with the USDA and DGA nutrition guidelines during the instruction of a dental school nutrition course.

2. Materials and Methods

2.1. Human Subjects

The protocol for this study titled "Retrospective analysis of health status of dental student population" was reviewed and approved by the Office for the Protection of Research Subjects (OPRS) and Institutional Review Board (IRB) of the University of Nevada, Las Vegas (UNLV), on 21 May 2020 [Protocol 1607120-2]. Informed consent was waived due to the exemption to human subject research under the Basic HHS Policy for Protection of Human Research Subjects, (46.101) Subpart A (b) regarding IRB exemption for research involving the use of education tests (cognitive, diagnostic, aptitude, achievement) in which the subjects cannot be identified directly or through identifiers.

Briefly, this study involved a retrospective review of voluntary student responses previously collected as part of the Clinical Nutrition course at UNLV-SDM for first-year dental students. All student responses were anonymous with no personal identifying information; only basic demographic information (age, sex, race/ethnicity) was collected with each set of dietary and exercise behaviors.

2.2. Diet and Exercise Survey

The voluntary student diet and exercise questionnaire consisted of N = 17 questions, which corresponded to the basic parameters of the current DGA recommendations. These included questions regarding fruit and vegetable intake, sugar-sweetened beverages, and the frequency and intensity of physical activity.

2.3. Statistical Analysis

Each of the diet and exercise survey responses were tabulated and basic descriptive statistics associated with these respondents were reported with summary statistics for the percentage of responses from each question. Differences between dental (DMD) student responses and the Dietary Guidelines for Americans (DGA) were assessed through chi-squared analysis using online software from GraphPad (San Diego, CA, USA).

3. Results

This NHANES-based survey was administered over multiple years to first-year dental students during a nutrition course, with a total of n = 327 students receiving the voluntary survey (Table 1). In brief, a total of n = 299 students participated and completed the survey, yielding an overall response rate of 91.4%. The percentage of males and females in the survey (42% and 58%, respectively) was not significantly different from the overall student population from which the samples were taken (41%, 59%, respectively), $p = 0.8389$. In addition, the percentage of students identifying as White/Caucasian/non-minority among the study sample was 40.5%, which was not significantly different from the overall student population (48%), $p = 0.1612$. Most of these minority students self-identified as Asian.

Table 1. Demographic characteristics of dental student participants.

	Respondents (n = 299)	Total Student Population	Statistical Analysis
Females	n = 126/299 (42.1%)	41%	$\chi^2 = 0.041$, d.f. = 1
Males	n = 173/299 (57.9%)	59%	$p = 0.8389$
Caucasian/White	n = 121/299 (40.5%)	48%	$\chi^2 = 1.963$, d.f. = 1
Minority/non-White	n = 178/299 (59.5%)	52%	$p = 0.1612$
Asian	n = 123/299 (41.1%)	40%	
Hispanic/Black/Other	n = 55/299 (18.4%)	12%	

The estimate of overall fruit servings per day (0.69) was significantly lower than the DGA recommendations of 2.0. In addition, fruit consumption among 18–30-year-old females (0.5 servings) and males (0.4 servings) was also significantly lower than the DGA recommendations. Analysis of the data from UNLV-SDM dental students found no significant differences between males and females, $p = 0.899$. In addition, fruit consumption among females and males (0.8 servings per day) was significantly higher than the U.S. population in general and young adults (18–30), more specifically, $p = 0.031$ (Figure 1).

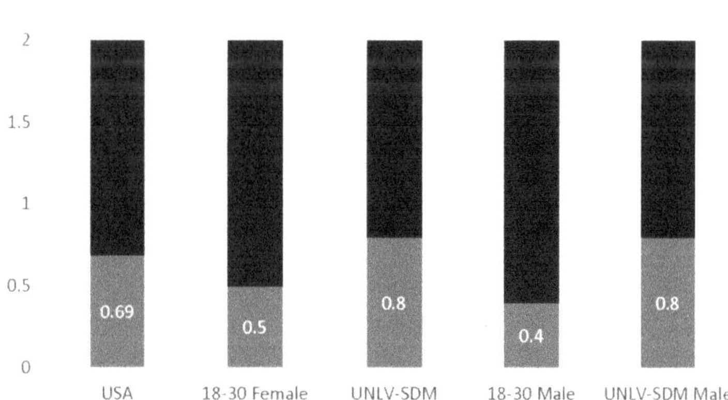

Figure 1. DGA fruit consumption analysis. Analysis of UNLV-SDM dental students' fruit consumption among females and males, which was significantly higher than the U.S. population in general and young adults (18 to 30-year olds), more specifically, $p = 0.031$, but no significant differences were found between males and females, $p = 0.899$, and did not meet the DGA recommendations.

The estimate of overall vegetable servings per day (1.22) was significantly lower than the DGA recommendations of 2.5. In addition, vegetable consumption among 18–30-year-old females (1.51 servings) and males (1.31 servings) was also significantly lower than the DGA recommendations (Figure 2). Analysis of the data from UNLV-SDM dental students found significant differences between males and females. Reported vegetable consumption among females (1.0 servings per day) was significantly higher than males (0.6 servings per day), $p = 0.022$—and lower than the U.S. population in general and young adults (18–30), more specifically, $p = 0.018$.

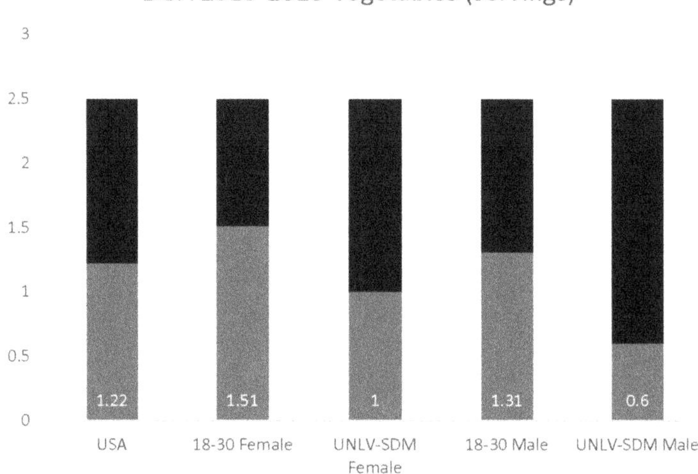

Figure 2. DGA vegetable consumption analysis. Analysis of UNLV-SDM dental students revealed significant differences, with consumption among females significantly higher than males, $p = 0.022$—although this was lower than the U.S. population in general and 18 to 30-year-olds, more specifically, $p = 0.018$, and did not meet the DGA recommendations.

The estimate of overall dairy consumption (1.9 cups per day) was significantly lower than the DGA recommendation of 3.0 cups. In addition, dairy consumption among 18–30-year-old females (1.4 cups) and males (1.9 cups) was also significantly lower than the DGA recommendations (Figure 3). Analysis of the data from UNLV-SDM dental students also found significant differences between males and females, with reported dairy consumption among females (1.7 cups per day) significantly lower than males (2.4 cups per day), $p = 0.0014$—and different from the U.S. population in general and young adults (18–30), more specifically, $p = 0.0388$.

Finally, the estimates of overall whole grain consumption (0.72 ounces per day) were significantly lower than the DGA recommendations of 3.0 ounces (Figure 4). In addition, whole grain consumption among 18–30-year-old females (1.4 ounces) and males (1.7 ounces) was also significantly lower than the DGA recommendations. Analysis of the data from UNLV-SDM dental students also found significant differences between males and females; the reported whole grain consumption among females (1.1 ounces per day) was not significantly higher than males (0.9 ounces per day), $p = 0.3687$, but was higher than the U.S. population in general and significantly lower than estimated among young adults (18–30 years old), more specifically, $p = 0.0026$.

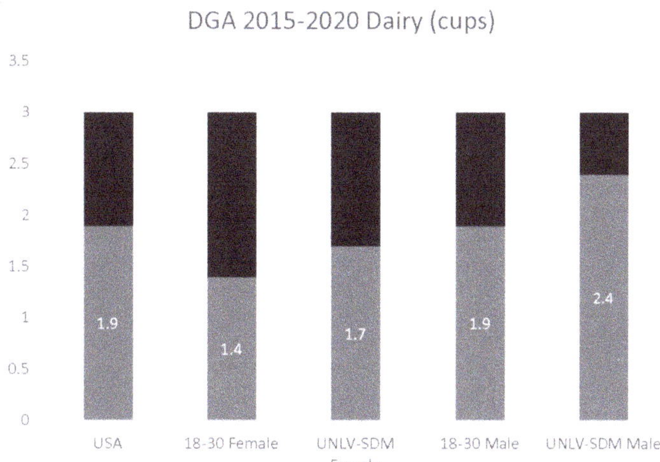

Figure 3. DGA dairy consumption analysis. UNLV-SDM dental student females consumed significantly less than males, $p = 0.0014$—although this was higher than observed among 18 to 30-year-olds, $p = 0.0388$, but still did not meet the DGA recommendations.

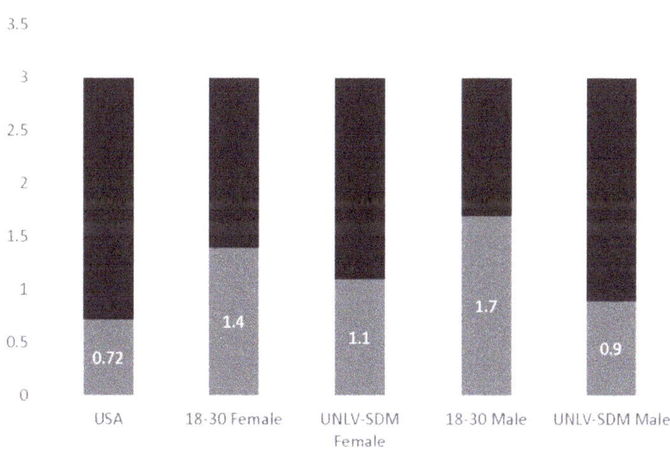

Figure 4. DGA whole grain consumption analysis. UNLV-SDM dental student females consumed nearly the same amount as males, $p = 0.3687$—although this was lower than observed among young adults between 18 and 30 years old, $p = 0.0026$, and did not meet the DGA recommendations.

4. Discussion

The primary objective of this study was to assess specific components of dietary consumption among dental students to compare with the DGA recommendations. Despite the highly educated nature of this study cohort, these results clearly demonstrated that dental students are no more likely to follow the DGA guidelines than other 18–30-year-olds in the United States. These data may also suggest that more in-depth integration of nutrition education, screening, counseling and referral may be needed to improve dental students' knowledge, awareness and compliance with DGA recommendations and the subsequent incorporation into dental practice [29,30].

The results of this study may become increasingly important as other studies confirm the role of proper diets in maintaining oral health and the prevention of oral disease, such as the role of dental erosion and caries associated with the intake of sugar-sweetened beverages and other beverages with a strong acidic content [31,32]. In fact, many studies have specifically examined the role of diet, the maintenance of oral health, and the prevention of disease, although have increasingly focused on the consumption of extrinsic (added) dietary sugars and the relationship with coronal dental caries [33,34]. However, prominent calls for the inclusion of dietary advice into dental practice have not yet become fully integrated due to the lack of standardization in dental education regarding dietary consumption patterns, how these compare with DGA recommendations, and the influence of these behaviors on oral and systemic health [35].

This study may also be important to compare and contrast with the current status of dietary studies in dental education, which tend to focus more specifically on dietary knowledge, practices and screening, specific to caries development, progression and prevention—such as the frequency of consumption and total levels of dietary sugar intake [36,37]. Although an understanding of the relationship between sugar-sweetened beverages and sugar-rich diets with dental caries is an essential component of the dental curriculum, the understanding of proper nutrition and positive dietary practices, such as the consumption of fruits, vegetables, whole grain and dairy and their role in maintaining and preventing oral diseases is also critically important, such as the role of dietary vitamin C and B12 in preventing gingival bleeding and periodontal disorders by maintaining collagen and extracellular matrix integrity [38–40]. Indeed, many other oral conditions, including periodontal disease, disorders of the oral mucosa and infectious agents, are also mediated by dietary behaviors and could be improved with dental provider recommendations and targeted dietary counseling and education [41].

Despite the significance of these results, there are some limitations associated with this study that should be addressed and considered. First, this was a retrospective, cross-sectional study, and therefore did not address any potential changes in dietary behavior following the completion of the nutrition course or DGA modules [42,43]. No data were collected from alumni or graduates, which could potentially demonstrate that this curricular component may positively influence dental student dietary choices and behaviors. In addition, this study did not fully assess or estimate the dietary consumption and intake of other items associated with poor health outcomes and negative health behaviors, such as added salt, sugar and fat, or low-nutrient-dense snack foods containing these ingredients [44]. Incorporation of these items into a more comprehensive dietary assessment may facilitate integration of these data into additional areas of the dental school curriculum, such as dental public health, caries and periodontology concepts.

However, many new innovations have been developed to teach and integrate nutrition education in medical and dental curricula in recent years [45]. For example, a new interactive teaching and learning platform, "Health Meets Food", features specifically designed online interactive course modules, continuing education credits and online videos to complement and enhance applied nutrition education in clinical training programs, including medicine and dentistry [46,47]. It has been demonstrated that these interactive courses and education modules may improve and achieve dietary sodium recommendations among cardiovascular patients, as well as reducing heart-failure-associated readmissions and improving HbA1c, blood pressure and cholesterol levels for patients with adult onset or Type II diabetes [48–50].

These innovations rely on the ability to identify dietary and culinary deficiencies among graduate and professional students during their clinical education and curriculum in order to appropriately integrate their training towards healthy cooking and eating—an important first step before these recommendations can be taught to their patients [51,52]. The ability to then supplement and apply this training towards specific health conditions, such as nutrition for cancer prevention and supplemental treatment, then becomes feasible [53]. These (and other) studies have clearly demonstrated the potential to significantly modify not only the attitudes, behaviors, and knowledge of graduate and professional healthcare students during their training, but also to influence the integration of these attitudes, knowledge and behavior towards their clinical training and recommendations during patient care [54–57].

5. Conclusions

This study may be among the first to evaluate the dietary intake of U.S. dental students for comparison with the DGA for positive health behaviors, including the consumption of fruits, vegetables, dairy and whole grains. The results of this study highlight the need for the curricular integration of diet and nutrition into dental and healthcare curricula due to the low levels of adherence among highly educated doctoral-level students in training. Future studies may be needed to evaluate the impact of these educational initiatives and measure any changes in dietary behaviors following the completion of these modules and courses.

Author Contributions: C.F., K.K. and J.M.P. were responsible for the overall project design. C.D. and B.H. were responsible for data generation. All authors were responsible for analysis and the writing of this manuscript. All authors have read and agreed to the published version of the manuscript.

Funding: No external funding was obtained for this study. The authors would like to acknowledge the Office of Research and the Department of Biomedical Sciences at the University of Nevada, Las Vegas, School of Dental Medicine—for support of this project. Karl Kingsley is a co-investigator with the National Institute of Health (NIH) grant R15DE028431.

Institutional Review Board Statement: The study was conducted according to the guidelines of the Declaration of Helsinki, and approved exempt by the Office for the Protection of Research Subjects (OPRS) and Institutional Review Board (IRB) at the University of Nevada, Las Vegas (UNLV) on 21 May 2020 under Protocol 1607120-2 "Retrospective analysis of health status of dental student population".

Informed Consent Statement: Informed consent was waived due to the exemption to human subject research under the Basic HHS Policy for Protection of Human Research Subjects, (46.101) Subpart A (b) regarding IRB exemption for research involving the use of education tests (cognitive, diagnostic, aptitude, achievement) in which the subjects cannot be identified directly or through identifiers.

Data Availability Statement: The data presented in this study are available on request from the corresponding author. The data are not publicly available due to the study protocol data protection parameters requested by the IRB and OPRS for the initial study approval.

Acknowledgments: This study is part of a Graduate Certificate Program in Pediatric Dentistry for CF. In addition, preliminary data from this study have been submitted for presentation to the American Association for Dental Research (AADR) 2021 conference.

Conflicts of Interest: The authors declare no conflict of interest.

References

1. Locke, A.; Schneiderhan, J.; Zick, S.M. Diets for Health: Goals and Guidelines. *Am. Fam. Physician* **2018**, *97*, 721–728.
2. National Academies of Sciences, Engineering, and Medicine; Health and Medicine Division; Food and Nutrition Board; Committee to Review the Process to Update the Dietary Guidelines for Americans. *Redesigning the Process for Establishing the Dietary Guidelines for Americans*; National Academies Press: Washington, DC, USA, 2017.
3. Slavin, J.L.; Lloyd, B. Health benefits of fruits and vegetables. *Adv. Nutr.* **2012**, *3*, 506–516. [CrossRef]
4. Wolfenden, L.; Barnes, C.; Lane, C.; McCrabb, S.; Brown, H.M.; Gerritsen, S.; Barquera, S.; Véjar, L.S.; Munguía, A.; Yoong, S.L. Consolidating evidence on the effectiveness of interventions promoting fruit and vegetable consumption: An umbrella review. *Int. J. Behav. Nutr. Phys. Act.* **2021**, *18*, 11. [CrossRef]
5. Sacks, F.M.; Lichtenstein, A.H.; Wu, J.H.Y.; Appel, L.J.; Creager, M.A.; Kris-Etherton, P.M.; Miller, M.; Rimm, E.B.; Rudel, L.L.; Robinson, J.G.; et al. Dietary Fats and Cardiovascular Disease: A Presidential Advisory From the American Heart Association. *Circulation* **2017**, *136*, e1–e23. [CrossRef]
6. Chiavaroli, L.; Viguiliouk, E.; Nishi, S.K.; Blanco Mejia, S.; Rahelić, D.; Kahleová, H.; Salas-Salvadó, J.; Kendall, C.W.; Sievenpiper, J.L. DASH Dietary Pattern and Cardiometabolic Outcomes: An Umbrella Review of Systematic Reviews and Meta-Analyses. *Nutrients* **2019**, *11*, 338. [CrossRef] [PubMed]
7. Pallazola, V.A.; Davis, D.M.; Whelton, S.P.; Cardoso, R.; Latina, J.M.; Michos, E.D.; Sarkar, S.; Blumenthal, R.S.; Arnett, D.K.; Stone, N.J.; et al. A Clinician's Guide to Healthy Eating for Cardiovascular Disease Prevention. *Mayo Clin. Proc. Innov. Qual. Outcomes* **2019**, *3*, 251–267. [CrossRef] [PubMed]

8. Quader, Z.S.; Cogswell, M.E.; Fang, J.; Coleman King, S.M.; Merritt, R.K. Changes in primary healthcare providers' attitudes and counseling behaviors related to dietary sodium reduction, DocStyles 2010 and 2015. *PLoS ONE* **2017**, *12*, e0177693. [CrossRef]
9. Jahns, L.; Davis-Shaw, W.; Lichtenstein, A.H.; Murphy, S.P.; Conrad, Z.; Nielsen, F. The History and Future of Dietary Guidance in America. *Adv. Nutr.* **2018**, *9*, 136–147. [CrossRef]
10. Mosher, A.L.; Piercy, K.L.; Webber, B.J.; Goodwin, S.K.; Casavale, K.O.; Olson, R.D. Dietary Guidelines for Americans: Implications for Primary Care Providers. *Am. J. Lifestyle Med.* **2014**, *10*, 23–35. [CrossRef] [PubMed]
11. Quan, M. Addressing Nutritional Gaps: Simple Steps for the Primary Care Provider. *J. Fam. Pract.* **2020**, *69* (Suppl. 7), S2–S7. [CrossRef] [PubMed]
12. AuYoung, M.; Linke, S.E.; Pagoto, S.; Buman, M.P.; Craft, L.L.; Richardson, C.R.; Hutber, A.; Marcus, B.H.; Estabrooks, P.; Sheinfeld Gorin, S. Integrating Physical Activity in Primary Care Practice. *Am. J. Med.* **2016**, *129*, 1022–1029. [CrossRef]
13. Habib-Mourad, C.; Ghandour, L.A.; Maliha, C.; Awada, N.; Dagher, M.; Hwalla, N. Impact of a one-year school-based teacher-implemented nutrition and physical activity intervention: Main findings and future recommendations. *BMC Public Health* **2020**, *20*, 256. [CrossRef] [PubMed]
14. Thomas, D.T.; Erdman, K.A.; Burke, L.M. Position of the Academy of Nutrition and Dietetics, Dietitians of Canada, and the American College of Sports Medicine: Nutrition and Athletic Performance. *J. Acad. Nutr. Diet.* **2016**, *116*, 501–528. [CrossRef] [PubMed]
15. Akabas, S.R.; Chouinard, J.D.; Bernstein, B.R. Nutrition and physical activity in health promotion and disease prevention: Potential role for the dental profession. *Dent. Clin.* **2012**, *56*, 791–808.
16. Marshall, T.A. Translating the new dietary guidelines. *J. Am. Dent. Assoc.* **2006**, *137*, 1258–1260. [CrossRef]
17. Touger-Decker, R.; Mobley, C.C.; American Dietetic Association. Position of the American Dietetic Association: Oral health and nutrition. *J. Am. Diet. Assoc.* **2007**, *107*, 1418–1428.
18. American Academy of Pediatric Dentistry Clinical Affairs Committee; American Academy of Pediatric Dentistry Council on Clinical Affairs. Policy on dietary recommendations for infants, children, and adolescents. *Pediatr. Dent.* **2005**, *27* (Suppl. 7), 36–37.
19. American Academy on Pediatric Dentistry Clinical Affairs Committee; American Academy on Pediatric Dentistry Council on Clinical Affairs. Policy on dietary recommendations for infants, children, and adolescents. *Pediatr. Dent.* **2008**, *30* (Suppl. 7), 47–48.
20. Sim, C.J.; Iida, H.; Vann, W.F., Jr.; Quinonez, R.B.; Steiner, M.J. Dietary recommendations for infants and toddlers among pediatric dentists in North Carolina. *Pediatr. Dent.* **2014**, *36*, 322–328.
21. Crowley, J.; Ball, L.; Hiddink, G.J. Nutrition in medical education: A systematic review. *Lancet Planet. Health* **2019**, *3*, e379–e389. [CrossRef]
22. Blunt, S.B.; Kafatos, A. Clinical Nutrition Education of Doctors and Medical Students: Solving the Catch 22. *Adv. Nutr.* **2019**, *10*, 345–350. [CrossRef] [PubMed]
23. Glen, M. Nutrition Education in Medical Training. *JAMA* **2019**, *322*, 784. [CrossRef]
24. Hark, L.A.; Deen, D. Position of the Academy of Nutrition and Dietetics: Interprofessional Education in Nutrition as an Essential Component of Medical Education. *J. Acad. Nutr. Diet.* **2017**, *117*, 1104–1113. [CrossRef]
25. Ray, S. The NNEdPro Global Centre for Nutrition and Health: A Consolidated Review of Global Efforts Towards Medical and Healthcare-Related Nutrition Education. *Nestle Nutr. Inst. Workshop Ser.* **2019**, *92*, 143–150.
26. DiMaria-Ghalili, R.A.; Mirtallo, J.M.; Tobin, B.W.; Hark, L.; Van Horn, L.; Palmer, C.A. Challenges and opportunities for nutrition education and training in the health care professions: Intraprofessional and interprofessional call to action. *Am. J. Clin. Nutr.* **2014**, *99* (Suppl. 5), 1184S–1193S. [CrossRef]
27. Johnson, D.L.; Gurenlian, J.R.; Freudenthal, J.J. A Study of Nutrition in Entry-Level Dental Hygiene Education Programs. *J. Dent. Educ.* **2016**, *80*, 73–82. [CrossRef]
28. Khan, S.Y.; Holt, K.; Tinanoff, N. Nutrition Education for Oral Health Professionals: A Must, Yet Still Neglected. *J. Dent. Educ.* **2017**, *81*, 3–4. [CrossRef]
29. Touger-Decker, R. Role of nutrition in the dental practice. *Quintessence Int.* **2004**, *35*, 67–70.
30. Touger-Decker, R.; Barracato, J.M.; O'Sullivan-Maillet, J. Nutrition education in health professions programs: A survey of dental, physician assistant, nurse practitioner, and nurse midwifery programs. *J. Am. Diet. Assoc.* **2001**, *101*, 63–69. [CrossRef]
31. Moynihan, P.; Petersen, P.E. Diet, nutrition and the prevention of dental diseases. *Public Health Nutr.* **2004**, *7*, 201–226. [CrossRef] [PubMed]
32. Mazur, M.; Bietolini, S.; Bellardini, D.; Lussi, A.; Corridore, D.; Maruotti, A.; Ottolenghi, L.; Vozza, I.; Guerra, F. Oral health in a cohort of individuals on a plant-based diet: A pilot study. *Clin. Ter.* **2020**, *171*, e142–e148.
33. Moynihan, P. The interrelationship between diet and oral health. *Proc. Nutr. Soc.* **2005**, *64*, 571–580. [CrossRef]
34. Sheiham, A. Dietary effects on dental diseases. *Public Health Nutr.* **2001**, *4*, 569–591. [CrossRef]
35. Moynihan, P.J. Dietary advice in dental practice. *Br. Dent. J.* **2002**, *193*, 563–568. [CrossRef] [PubMed]
36. Moynihan, P.J. The role of diet and nutrition in the etiology and prevention of oral diseases. *Bull. World Health Organ.* **2005**, *83*, 694–699.
37. Hujoel, P.P.; Lingström, P. Nutrition, dental caries and periodontal disease: A narrative review. *J. Clin. Periodontol.* **2017**, *44*, S79–S84. [CrossRef] [PubMed]

38. Soares, R.C.; da Rosa, S.V.; Moysés, S.T.; Rocha, J.S.; Bettega, P.V.C.; Werneck, R.I.; Moysés, S.J. Methods for prevention of early childhood caries: Overview of systematic reviews. *Int. J. Paediatr. Dent.* **2020**, *31*, 394–421. [CrossRef]
39. Von Philipsborn, P.; Stratil, J.M.; Burns, J.; Busert, L.K.; Pfadenhauer, L.M.; Polus, S.; Holzapfel, C.; Hauner, H.; Rehfuess, E. Environmental interventions to reduce the consumption of sugar-sweetened beverages and their effects on health. *Cochrane Database Syst. Rev.* **2019**, *6*, CD012292. [CrossRef]
40. Moynihan, P.; Tanner, L.M.; Holmes, R.D.; Hillier-Brown, F.; Mashayekhi, A.; Kelly, S.A.M.; Craig, D. Systematic Review of Evidence Pertaining to Factors That Modify Risk of Early Childhood Caries. *JDR Clin. Trans. Res.* **2019**, *4*, 202–216. [CrossRef] [PubMed]
41. Gondivkar, S.M.; Gadbail, A.R.; Gondivkar, R.S.; Sarode, S.C.; Sarode, G.S.; Patil, S.; Awan, K.H. Nutrition and oral health. *Dis. Mon.* **2019**, *65*, 147–154. [CrossRef]
42. Levin, K.A. Study design III: Cross-sectional studies. *Evid. Based Dent.* **2006**, *7*, 24–25. [CrossRef] [PubMed]
43. Dufault, B.; Klar, N. The quality of modern cross-sectional ecologic studies: A bibliometric review. *Am. J. Epidemiol.* **2011**, *174*, 1101–1107. [CrossRef] [PubMed]
44. Yoo, A.R.; Son, P.H.; Kingsley, K.; Polanski, J. Dietary Habits And Anthropometric Measures Of A Dental Student Population. *Eur. J. Nutr. Food Saf.* **2021**, *13*, 95–102. [CrossRef]
45. Van Horn, L.; Lenders, C.M.; Pratt, C.A.; Beech, B.; Carney, P.A.; Dietz, W.; DiMaria-Ghalili, R.; Harlan, T.; Hash, R.; Kohlmeier, M.; et al. Advancing Nutrition Education, Training, and Research for Medical Students, Residents, Fellows, Attending Physicians, and Other Clinicians: Building Competencies and Interdisciplinary Coordination. *Adv. Nutr.* **2019**, *10*, 1181–1200. [CrossRef]
46. Magallanes, E.; Sen, A.; Siler, M.; Albin, J. Nutrition from the kitchen: Culinary medicine impacts students' counseling confidence. *BMC Med. Educ.* **2021**, *21*, 88. [CrossRef]
47. Lawrence, J.C.; Knol, L.L.; Clem, J.; de la, O.R.; Henson, C.S.; Streiffer, R.H. Integration of Interprofessional Education (IPE) Core Competencies Into Health Care Education: IPE Meets Culinary Medicine. *J. Nutr. Educ. Behav.* **2019**, *51*, 510–512. [CrossRef]
48. Razavi, A.C.; Dyer, A.; Jones, M.; Sapin, A.; Caraballo, G.; Nace, H.; Dotson, K.; Razavi, M.A.; Harlan, T.S. Achieving Dietary Sodium Recommendations and Atherosclerotic Cardiovascular Disease Prevention through Culinary Medicine Education. *Nutrients* **2020**, *12*, 3632. [CrossRef]
49. Razavi, A.C.; Monlezun, D.J.; Sapin, A.; Sarris, L.; Schlag, E.; Dyer, A.; Harlan, T. Etiological Role of Diet in 30-Day Readmissions for Heart Failure: Implications for Reducing Heart Failure-Associated Costs via Culinary Medicine. *Am. J. Lifestyle Med.* **2019**, *14*, 351–360. [CrossRef]
50. Monlezun, D.J.; Kasprowicz, E.; Tosh, K.W.; Nix, J.; Urday, P.; Tice, D.; Sarris, L.; Harlan, T.S. Medical school-based teaching kitchen improves HbA1c, blood pressure, and cholesterol for patients with type 2 diabetes: Results from a novel randomized controlled trial. *Diabetes Res. Clin. Pract.* **2015**, *109*, 420–426. [CrossRef]
51. Leong, B.; Ren, D.; Monlezun, D.J.; Ly, D.; Sarris, L.; Harlan, T.S. Teaching 3rd & 4th year medical students how to cook: An innovative approach to balance lifestyle modification and medication therapy in chronic disease management. *Med. Sci. Educ.* **2014**, *24*, 43.
52. Birkhead, A.; Foote, S.; Monlezun, D.J.; Loyd, J.; Joo, E.; Leong, B.; Sarris, L.; Harlan, T. Medical student-led community cooking classes: A novel preventative medicine model easy to swallow. *Am. J. Prev. Med.* **2014**, *46*, e41–e42. [CrossRef]
53. Monlezun, D.J.; Tsai, P.; Sarris, L.; Harlan, T. Recipe for cancer education: A novel integrated cooking and nutrition education curriculum for medical students and physicians in dietary preventive and supplemental treatment for pancreatic cancer. *J. Med. Pers.* **2014**, *12*, 125–128. [CrossRef]
54. Arman, D.; Monlezun, D.J.; Peters, B.; Urday, P.; Cutler, H.; Pellicore, D.; Lim, H.J.; Sarris, L.; Harlan, T.S. CHOP-International: An open access nutrition education tool for physicians, resident doctors, and medical and public health students. *J. Med. Pers.* **2015**, *13*, 118–124. [CrossRef]
55. Razavi, A.C.; Monlezun, D.J.; Sapin, A.; Stauber, Z.; Schradle, K.; Schlag, E.; Dyer, A.; Gagen, B.; McCormack, I.G.; Akhiwu, O.; et al. Multisite Culinary Medicine Curriculum Is Associated With Cardioprotective Dietary Patterns and Lifestyle Medicine Competencies Among Medical Trainees. *Am. J. Lifestyle Med.* **2020**, *14*, 225–233. [CrossRef] [PubMed]
56. Razavi, A.C.; Sapin, A.; Monlezun, D.J.; McCormack, I.G.; Latoff, A.; Pedroza, K.; McCullough, C.; Sarris, L.; Schlag, E.; Dyer, A.; et al. Effect of culinary education curriculum on Mediterranean diet adherence and food cost savings in families: A randomised controlled trial. *Public Health Nutr.* **2020**, *23*, 2297–2303.
57. Downer, S.; Berkowitz, S.A.; Harlan, T.S.; Olstad, D.L.; Mozaffarian, D. Food is medicine: Actions to integrate food and nutrition into healthcare. *BMJ* **2020**, *369*, m2482. [CrossRef] [PubMed]

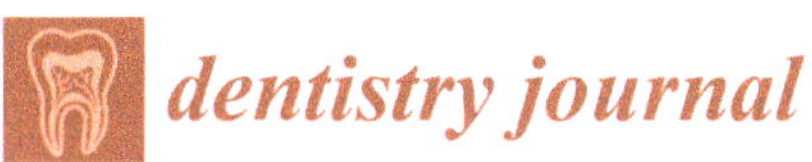 MDPI

Article

Evaluating Classification Consistency of Oral Lesion Images for Use in an Image Classification Teaching Tool

Yuxin Shen, Minn N. Yoon, Silvia Ortiz, Reid Friesen and Hollis Lai *

Department of Dentistry, Faculty of Medicine and Dentistry, University of Alberta, Edmonton, AB T6G 1C9, Canada; shen3@ualberta.ca (Y.S.); minn.yoon@ualberta.ca (M.N.Y.); ssortiz@ualberta.ca (S.O.); rtfriese@ualberta.ca (R.F.)

* Correspondence: hollis1@ualberta.ca; Tel.: +1-780-492-8735

Abstract: A web-based image classification tool (DiLearn) was developed to facilitate active learning in the oral health profession. Students engage with oral lesion images using swipe gestures to classify each image into pre-determined categories (e.g., left for refer and right for no intervention). To assemble the training modules and to provide feedback to students, DiLearn requires each oral lesion image to be classified, with various features displayed in the image. The collection of accurate meta-information is a crucial step for enabling the self-directed active learning approach taken in DiLearn. The purpose of this study is to evaluate the classification consistency of features in oral lesion images by experts and students for use in the learning tool. Twenty oral lesion images from DiLearn's image bank were classified by three oral lesion experts and two senior dental hygiene students using the same rubric containing eight features. Classification agreement among and between raters were evaluated using Fleiss' and Cohen's Kappa. Classification agreement among the three experts ranged from identical (Fleiss' Kappa = 1) for "clinical action", to slight agreement for "border regularity" (Fleiss' Kappa = 0.136), with the majority of categories having fair to moderate agreement (Fleiss' Kappa = 0.332–0.545). Inclusion of the two student raters with the experts yielded fair to moderate overall classification agreement (Fleiss' Kappa = 0.224–0.554), with the exception of "morphology". The feature of clinical action could be accurately classified, while other anatomical features indirectly related to diagnosis had a lower classification consistency. The findings suggest that one oral lesion expert or two student raters can provide fairly consistent meta information for selected categories of features implicated in the creation of image classification tasks in DiLearn.

Keywords: dental education; dental hygiene education; educational technology; classification consistency; oral lesion

Citation: Shen, Y.; Yoon, M.N.; Ortiz, S.; Friesen, R.; Lai, H. Evaluating Classification Consistency of Oral Lesion Images for Use in an Image Classification Teaching Tool. *Dent. J.* **2021**, *9*, 94. https://doi.org/10.3390/dj9080094

Academic Editor: Patrick R. Schmidlin

Received: 2 July 2021
Accepted: 4 August 2021
Published: 12 August 2021

1. Introduction

Exposure to oral lesion images is an important component of dental education and oral pathology education. In traditional classroom settings, lecturers show an image of oral lesions and discuss the feature of an image iteratively. The process of interpreting a diagnostic image is generally divided into three phases [1], namely: (1) psycho-physical, which identifies the appropriate examination technique and human anatomical system; (2) psychological, which provides a higher cognitive process in organizing the images into precepts; and (3) nosological, which integrates the medical knowledge required to produce a diagnosis.

To effectively train students to produce a diagnosis based on diagnostic images, students are required to process the image, incorporating an array of information such as the location, size, opacity, medical history, demographic information, and underlying histology [2]. While students are often given longitudinal case information, this inductive approach trains students through a step-by-step manner, drawing on their nuanced understanding of clinical information, features of the image, and a cognitive understanding to interpret the image [3]. Students beginning in the profession often do not possess the aptitude to follow the process required for integrating all of the necessary information. Rather than focusing on interpreting entire cases at the outset, our study will focus on providing students with opportunities to familiarize themselves with the definitions, signs, and features associated with various abnormalities; features that are required to interpret images in the nosological phase [3].

Studies have demonstrated varying effects in diagnostic training in image-based areas such as radiography. Specifically, students who received training on pathophysiological information had a better diagnostic accuracy than students who were trained using feature lists [4]. The preference of a pathophysiological primer suggests novice learners need to be exposed to the features and anatomical cues. This process is supported by the development of domain expertise knowledge [5], where expertise is developed through exposure to domain related categories, cues, and knowledge that are related to the presented visual features.

Incorporating computer-assisted instruction (CAI) to complement other forms of traditional instruction is advantageous as it allows students to learn independently and have the learning reinforced with immediate feedback. Using CAI has been shown to be equivalent in cognitive performance and superior in clinical performance compared with traditional didactic instruction [6]. Moreover, the students required comparable amounts of learning time but progressed on an individual basis while receiving immediate feedback to reinforce their learning. Research has also found that a blended learning approach (teaching method that uses asynchronous learning to complement synchronous learning events) to teaching radiology led to superior student performance when compared with traditional approaches [2].

Overview of DiLearn

Spaced education is a pedagogical approach that focuses on the repetition of tasks that are separated or spaced through time to leverage the spacing effect in learning [7–9]. Students who are instructed in this method have yielded longer retention [7], and the immediate feedback provided electronically has shown to improve self-assessment [8].

To emulate this learning approach in the electronic environment, DiLearn organizes learning by modules. Each module contains a collection of images and is designed to train students on a defined topic through three stages, namely: learning, training, and assessment. In the learning phase—students are presented with images and are required to determine what clinical action is required (e.g., intervene by referring to a specialist). Students receive immediate feedback after an action (outline the type of feedback: correct, incorrect, information related to the features of the image). In the training phase, students undergo the same classification task with different images, with the only difference being that feedback is presented at the end of the exercise (e.g., total number correct) with a chance to review selections. Students have unlimited attempts at modules, and the modules are assembled randomly from a bank of images. After students have achieved a certain level of correct classification in the training phase, they are then allowed to attempt the assessment phase, where they complete the same classification task with a novel set of images and without immediate feedback.

To create the learning modules, a large collection of images related to different presentations and diagnoses of oral lesions were needed. Each image then required meta-information, or tags based on a taxonomy of clinical features. Figure 1 illustrates examples of tags associated with images. The information provided in the tags can be used by instructors to define the classification students will choose in each module, or to balance the presentation of a specific feature presented in each module through searching and filtering (e.g., images of lesions on tongues; red lesions).

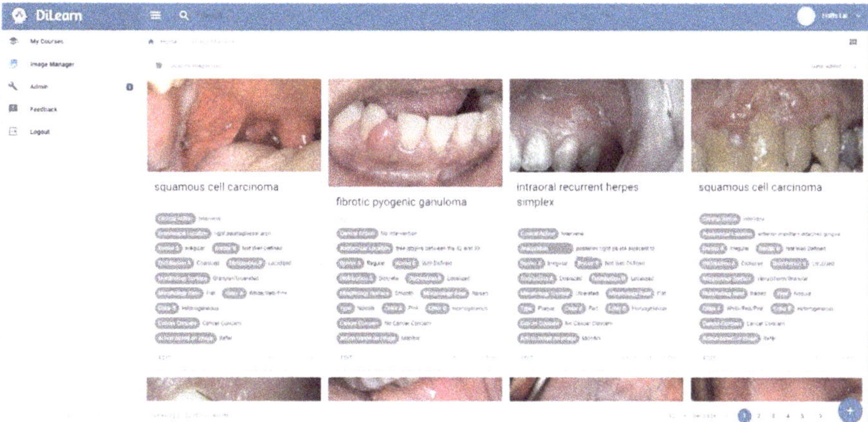

Figure 1. An image bank with its corresponding tags.

After a module is assembled, it can be administered to students to complete. Figure 2 illustrates how images can be assigned to a stage. The application requires university authentication to verify student identity. Figure 3 presents the smartphone interface for how the learning modules can be completed by students. Students will be presented with an oral lesion image; they are given the choice of either swiping left to choose the action of "refer" or swiping right to choose the action of "no intervention". Given the importance of the meta-information and tags associated with each image, which are needed to develop learning modules and for providing the suggested action when presented with an oral lesion image in the student interface, the creation and validation of this meta-information structure is the focus of this study.

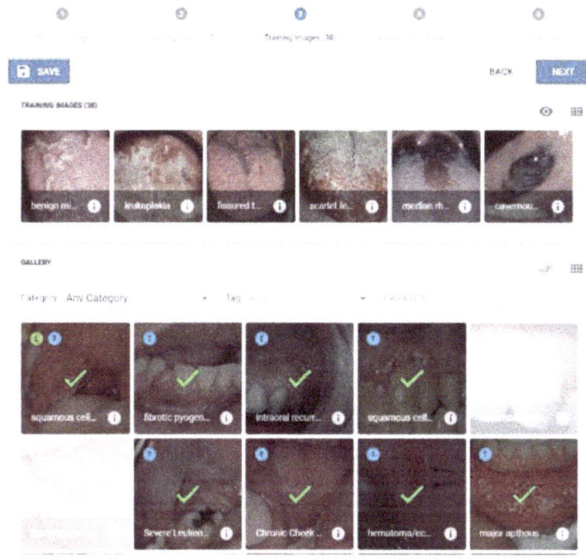

Figure 2. The selected images assigned to a stage.

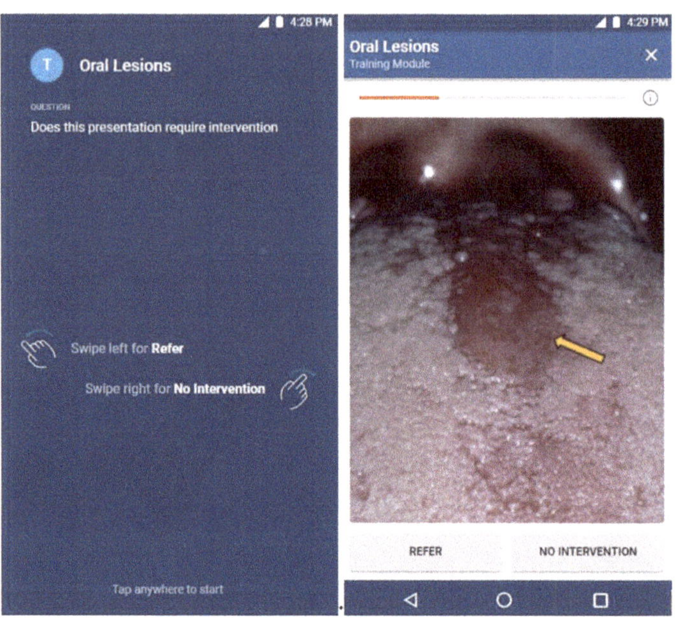

Figure 3. Screen captures of the student interface.

2. Materials and Methods

This study was approved at the University of Alberta by the Research Ethics Board (Pro00066469). To develop and evaluate a taxonomy for teaching oral lesions, the study was separated into two phases. In the first phase, a taxonomy of oral lesion descriptions was created. Two content experts were tasked to provide a list of features required to describe oral lesions in order to help students learn about oral pathology. Each expert was asked to inductively provide the features they commonly identify and distinguish in order to diagnose the presentation of an oral lesion. After the two experts provided their individual lists, they compared the two list of categories and features, and agreed on a single taxonomy of clinical features that could be used to describe an oral lesion, and used as tags for classifying the images. A glossary of terms was then developed that operationalized each feature using descriptive characteristics.

In the second phase, five participants were recruited for the study—three oral pathology specialists with expertise in oral cancer lesions and two senior dental hygiene students with training in oral lesions. A set of 20 oral lesion images was selected from DiLearn's image bank. The five raters classified the 20 oral lesion images using the taxonomy developed in phase one. Responses were recorded and compiled into Microsoft Excel, after which the coded data were imported into IBM SPSS Version 23. Three levels of statistical analyses were carried out to evaluate the classification agreement among the three oral lesion experts, between the student raters, and among all five raters. Fleiss' Kappa of the three oral lesion experts was computed to determine the overall agreement among the experts. The Cohen's Kappa between the two student raters was used to determine the classification agreement between the student raters. With the inclusion of the student raters, an overall Fleiss' Kappa of the five raters was computed to evaluate how the incorporation of the student raters contributed to the overall classification agreement. Cohen's and Fleiss' Kappa were chosen because of the categorical nature of the tags, and were interpreted based on Landis' and Koch's guidelines [10].

3. Results

In the first phase, two of the three content experts described and agreed on eight features for describing oral lesions. The eight features included clinical action, anatomical location, border, configuration, color, type, morphology, and localization. Each category then contained different definitions that described the morphological features of the lesion in the image. An example of the definitions for each category described in the taxonomy is provided in Table 1.

Table 1. A description of the taxonomy and the keys used to code each image.

Category	Description
Clinical Action	intervene (1), or monitor or no intervention (0)
Border Regularity	regular (1) or irregular (2)
Border Definition	defined (3) or ill-defined (4)
Anatomical Location	tongue (1), gingiva (2), mucosa (3), palate (4), floor of mouth (5), lip (6), interdental papilla (7), vestibule (8), or alveolar bone (9)
Configuration	discrete (1), coalesced (2) multiple (3), or no applicable terms (4)
Color	white (1), yellow (2), pink (3), or red (4)
Type	exophytic (1), plaque (2), submucosal mass (3), macule (4), or ulcer (5)
Morphology	granular (1), smooth (2), ulcerated (3), verruciform (4), fissured (5), or lobulated (6)
Localization	localized (1) or non-localized (2)

In the second phase, all five raters tagged a collection of 20 images from DiLearn's image bank using the eight features provided in phase one. The category of the highest importance was clinical action, as this category provided the suggested intervention in the DiLearn's student interface. Fleiss' Kappa on clinical action among all three experts was calculated to be 1, showing perfect classification consistency among all three experts. Consistency between the two students for intervention was measured at 0.33 using Cohen's Kappa, demonstrating a fair agreement between the students. Fleiss' Kappa on clinical action decreased from 1 to 0.52 with the addition of the two student raters. Even with the decrease in Fleiss' Kappa, there was still moderate agreement for clinical action after the inclusion of the two student raters.

Overall, classification consistency among the three experts ranged from perfect for clinical action to slight agreement for border regularity, with the majority of categories having moderate to fair agreement, as seen in Table 2. There was moderate agreement among the three experts for the anatomical location, color, and morphology, with Fleiss' Kappa calculated to be 0.46, 0.55, and 0.54, respectively. Fleiss' Kappa showed fair agreement for border definition, configuration, type, and localization.

The agreement between the two students ranged from substantial to poor. There was substantial agreement between the two students for color, as demonstrated by a Cohen's Kappa of 0.70. Moderate to fair agreements between student raters were measured for the categories of clinical action, border regularity, anatomical location, configuration, type, and localization. A poor agreement was measured for morphology.

The overall Fleiss' Kappa was calculated to evaluate the effect the student raters had on the classification consistency and to compare the student raters with the expert raters. After the inclusion of student raters, there was moderate to fair agreement for all of the categories, except for morphology. For the categories of border regularity, anatomical location, configuration, color, and type, the addition of the two student raters increased the Fleiss' Kappa, suggesting an increase in agreement with the addition of the two less experienced raters. For the categories clinical action, border definition, morphology, and localization, the addition of the two student raters decreased the overall agreement, as demonstrated by a decrease in Fleiss' Kappa.

Table 2. Fleiss' and Cohen's Kappa evaluating the classification agreement of 20 oral lesion images by three experts and two students.

	Fleiss' Kappa		Cohen's Kappa
	Experts	**Overall**	**Between Two Students**
Clinical Action	1	0.523	0.327
Border Regularity	0.136	0.224	0.348
Border Definition	0.347	0.256	0.097
Anatomical Location	0.464	0.539	0.571
Configuration	0.332	0.368	0.568
Color	0.545	0.554	0.695
Type	0.392	0.441	0.490
Morphology	0.537	0.146	−0.019
Localization	0.392	0.391	0.211

4. Discussion

Oral cancer screening is often a routine part of the dental examination of patient, especially when examining those with risk factors for oral cancer. An oral cancer screening program in Taiwan targeting high-risk individuals demonstrated the effectiveness of reducing later stage oral cancers and oral cancer mortality [11]. The effectiveness of the oral visual screening in reducing mortality in high-risk individuals was corroborated by a randomized control trial in India [12]. A study by Hassona et al. showed that dental students' ability to recognize oral lesions of concern was significantly correlated with oral cancer knowledge and knowledge about potentially malignant oral disorders [13]. To improve students' future diagnostic ability and their ability to complete oral cancer screening, there is a need for increasing students' exposure to oral lesions and for improving the educational methods used to deliver the content on oral cancer and oral lesions.

Tools and technology for active learning in health profession education are currently in high demand. In Saxena et al.'s article from 2009, crossword puzzles were introduced to the undergraduate medical curriculum to help students review and reinforce concepts and vocabulary learned in a pathology class [14]. Specially constructed content-relevant digital games were constructed by Kanthan et al., and helped improve academic performance in undergraduate pathology courses [15]. However, few tools have been created specifically for undergraduate dental and dental hygiene curriculums to learn oral pathology and oral medicine. There are even fewer tools that have been developed based on learning theories, and these tools are seldom evaluated. By introducing a new tool for image classification such as DiLearn, faculties from dentistry and dental hygiene can integrate active learning into oral pathology, which is traditionally delivered in a didactic format. The development of this learning tool also has the potential to integrate learning for students in other disciplines. Student performance data collected in the coming year should allow for an analysis of student learning to illustrate the learning curve of a given classification for diagnosis, a challenge that has not yet been done, despite the abundant research conducted on competency education in the health profession. Such learning curve information can be used to determine the appropriate amount of instruction and exposure required to master a specific oral pathology.

The validation evidence demonstrated in this study shows how the three experts can provide relatively consistent meta-information for the tagging of the 20 images as reflected by the fair to perfect agreement for all categories, with the exception of border regularity. The three experts reached consensus when categorizing clinical action, which is one of the more important categories in DiLearn, as this category provides the suggested action in the DiLearn's student interface and will also be used to track student progress. The lower Fleiss' Kappa for some categories can be explained partly by the lack of a definitive key or descriptors for each taxonomical category. For instance, when describing border, two of the expert raters chose one descriptor from "regular", "irregular", "well defined", and "not well defined" to describe the border of the pathological lesions, while the other expert chose one descriptor from "regular" and "irregular" and one descriptor from "well defined" and "not well defined" to describe the border of the pathological lesions. It is suggested that the introduction of a multiple-choice format with set descriptors for each category be implemented for future classification tasks, as this strategy will likely increase the overall agreement between and among raters.

The agreement between the two student raters ranged from substantial to poor, with the majority of categories having moderate to fair agreement. The two students had the most agreement when classifying anatomical location and color, and the least agreement when classifying morphology, perhaps reflecting that the student raters were more comfortable when classifying categories such as anatomical location and color than morphology. The negative Cohen's Kappa for morphology reflects that the students were not beating chance when it came to categorizing morphology. A negative Kappa value for morphology may suggest that students were less experienced with the characterization of morphology, or that the two student raters may have a different interpretation of the tags used for morphology.

Lastly, the effect the two student raters had on classification agreement was examined by comparing the Fleiss' Kappa for the three experts with the Fleiss' Kappa after the inclusion of the student raters. The inclusion of the two student raters increased the Fleiss' Kappa for border regularity, anatomical location, configuration, color, and type. For the categories clinical action, border definition, morphology, and localization, the addition of the two student raters decreased the overall classification agreement. Though it has to be noted that clinical action had an initial Fleiss' Kappa of 1, and the 0.001 decrease in Fleiss' Kappa for localization was likely of negligible significance. With the exception of morphology, the inclusion of the two student raters did not have a negative impact on the overall classification agreement. On the contrary, the overall classification agreement increased in some cases when more raters were involved in the classification task.

One of the most important categories for DiLearn is the category of clinical action, as the tags associated with clinical action will be used in the student interface (Figure 3). In the student interface, students are presented with an oral lesion image and are given the choice to swipe left for "refer" or swipe right for "no intervention". The three oral lesion experts had a Fleiss' Kappa of 1 for the category of clinical action (the three oral lesion experts agreed on the clinical action when presented with an oral lesion image), suggesting only one oral lesion expert is needed for tagging the category of clinical action. With the inclusion of the two student raters, the overall Fleiss' Kappa reduced to 0.523 for the category of clinical action, suggesting that the two student raters can still provide fairly consistent meta-information for tagging the category of clinical action. Given the time and effort required for subject matter experts to provide tags and to assemble the learning modules, and the relative agreement when more raters participate in the tagging task, a future study should investigate whether increasing the number of students in tagging may provide meta-information with similar precision when compared with experts.

5. Conclusions

With an increasing need to provide students with exposure to various presentations of oral pathologies, learning tools like DiLearn have the potential to facilitate an independent learning process. It must be noted, however, that the collection of accurate meta-information is a crucial step for enabling the self-directed active learning approach taken in DiLearn. The learning process of each module and the feedback provided to the students are reliant on accurate diagnostic outcomes. Validation evidence presented in this study suggests one oral lesion expert or two student raters can provide fairly consistent meta-information for select category of features implicated in the creation of the classification tasks, especially for the category of clinical action. The inclusion of the two student raters did not significantly alter the overall classification agreement, but future investigations should be carried out to investigate whether increasing the number of students in tagging may provide meta-information with similar precision as for the experts.

Author Contributions: Conceptualization, M.N.Y., R.F. and H.L.; methodology, validation, and investigation, Y.S., M.N.Y., S.O., R.F. and H.L.; software, H.L.; formal analysis, Y.S. and S.O.; writing—original draft preparation, Y.S. and H.L.; writing—review and editing, resources, project administration, and funding acquisition Y.S., M.N.Y., S.O., R.F. and H.L.; supervision, M.N.Y., R.F. and H.L. All authors have read and agreed to the published version of the manuscript.

Funding: This research was funded by the University of Alberta Department of Dentistry's Summer Research Program and the Education Research Scholarship Unit.

Institutional Review Board Statement: The study was conducted according to the guidelines of the Declaration of Helsinki and was approved by the University of Alberta research ethics board on 4 July 2019. The project identification code is Pro00066469.

Informed Consent Statement: Informed consent was obtained from all of the subjects involved in the study.

Data Availability Statement: The data presented in this study are available on request from the corresponding author.

Acknowledgments: We would like to express a special thank you to Jerry Bouquot for his generosity in allowing us to use his large database of oral pathology images collected over the tenure of his career. Many thanks to M. Lorencs, C. Surgin, and the CMPUT401 Team on the development of the software. We also thank the students who helped with the development of the project (A. Howery, R. Lowry, M. Howey, and C. Dinel). Thank you to McGaw and Parashar for contributing their expertise.

Conflicts of Interest: The authors declare no conflict of interest.

References

1. Blesser, B.; Ozonoff, D. A model for the radiologic process. *Radiology* **1972**, *103*, 515–521. [CrossRef] [PubMed]
2. Kavadella, A.; Tsiklakis, K.; Vougiouklakis, G.; Lionarakis, A. Evaluation of a blended learning course for teaching oral radiology to undergraduate dental students. *Eur. J. Dent. Educ.* **2010**, *16*, E88–E95. [CrossRef] [PubMed]
3. Baghdady, M.T.; Carnahan, H.; Lam, E.W.N.; Woods, N.N. Dental and dental hygiene students' diagnostic accuracy in oral radiology: Effect of diagnostic strategy and instructional method. *J. Dent. Educ.* **2014**, *78*, 1279–1285. [CrossRef] [PubMed]
4. Baghdady, M.T.; Pharoah, M.J.; Regehr, G.; Lam, E.W.N.; Woods, N.N. The role of basic sciences in diagnostic oral radiology. *J. Dent. Educ.* **2009**, *73*, 1187–1193. [CrossRef] [PubMed]
5. Crowley, R.S.; Naus, G.J.; Stewart, I.J.; Friedman, C.P. Development of visual diagnostic expertise in pathology: An information-processing study. *J. Am. Med. Inform. Assoc.* **2003**, *10*, 39–51. [CrossRef] [PubMed]
6. Rohlin, M.; Di, O.; Hirschmann, P.N.; Matteson, S. Global trends in oral and maxillofacial radiology education. *Oral Surg. Oral Med. Oral Pathol. Oral Radiol. Endod.* **1995**, *80*, 517–526. [CrossRef]
7. Al-Rawi, W.; Easterling, L.; Edwards, P.C. Development of a mobile device optimized cross platform-compatible oral pathology and radiology spaced repetition system for dental education. *J. Dent. Educ.* **2015**, *79*, 439–447. [CrossRef] [PubMed]
8. Tshibwabwa, E.; Mallin, R.; Fraser, M.; Tshibwabwa, M.; Sanii, R.; Rice, J.; Cannon, J. An integrated interactive-spaced education radiology curriculum for preclinical students. *J. Clin. Imaging Sci.* **2017**, *7*, 22. [CrossRef] [PubMed]
9. Ebbinghaus, H. Memory: A contribution to experimental psychology. *Ann. Neurosci.* **2013**, *20*, 155. [CrossRef] [PubMed]
10. Landis, J.R.; Koch, G.G. The measurement of observer agreement for categorical data. *Biometrics* **1977**, *33*, 159–174. [CrossRef] [PubMed]
11. Chuang, S.-L.; Su, W.W.-Y.; Chen, S.L.-S.; Yen, A.M.-F.; Wang, C.-P.; Fann, J.C.-Y.; Chiu, S.Y.-H.; Lee, Y.-C.; Chiu, H.-M.; Chang, D.-C.; et al. Population-based screening program for reducing oral cancer mortality in 2,334,299 Taiwanese cigarette smokers and/or betel quid chewers. *Cancer* **2017**, *123*, 1597–1609. [CrossRef] [PubMed]
12. Sankaranarayanan, R.; Ramadas, K.; Thomas, G.; Muwonge, R.; Thara, S.; Mathew, B.; Rajan, B. Effect of screening on oral cancer mortality in Kerala, India: A cluster-randomised controlled trial. *Lancet* **2005**, *365*, 1927–1933. [CrossRef]
13. Hassona, Y.; Scully, C.; Abu Tarboush, N.; Baqain, Z.; Ismail, F.; Hawamdeh, S.; Sawair, F. Oral cancer knowledge and diagnostic ability among dental students. *J. Cancer Educ.* **2015**, *32*, 566–570. [CrossRef] [PubMed]
14. Saxena, A.; Nesbitt, R.; Pahwa, P.; Mills, S. Crossword puzzles: Active learning in undergraduate pathology and medical education. *Arch. Pathol. Lab. Med.* **2009**, *133*, 1457–1462. [CrossRef] [PubMed]
15. Kanthan, R.; Senger, J.L. The impact of specially designed digital games-based learning in undergraduate pathology and medi-cal education. *Arch. Pathol. Lab. Med.* **2011**, *135*, 135–142. [CrossRef] [PubMed]

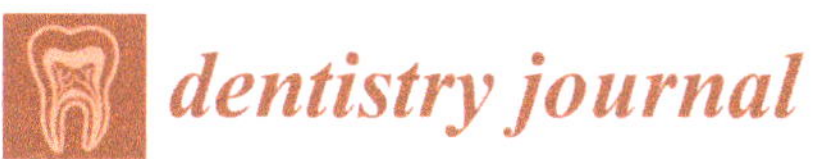

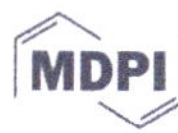

Article

Biomedical Courses Should Also Be Designed for Dental Students: The Perceptions of Dental Students

Fanny Mussalo [1,*], Terhi Karaharju-Suvanto [1], Päivi Mäntylä [2,3] and Eeva Pyörälä [4]

1 Department of Oral and Maxillofacial Diseases, University of Helsinki and Helsinki University Hospital, 00014 Helsinki, Finland; terhi.karaharju-suvanto@helsinki.fi
2 Institute of Dentistry, University of Eastern Finland, 70211 Kuopio, Finland; paivi.mantyla@uef.fi
3 Oral and Maxillofacial Clinic, Kuopio University Hospital, 70029 Kuopio, Finland
4 Center for University Teaching and Learning, University of Helsinki, 00014 Helsinki, Finland; Eeva.pyorala@helsinki.fi
* Correspondence: fanny.mussalo@helsinki.fi

Abstract: Introduction: It can be challenging integrating biomedical sciences into dentistry programs. The aim was to examine students' perceptions of how joint biomedical courses with medical students and courses tailored for dental students supported their clinical studies. Materials and methods: The target group was clinical phase dental students. Cross-sectional survey data were collected using a questionnaire, which consisted of questions covering biomedical and clinical study content and learning methods. Results: A total of 110 (82%) students completed the survey. Students had difficulty recognising the relevance of joint biomedical courses for clinical work, but when the link was clear, their interest in the content increased. The closer the respondents were to graduation, the less relevance they expressed the biomedical sciences had. Almost all students (95%) wanted more dental content for the early study years. Discussion: The student perspective provides valuable information for the development of biomedical courses. Students should be offered customised courses that include dental content and perspectives on clinical work, whenever suitable to the didactic content of the basic science course. Our study shows that the dental perspective needs greater integration with the biomedical content. This also supports interprofessional learning and appreciation for the other field's contribution to human health

Keywords: dental students; biomedical sciences; vertical integration; curriculum reform; interprofessional learning

Citation: Mussalo, F.; Karaharju-Suvanto, T.; Mäntylä, P.; Pyörälä, E. Biomedical Courses Should Also Be Designed for Dental Students: The Perceptions of Dental Students. *Dent. J.* **2021**, *9*, 96. https://doi.org/10.3390/dj9080096

Academic Editors: Jelena Dumancic and Božana Lončar Brzak

Received: 28 June 2021
Accepted: 12 August 2021
Published: 16 August 2021

1. Introduction

Globally, in most dental education units, dentistry programs are generally started with so-called preclinical courses lasting one to two years, focusing on biomedical content. Often these are carried out as shared learning for dental and medical students, and with medical students representing the majority, much of the material and assignments are primarily designed for them [1,2]. Most dental educators agree that biomedical knowledge forms an important part of the dental curriculum and provides enough life sciences evidence for the clinical practice in dentistry [3–5]. Studying biomedical sciences jointly with medical students requires attentive curriculum planning and good communication between teaching faculties, so that learning is effective for both groups, and marginalisation of dental students is reduced [6].

Recent research has shown that dental students were overwhelmed [7,8] and demotivated [6,9] by the abundance of biomedical study content, and emphasising the dental context could engage and enhance the dental curriculum [10]. Several studies have pointed out that dental students had difficulty recognising the link between biomedical courses and dental clinical practice [11,12]. In terms of motivation, it would be important to specify the relevance of the biomedical courses for the students [7,10]. In addition, the design of dental content influenced students' motivation, effectiveness and stress levels [13]. Interactive, small-group case-based activities effectively increased students' comfort levels and readiness to initiate clinical procedures [14]. First-year dental students have been found to be more interested in clinical than biomedical topics [15]. However, an important finding is that students who studied jointly with medical students expressed that they were better qualified to treat dental patients with medical conditions [12].

Interprofessional learning aims to bring together different professionals to learn with, from and about one another to collaborate more effectively in the delivery of safe, high-quality care for patients [16]. Health education has actively sought to promote interprofessional learning for more than two decades. A systematic review [17] revealed that learners responded positively to this type of learning and their attitudes and perceptions, as well as their collaboration and skills, improved in interprofessional learning. Less evidence was found for the effects on behaviour and patient care. Interprofessional learning should be tailored so that its contents and practices are relevant and of interest to all learners, and all students participating should feel equally valued [17]. In many dental education units, medical and dental students learn biomedicine together, but there is still little evidence of the positive effects of interprofessional learning in this style of teaching.

In 2020, the Association for Dental Education in Europe (ADEE) published a new consensus report on biomedical study content in European dental degree programs [3]. The consensus group claimed that progress had been made both in integrating courses horizontally between the disciplines and vertically over the successive study years. The report suggested that the so-called "2 + 3 model", in which the degrees were divided into two preclinical and three clinical years, was no longer generally recommended. Instead, it was increasingly typical for degree programs to address the clinical topics in the early years and correspondingly bring in the elements of basic research into the clinical years. Involving dental students' views is valuable in evaluating the success of integration. Of particular interest are their views on whether biomedical content has supported their clinical learning and the requirements of clinical work, and thus meets the prerequisites of a high-quality dental curriculum.

Students are important stakeholders in developing dental education [18]. They provide feedback on the quality of their education in course evaluations as well as in post-graduation surveys evaluating the working-life relevance of what they had studied. They also identify both formal and informal learning requirements, that is, what is written in the syllabus and what they are actually required to pass the courses.

At the University of Helsinki, the dental programs are conducted within the Faculty of Medicine, in which there are degree programs for both medical and dental students. The first two years of biomedical sciences are common for both medical and dental students. Many dental degree programs face the same challenge of how to integrate biomedical sciences into the dental curriculum. This study explores this issue from the perspective of clinical phase dental students. The aim of the study was to examine the early-stage biomedical courses from the students' perspective and provide research-based recommendation for revising a dental curriculum. We hope to shed light on the aim by answering the following research questions:

(1) How did dental students in the clinical phase evaluate the relevance of the joint biomedical courses with medical students and the separate preclinical courses designed for dental students?
(2) How did the evaluation of preclinical courses vary between the third-, fourth- and fifth-year dental students?
(3) What learning content (dental theoretical disciplines and elements) did the dental students propose should be added to the first two years of study?

2. Materials and Methods

2.1. Study Content

In 2000, a major curriculum reform was implemented in the dental and medical education at the University of Helsinki. The curriculum introduced continued as it was until 2016, largely based on the educational approaches adopted at that time. Before this reform, the first two years consisted of a significant proportion of lectures. Most of these lectures were replaced by problem-based learning (PBL) tutorials in groups of seven or eight medical students and one or two dental students. The key learning principles of PBL are that learning is based on real-life problems, and student learning is constructive, self-directed, collaborative and context-based [19]. A well-designed PBL promotes scientific attitude and offers students the opportunity to learn clinical topics from the beginning of their education [20]. However, in PBL tutorials at the University of Helsinki, there were no cases designed for dental students, and aspects of oral health were not included in the learning tasks or materials. Biomedical study courses were built around the physiology and anatomy of organ systems, which was a common way to teach these contents around the globe [1]. Basic science subjects were taught in entities within an integrative strategy. Other learning methods used were lectures, seminars, demonstrations and dissections. Dental and medical students attended the same lectures and sitting exams and were assessed in the same way. Thus, the 2000 curriculum reform was done in part at the expense of dental students. In 2016, when the data for this study were collected, the faculty members were in a situation in which they had sufficient experience of the challenges of the 2000 curriculum and were ready to design and implement a new curriculum.

Most of the professional dental content and clinical skills were taught during an intensive, stressful [21] three-year clinical phase at the dental department and the student clinic. The main learning methods used in these courses were lectures, self-directive learning, digital learning, clinical work under supervision, skills laboratory, peer-to-peer practices and procedures, patient care practice in pairs and comprehensive longitudinal patient care. The detailed content of the dental curriculum is presented in Appendix A.

2.2. Study Design, Participants and Questionnaire

The questionnaire (Appendix B) was addressed to the 134 clinical phase dental students at the University of Helsinki in April 2016. Data were collected among third-, fourth- and fifth-year dental students after lectures with a paper questionnaire. It consisted of multiple-choice and open-ended questions on nine different sections covering preclinical and clinical courses, curriculum content, learning outcomes and methods used for learning and assessment.

In this study, we analysed two of the nine sections of the questionnaire. We explored the items in which students were asked to evaluate how the preclinical courses laid a foundation for the dental clinical courses. Students were asked to rate the courses on a 5-point Likert scale. In addition, we analysed the responses to a question in which students were asked for suggestions on what topics should be added to the preclinical phase. Data from the other sections of the survey were used in other research and in the development of the dental curriculum.

2.3. Ethics

The research was carried out in accordance with the guidelines of the Declaration of Helsinki and the Finnish National Advisory Board on Research Ethics. Students were informed by email about the study prior to data collection. In the beginning of the questionnaire, the students were informed about the aims of the study, the contact information of the researchers and that answering was voluntary and anonymous (Appendix B). In the end of the questionnaire, students were asked to express their informed consent to participate in the study. The responses were collected and analysed anonymously, and the confidentiality was guaranteed throughout the process.

2.4. Statistical Analysis

SPSS 27.0 (IBM Corporation) was used in the analysis. The nonparametric Kruskal–Wallis one-way analysis of variance was used to test the statistical significance of differences between the categorical variables. Participants were clustered into groups based on their demographic background variables (age, gender, academic study year, previous studies). The Kruskal–Wallis test qualified for the five-level psychometric scale assuming that the variables were ultimately continuous. The cut-off p-value used was 0.05. To measure the reliability and internal consistency of the Likert scale used, the Cronbach's alpha was calculated. A value for Cronbach alpha over 0.9 indicates a very good level of reliability.

3. Results

A total of 110 (82%) students completed the questionnaire. From the third study year 37 students (80%) responded, from the fourth study year 40 (77%) responded, and from the fifth study year 33 (77%) students responded. All respondents answered the multiple-choice questions in which they evaluated study-related aspects, and 62% answered open-ended questions.

3.1. Participant Background Information

The background data of the respondents are presented in Table 1: 71% were women and 29% men. Three-quarters of the respondents were under 30 years of age, and a quarter (27%) of them were older. Sixty percent of respondents had previous academic studies, and 40% had an academic degree.

Table 1. Background information on the respondents (n = 110).

Age		N	%
	Over 30	30	27
	Under 30	78	71
	Not mentioned	2	2
Gender			
	Female	78	71
	Male	26	24
	Not mentioned	6	5
Study year			
	3rd	37	34
	4th	40	36
	5th	33	30
Previous studies			
	Academic degree	28	25
	Academic studies	39	35
	Healthcare studies	4	4
	Other previous studies	1	1
	No previous studies	37	34

3.2. Relevance of the Preclinical Studies

Students were asked to rate each preclinical course in the first two study years on how it laid the foundation for clinical dental education. The Cronbach's alpha for the evaluations on the biomedical study courses was 0.900 and 0.942 for the study courses tailored for dental students.

Of the joint biomedical study courses with medical students (Table 2), the best evaluation from all respondents (n = 110) was given to the course covering pharmacology of antibiotics and protection against microbes with the mean (M) of 3.7 and standard deviation (SD) of 0.9. The lowest evaluation was given to molecular biology (M = 2.5, SD = 1.1) and the course covering endocrinology and the human reproductive system (M = 2.6, SD = 1.0).

In most courses, the evaluations remained relatively similar, with the M ranging from 2.7 to 3.4.

Table 2. Students' responses to the question asking them to evaluate how common biomedical courses had laid the foundation for dental clinical courses. Mean values (M) and standard deviations (SD) of the course evaluations.

Study Course	3rd–5th N = 110 M (SD)	3rd N = 37 M (SD)	4th N = 40 M (SD)	5th N = 33 M (SD)	*p*-Value
Dealing with an emergency or crisis situation	3.3 (0.9)	3.6 (1.0)	3.2 (0.8)	3.2 (0.9)	0.070
Medical biochemistry and pharmacology	3.3 (0.9)	3.5 (1.1)	3.2 (0.9)	3.3 (0.8)	0.380
Cellular biology and basic tissues	3.2 (0.9)	3.3 (0.8)	3.2 (0.9)	3.0 (1.0)	0.141
Metabolism and its regulation	2.8 (0.9)	2.8 (0.9)	2.7 (0.9)	2.9 (1.0)	0.435
Molecular biology	2.5 (1.1)	2.5 (1.0)	2.5 (0.9)	2.5 (1.1)	0.939
Embryology	2.7 (0.9)	2.7 (0.9)	2.6 (0.9)	2.7 (1.0)	0.739
Neurobiology	3.2 (0.8)	3.5 (0.7)	3.2 (0.7)	2.8 (0.9)	<0.001 *
Physiology and anatomy of the musculoskeletal system	3.2 (1.0)	3.5 (0.9)	3.2 (1.0)	3.0 (0.9)	0.108
Heart, circulatory system and kidney	3.4 (0.9)	4.0 (0.7)	3.2 (0.8)	3.1 (0.9)	<0.001 *
The surrounding environment, body's defence and protection	3.7 (0.9)	4.1 (0.8)	3.7 (1.0)	3.4 (0.9)	0.007 *
The respiratory system	3.0 (0.9)	3.3 (0.9)	2.9 (0.9)	2.8 (0.9)	0.033 *
The digestive system and nutrition	3.3 (1.0)	3.8 (0.9)	3.2 (0.8)	2.9 (0.9)	<0.001 *
Endocrinology and genitals	2.6 (1.0)	2.8 (0.9)	2.6 (1.0)	2.5 (1.0)	0.432
Study courses overall mean	3.1	3.4	3.1	3.0	

* The differences between the evaluations between the groups is statistically significant. Cronbach α for the scale used 0.900. Scale: 1 = Not at all, 2 = Slightly, 3 = Moderately, 4 = Well, 5 = Very well.

Of the study courses tailored specifically for dental students (Table 3), the best evaluation from all respondents (N = 110) was given to the course that covers the scope of basic level information on clinical dental disciplines (M = 4.1, SD = 0.8), and the lowest evaluations were given to the courses covering professionalism (M = 2.9, SD = 1.0 and M = 3.1, SD = 1.0). Most of the courses received relatively similar evaluations, with the M ranging between 3.3 (SD = 1.0) and 3.7 (SD = 0.9).

Table 3. Students' responses to the question asking them to evaluate how the courses tailored specifically for the dental students had laid a foundation for the clinical courses in dentistry. Mean values (M) and standard deviations (SD) of the course evaluations.

Study Course	3rd–5th N = 110 M (SD)	3rd N = 37 M (SD)	4th N = 40 M (SD)	5th N = 33 M (SD)	*p*-Value
Professionalism—study course 1	2.9 (1.0)	3.2 (0.9)	2.7 (0.9)	2.9 (1.1)	0.060
Interaction with a paediatric patient	3.3 (1.0)	3.7 (0.9)	3.2 (0.9)	3.1 (1.1)	0.038 *
Professionalism—study course 2	3.1 (1.0)	3.5 (0.9)	2.9 (0.9)	3.0 (1.1)	0.052
Paediatric dentistry	3.7 (0.9)	3.8 (0.9)	3.8 (0.9)	3.6 (0.9)	0.595
Face, mouth and teeth	4.1 (0.8)	4.6 (0.5)	4.0 (0.9)	3.8 (0.8)	<0.001 *
Feel the clinic	3.7 (1.2)	4.0 (1.2)	3.1 (1.2)	3.9 (1.0)	0.034 *
Study courses overall mean	3.5	4.0	3.8	3.7	

* The differences between the evaluations between the groups is statistically significant. Cronbach α for the scale used 0.942. Scale: 1 = Not at all, 2 = Slightly, 3 = Moderately, 4 = Well, 5 = Very well.

Courses tailored specifically for dental students (M = 3.5) received somewhat higher ratings from respondents than joint biomedical courses for medical and dental students (M = 3.1).

3.3. Evaluation of Preclinical Courses by Academic Year

Respondents were gathered into groups based on their academic study year to find out whether there was a difference on how they evaluated the study courses.

Third-year students who were at the beginning of their clinical phase rated 79% of the biomedical study courses higher than the fourth- and fifth-year students. The result was statistically significant in half (53%) of the courses. The study courses for which the evaluations were statistically significant covered the following subjects (p-value): neurobiology (<0.001), the cardiovascular system (<0.001), pharmacology of antibiotics and protection against microbes (0.007), the respiratory system (0.033) and the digestive system and nutrition (<0.001).

3.4. Adding Dental Content to the Preclinical Phase

Participants were able to suggest which dental theoretical subjects and dental elements they would like to add to the first two study years.

Almost all students (95%) wanted more dental content, both theoretical and clinical in the first two study years. Most students wanted simulations, e.g., skills lab and peer-to-peer procedures (88%), observation of clinical work of dental students (81%) and visits to dental care units (60%). Students also wanted the following theoretical content for the early study years: cariology and endodontics (65%), dental public health (60%) and periodontology (55%). The elements and dental theoretical subjects that students wanted to add to the first two study years are presented in Figures 1 and 2. In the open-ended answers, students wished that the curriculum would include, among other things, observation of a specialised dentist, practise of patients' self-care with actors and work as a dental assistant.

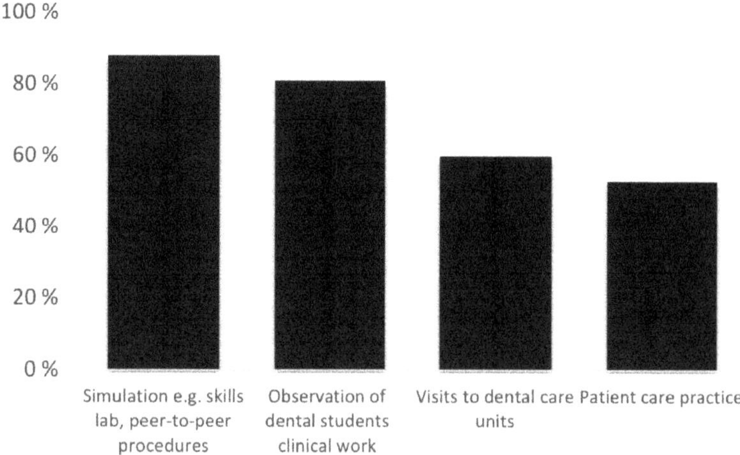

Figure 1. Elements proposed for the preclinical study phase of the dental curriculum (n = 110).

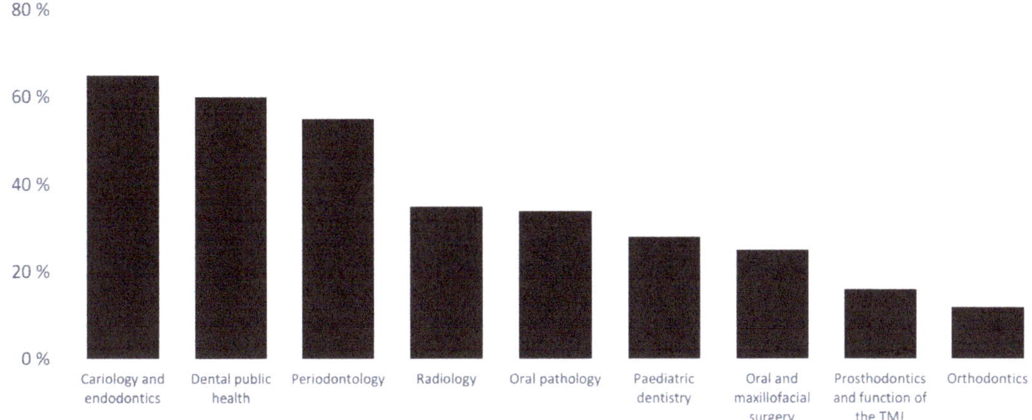

Figure 2. Dental theoretical subjects suggested for the preclinical study phase (n = 110).

4. Discussion

Dental units see biomedical study content as an important part of the degree program, but they face challenges in providing these courses in a way that interests and motivates dental students [3–5]. This is particularly the case for education units with both dental and medical degree programs, in which these studies are conducted mainly as joint courses that are primarily designed for medical students [1,2,10–12]. Research has found that in this type of dental unit, coordination between the basic sciences and dental subjects has been deficient [22].

This study was conducted in a university in which both medical and dental students are trained, and where dental students are clearly the minority. The aim of the study was to examine dental students' perceptions of how joint biomedical courses and courses specifically tailored for dental students supported their clinical phase learning, and what they suggested should be added to their first few study years. The main findings of the study were as follows: (1) Dental students wanted more tailor-made dental courses in the first years of study. (2) The dental perspective should be integrated into joint courses with medical students. (3) The closer the respondents (third-, fourth- and fifth-year dental students) were to graduation, the less important they considered biomedical topics.

Research on dental education has shown that biomedical courses form an extensive part of the degree program [10]. Consistent with previous studies, we observed that students had difficulty recognising the relevance of joint biomedical courses for clinical work in dentistry [11,12], but when the link was clear, it increased their interest in the course content [7,8,10]. For example, courses that included pharmacology of antibiotics were graded more highly than courses covering embryology, molecular biology and genitals.

Studies have shown that dental students have felt themselves marginalised in the joint courses [7–9,21]. Our study demonstrated lost opportunities for interprofessional learning in dental education. The medical and dental students were learning biomedical sciences side by side for two years, but they were not learning with and from one another [16]. For joint biomedical courses to be mutually inspiring, they should be tailored so that course content includes both medical and dental topics and supports the active participation of both groups. Furthermore, all students should feel equally valued [17]. Without adequate planning, PBL alone did not guarantee students this opportunity. We need more research on how common biomedical sciences could be taught so that interprofessional learning would have positive outcomes. Designing courses of this type requires careful review of course evaluations and collaboration between biomedical, dental and medical teachers and students to make the study contents meaningful for both student groups. Furthermore, well-planned and well-timed dental courses during the preclinical phase support and maintain students' motivation.

ADEE [23] suggests enhancing vertical integration, that is, including dental clinical material in the early years of study and adding biomedical subjects to clinical courses [3]. The results of our study were in line with ADEE suggestions and a previous study [15] which showed that students appreciated studies tailored specifically for dental students and agreed that more theoretical and practical content in dentistry could be included in the first two years of study in the curriculum. Students in this study proposed simulations, observation of dental students' clinical work, visits to dental units and theoretical content in cariology and endodontics, dental public health and periodontology. However, organising courses tailored specifically for dental students might be challenging for small dental education units.

Even though students were not able to see the connection between the biomedical learning content and their future work, they still saw the usefulness [12]. Furthermore, according to one study, dental students preferred learning basic sciences together with medical students [24]. Prevention and treatment of oral diseases requires dental practitioners to have adequate theoretical and clinical competence. Studies have increasingly shown an association between oral health and medical conditions [25,26]. To understand these processes, it is essential for dentists to understand the basic principles of biomedicine. For example, a solid theoretical knowledge of endocrinology is needed in the treatment of patients with diabetes [27], a medical condition that affects almost 8.5% of the world's population [28]. The emphasis on dental aspects in joint courses with medical students supports interprofessional learning and reminds of the importance of oral health for future physicians. If actively pursued by the faculty members, common learning of basic sciences develops connections and appreciation for the other field's contribution to human health.

The objective of a university degree is not only to prepare students for clinical work but also to provide them with competence for lifelong learning, scientific thinking and a possible career as a researcher. This is a viewpoint that students might not consider whilst evaluating their studies. Undergraduate students' views on their own education may not always provide the best course of action for designing an effective curriculum, and the perceptions of graduated dentists working in patient care and in research groups would complement the results of this study. Dentistry is a field in which research-based knowledge is growing rapidly as treatment techniques and practices evolve. The academic dental curriculum calls for a balance between the theoretical and clinical content taught.

In our study, we found that students studying in their last two years rated biomedical courses the lowest. Similar observations have been made in a recent study, in which undergraduate dental students found biomedical courses in some way relevant to their degree, but graduated dentists found them important only if they were heading for a scientific career [10]. This result supports the earlier observation that the more clinical work experience respondents had, the less relevant biomedical content seemed to be to them.

Strengths and Weaknesses of the Study

Even though the response rate expressed as percentages was high, including almost all clinical phase students at the time when the data were collected, the number of respondents was relatively small due to the small annual intake of dental students. In addition, our study analyses the situation in one dental education unit, and the results as such cannot be generalised to other units. However, we have described the content of our study, and the course structure is provided in Appendix A. Therefore, we assume that the units in which dental education is conducted in a relatively similar way can benefit from the results of our study.

It would have been interesting to collect data from the first- and second-year students and compare the results to the third-, fourth- and fifth-year students' evaluations. However, we thought it would be difficult for them to assess the clinical relevance of biomedical sciences. The collection of data over several years would have strengthened our results.

The curriculum was reformed after the data were collected, and therefore the study could not be repeated as such.

5. Conclusions

Students' perspectives on the basic biomedical sciences provide important information for developing the dental curriculum. Firstly, dental students should have study content designed for them specifically right from the start of their education. Secondly, the dental viewpoint should be incorporated into the joint courses with medical students and interprofessional learning promoted. Thirdly, as interest in biomedical sciences declined as studies progressed, these topics should be meaningfully integrated into the clinical phase of the undergraduate degree of dentistry.

Author Contributions: Conceptualization, F.M., T.K.-S., P.M. and E.P.; methodology, F.M., T.K.-S., P.M. and E.P.; investigation, F.M.; writing—original draft preparation, F.M., T.K.-S., P.M. and E.P. All authors have read and agreed to the published version of the manuscript.

Funding: This research received no external funding. Open access funding provided by the University of Helsinki Library.

Institutional Review Board Statement: The study was conducted according to the guidelines of the Declaration of Helsinki and the Finnish Research Ethics Board. In 2016, ethical review and approval were waived for this study, since at the time ethical evaluation was not required for collecting non-sensitive and non-invasive data among students at the University of Helsinki. The leaders of the program in dentistry as well as the target groups of the study were informed about the research and given the contact details of the researchers. Participation in the study was anonymous and voluntary. Confidentiality was guaranteed throughout the process.

Informed Consent Statement: Informed consent was obtained from all subjects involved in the study.

Data Availability Statement: The data presented in this study are available on request from the corresponding author.

Acknowledgments: The authors want to thank Jaakko Koivumäki, the senior researcher at the Finnish Dental Association, for help with the statistical analysis.

Conflicts of Interest: The authors declare no conflict of interest.

Appendix A

Table A1. Annex 1. Curriculum content and the number of ECTS (European Credit Transfer and Accumulation System) credits per study year at the University of Helsinki (for students who started their studies before the year 2015).

Study Year	Common Studies with the Medical Students	ECTS	Dental Studies	ECTS
1st	Dealing with an emergency or crisis situation, Medical biochemistry and pharmacology, Cellular biology and basic tissues, Metabolism and its regulation, Molecular biology, Embryology and part of Neurobiology	43/55 ECTS	Professionalism, Interaction with a paediatric patient, Face, mouth and teeth (basic anatomy and physiology), Working as a dental assistant for an upper year student	12/55 ECTS

Table A1. *Cont.*

Study Year	Common Studies with the Medical Students	ECTS	Dental Studies	ECTS
2nd	Neurobiology continues, Physiology and anatomy of the musculoskeletal system, Heart, circulatory system and kidney, The surrounding environment, Body's defence and protection, The respiratory system, The digestive system and nutrition and Endocrinology and genitals	45/53 ECTS	Paediatric dentistry, Dental public health, Medical microbiology	8/53 ECTS
3rd			20% of the studies consist of clinical work (patient care in pairs). Basic theoretical and clinical courses on periodontology, orthodontics, head and neck surgery, radiology, function of the TMJ, prosthodontics, cariology and endodontics.	58 ECTS
4th			40% of the studies consist of clinical work (procedures for patients, comprehensive longitudinal patient care). Theoretical courses of oral pathology, paediatric dentistry, prosthetics. Advanced courses on periodontology, head and neck surgery, orthodontics, radiology, orthodontics.	62 ECTS
5th			40% of the studies consist of clinical work (comprehensive longitudinal patient care). Refresher courses on all subjects and final written examinations	49 ECTS
6th			Six months of vocational training as a dental practitioner in a health centre	30 ECTS
	Language studies 6 ECTS Optional studies 10 ECTS	21/41 ECTS	Thesis 20 ECTS	41 ECTS

Appendix B

Annex 2. Questionnaire designed for the study. How has the teaching of the medical faculty supported my growth into becoming a dentist?

Study year ☐3rd ☐4th ☐5th
Age ☐Under 30 ☐Over 30
Gender ☐Female ☐Male
Previous studies (other than dental studies) ☐University degree ☐University studies
☐Health care studies
☐Other previous studies
Which studies ____________________________

Table A2. I Preclinical studies. Evaluate how the study courses of the first two study years have formed basis for the clinical phase studies. Circle the option "Not applicable" if you have not attended to the study course.

	Not at All	Slightly	Moderately	Well	Very Well	Not Applicable
Dealing with an emergency or crisis situation	1	2	3	4	5	0
Medical biochemistry and pharmacology	1	2	3	4	5	0
Cellular biology and basic tissues	1	2	3	4	5	0
Metabolism and its regulation	1	2	3	4	5	0
Molecular biology	1	2	3	4	5	0
Embryology	1	2	3	4	5	0
Neurobiology	1	2	3	4	5	0
Physiology and anatomy of the musculoskeletal system	1	2	3	4	5	0
Heart, circulatory system and kidney	1	2	3	4	5	0
The surrounding environment, body's defence and protection	1	2	3	4	5	0
The respiratory system	1	2	3	4	5	0
The digestive system and nutrition	1	2	3	4	5	0
Endocrinology and genitals	1	2	3	4	5	0

Table A3. II Studies designed specifically for dental students during the first two study years. Evaluate how the studies designed specifically for the dental students during the first two study years have formed basis for the clinical phase studies. Circle the option "Not applicable" if you have not attended to the study course.

	Not at All	Slightly	Moderately	Well	Very Well	Not Applicable
Professionalism—study course 1	1	2	3	4	5	0
Interaction with a paediatric patient	1	2	3	4	5	0
Professionalism—study course 2	1	2	3	4	5	0
Paediatric dentistry	1	2	3	4	5	0
Face, mouth and teeth	1	2	3	4	5	0
Feel the clinic	1	2	3	4	5	0

☐ Simulation, i.e., skills lab, demonstrations ☐ 1st ☐ 2nd
☐ Patient care ☐ 1st ☐ 2nd
☐ Observation of clinical work of dental students ☐ 1st ☐ 2nd
☐ Visits to dental care units ☐ 1st ☐ 2nd
☐ Professionalism –studies ☐ 1st ☐ 2nd
☐ Other, what?____

Dental theoretical subjects
☐ Radiology ☐ 1st ☐ 2nd
☐ Oral and maxillofacial surgery ☐ 1st ☐ 2nd
☐ Oral pathology ☐ 1st ☐ 2nd
☐ Periodontology ☐ 1st ☐ 2nd
☐ Cariology and endodontics ☐ 1st ☐ 2nd
☐ Paediatric dentistry ☐ 1st ☐ 2nd
☐ Prosthodontics and the function of TMJ ☐ 1st ☐ 2nd
☐ Orthodontics ☐ 1st ☐ 2nd
☐ Dental public health ☐ 1st ☐ 2nd

Table A4. III Learning methods. Evaluate how different learning methods support your learning. Circle the option "Not applicable" if you have not participated in the learning method.

	Not at All Useful	Slightly Useful	Moderately Useful	Very Useful	Extremely Useful	Not Applicable
Lectures	1	2	3	4	5	0
Small group teaching	1	2	3	4	5	0
PBL	1	2	3	4	5	0
Seminars	1	2	3	4	5	0
Peer-to-peer procedures	1	2	3	4	5	0
Skills lab	1	2	3	4	5	0
Demonstrations	1	2	3	4	5	0
Patient care practice in pairs	1	2	3	4	5	0
Before-class learning activities	1	2	3	4	5	0
Digital learning						
Digital applications	1	2	3	4	5	0
Videos	1	2	3	4	5	0
Thesis	1	2	3	4	5	0
Comprehensive longitudinal patient care	1	2	3	4	5	0
Procedures for patients	1	2	3	4	5	0
Self-directive learning	1	2	3	4	5	0

Which learning method(s) in the third year best supported the transition to clinical care practice (working with patients)?

____

Which learning method(s) best support the development of your clinical competence?

____

____

____

____

Explain how the curriculum content could be integrated so that teaching would form entities based on the patient's symptoms rather than the dental specialty.

____

____

____

____

____

IV Assessment of each dental specialty

What is the most important/first thing that comes to your mind from each dental specialty that benefits the dental clinical work?

Radiology ______________________________________

Oral and maxillofacial surgery ____________________________

Oral pathology ____________________________________

Periodontology ____________________________________

Cariology and endodontics ____________________________

Paediatric dentistry ________________________________

Prosthodontics and the function of TMJ ____________________

Orthodontics ______________________________________

Dental public health ________________________________

Table A5. V How has the learning of the following areas been implemented in the curriculum? What do you think about the following statements?

	Strongly Disagree	Disagree	Neutral	Agree	Strongly Agree
I have developed professionally during my education	1	2	3	4	5
I have sufficient communication and interaction skills to communicate with patients and their loved ones.	1	2	3	4	5
I have sufficient communication and interaction skills to communicate with healthcare professionals.	1	2	3	4	5
I have sufficient knowledge basis, computer skills, and critical thinking to tell the difference between a benign and pathological finding in the mouth.	1	2	3	4	5
I can gather the necessary clinical information about a patient's general health.	1	2	3	4	5
Without a problem, I can manage diagnostics and treatment planning.	1	2	3	4	5
In my work, I achieve and maintain oral health.	1	2	3	4	5
I am qualified to act as a promoter of oral health for both individuals and large groups.	1	2	3	4	5

Table A6. VI Assessment methods. Evaluate how different assessment methods support your learning. Circle the option "Not applicable" if you have not participated in the learning method.

	Not at All Useful	Slightly Useful	Moderately Useful	Very Useful	Extremely Useful	Not Applicable
Entrance examinations	1	2	3	4	5	0
Random tests	1	2	3	4	5	0
Examinations during study courses	1	2	3	4	5	0
Online examination	1	2	3	4	5	0
Course examination	1	2	3	4	5	0
Assessment of final lab work (e.g., during simulations)	1	2	3	4	5	0
Feedback from group work	1	2	3	4	5	0
Written feedback from teachers on clinical work	1	2	3	4	5	0
Oral feedback from teachers on clinical work	1	2	3	4	5	0
Final examinations on each dental specialty	1	2	3	4	5	0
Clinical competency assessments	1	2	3	4	5	0
Peer review	1	2	3	4	5	0
Self-evaluation	1	2	3	4	5	0

VII Self-evaluation.

Give a numeric assessment of your knowledge and skills as a dentist at the moment. ________

1 = Adequate (Clear gaps in skills that need to be improved in order to succeed the dentists' clinical work)

2 = Satisfactory (Minor deficiencies in skills that need to be improved in order to succeed in dentists' clinical work)

3 = Good (Competence is at a good level, I can manage dentists' clinical work)

4 = Commendable (Competence is systematic, I can manage dentists clinical work excellently)

5 = Excellent (Competence is systematic and extensive. I can manage patient care like an experienced dentist)

How has work experience with a dental assistant, dental technician and dental student benefitted you in developing your skills as a dentist? ________

1 = Very poorly

2 = Poorly

3 = Moderately

4 = Well

5 = Very well

0 = Not applicable

Was the teaching given during the autumn of the third study year have had time to be structured and utilized when you started caring for your own patients? _______

1 = Very poorly
2 = Poorly
3 = Moderately
4 = Well
5 = Very well

VIII Other feedback

What other feedback do you want to give about the dental studies?

____

IX Ideas on development

What ideas do you have for developing the dental studies?

____

X Informed consent

I give permission to use my answers in the research material ☐ Yes ☐ No

References

1. Haden, N.K.; Hendricson, W.D.; Kassebaum, D.K.; Ranney, R.R.; Weinstein, G.; Anderson, E.L.; Valachovic, R.W. Curriculum change in dental education, 2003-09. *J. Dent. Educ.* **2010**, *74*, 539–557. [CrossRef] [PubMed]
2. Best, L.; Walton, J.N.; Walker, J.; Von Bergmann, H. Reaching Consensus on Essential Biomedical Science Learning Objectives in a Dental Curriculum. *J. Dent. Educ.* **2016**, *80*, 122–129. [CrossRef]
3. Bennett, J.H.; Beeley, J.A.; Anderson, P.; Belfield, L.; Brand, H.S.; Didilescu, A.C.; Dymock, D.; Guven, Y.; Hector, M.P.; Holbrook, P.; et al. A core curriculum in the biological and biomedical sciences for dentistry. *Eur. J. Dent. Educ.* **2020**, *24*, 433–441. [CrossRef] [PubMed]
4. Geissberger, M.J.; Jain, P.; Kluemper, G.T.; Paquette, D.W.; Roeder, L.B.; Scarfe, W.C.; Potter, B.J. Realigning biomedical science instruction in predoctoral curricula: A proposal for change. *J. Dent. Educ.* **2008**, *72*, 135–141. [CrossRef] [PubMed]
5. Slavkin, H.C. Evolution of the Scientific Basis for Dentistry and Its Impact on Dental Education: Past, Present, and Future. *J. Dent. Educ.* **2012**, *76*, 28–35. [CrossRef] [PubMed]
6. Ajjawi, R.; Hyde, S.; Roberts, C.; Nisbet, G. Marginalisation of dental students in a shared medical and dental education programme. *Med. Educ.* **2009**, *43*, 238–245. [CrossRef]
7. Postma, T.C.; Bronkhorst, L. Second-year dental students' perceptions about a joint basic science curriculum. *Afr. J. Health Prof. Educ.* **2015**, *7*, 199. [CrossRef]
8. Komerik, N.; Sari, H.; Koray, M.; Hocaoglu, T.; Bas, B. Medical courses need to be tailored for dental students. *J. Contemp. Med. Educ.* **2014**, *2*, 79–84. [CrossRef]
9. Kristensen, B.T.; Netterstrom, I.; Kayser, L. Dental students' motivation and the context of learning. *Eur. J. Dent. Educ.* **2009**, *13*, 10–14. [CrossRef]
10. Youhanna, K.M.Y.; Adam, L.; Monk, B.C.; Loch, C. Dentistry students' experiences, engagement and perception of biochemistry within the dental curriculum and beyond. *Eur. J. Dent. Educ.* **2021**, *25*, 318–324. [CrossRef]
11. Lanning, S.K.; Wetzel, A.P.; Baines, M.B.; Byrne, B.E. Evaluation of a revised curriculum: A four-year qualitative study of student perceptions. *J. Dent. Educ.* **2012**, *76*, 1323–1333. [CrossRef]
12. Henzi, D.; Davis, E.; Jasinevicius, R.; Hendricson, W. In the students' own words: What are the strengths and weaknesses of the dental school curriculum? *J. Dent. Educ.* **2007**, *71*, 632–645. [CrossRef]
13. Miller, C.J.; Falcone, J.C.; Metz, M.J. A Comparison of Team-Based Learning Formats: Can We Minimize Stress While Maximizing Results? *J. Dent. Educ.* **2015**, *79*, 52–60. [CrossRef]
14. Chutinan, S.; Kim, J.Y.; Chien, T.; Meyer, H.Y.; Ohyama, H. Can an interactive case-based activity help bridge the theory-practice gap in operative dentistry? *Eur. J. Dent. Educ.* **2021**, *25*, 199–206. [CrossRef] [PubMed]

15. Henzi, D.; Davis, E.; Jasinevicius, R.; Hendricson, W.; Cintron, L.; Isaacs, M. Appraisal of the dental school learning environment: The students' view. *J. Dent. Educ.* **2005**, *69*, 1137–1147. [CrossRef] [PubMed]
16. CAIPE. Interprofessional Education—A Definition. 2002. Available online: https://www.caipe.org/resources/publications/caipe-publications/caipe-2002-interprofessional-education-today-yesterday-tomorrow-barr-h (accessed on 30 July 2021).
17. Reeves, S.; Fletcher, S.; Barr, H.; Birch, I.; Boet, S.; Davies, N.; McFadyen, A.; Rivera, J.; Kitto, S. A BEME systematic review of the effects of interprofessional education: BEME Guide No. 39. *Med. Teach.* **2016**, *38*, 656–668. [CrossRef] [PubMed]
18. Felten, P.; Abbot, S.; Kirkwood, J.; Long, A.; Lubicz-Nawrocka, T.; Mercer-Mapstone, L.; Verwoord, R. Reimagining the place of students in academic development. *Int. J. Acad. Dev.* **2019**, *24*, 192–203. [CrossRef]
19. Dolmans, D.H.J.M.; De Grave, W.; Wolfhagen, I.H.A.P.; Van Der Vleuten, C.P.M. Problem-based learning: Future challenges for educational practice and research. *Med. Educ.* **2005**, *39*, 732–741. [CrossRef]
20. Rohlin, M.; Petersson, K.; Svensäter, G. The Malmö model: A problem-based learning curriculum in undergraduate dental education. *Eur. J. Dent. Educ.* **1998**, *2*, 103–114. [CrossRef]
21. Koivumäki, J.; Auero, M.; Eerola, A.; Karaharju-Suvanto, T.; Kottonen, A.; Näpänkangas, R.; Pienihäkkinen, K.; Savanheimo, N.; Suominen, L.; Tuononen, T. Nuori hammaslääkäri 2014. Available online: https://www.hammaslaakariliitto.fi/sites/default/files/mediafiles/liiton_toiminta/nuori_hml_2014_verkkoon.pdf (accessed on 17 February 2021).
22. Martínez-Álvares, C.; Mariano, S.; Berthold, P. Basic sciences in the dental curriculum in Southern Europe. *Eur. J. Dent. Educ.* **2001**, *5*, 63–66. [CrossRef]
23. Manogue, M.; McLoughlin, J.; Christersson, C.; Delap, E.; Lindh, C.; Schoonheim-Klein, M.; Plasschaert, A. Curriculum structure, content, learning and assessment in European undergraduate dental education-update. *Eur. J. Dent. Educ.* **2011**, *15*, 133–141. [CrossRef] [PubMed]
24. Kuchenbecker Rösing, C.; Oppermann, R.V.; da Silva, D.T.; Deon, P.R.; Gjermo, P. Students´appraisal of their dental education related to basic sciences learning: A comparison of four curricula in Norway and Brazil. *Rev. Odonto. Ciênc.* **2008**, *23*, 234–237.
25. Pussinen, P.J.; Tuomisto, K.; Jousilahti, P.; Havulinna, A.S.; Sundvall, J.; Salomaa, V. Endotoxemia, Immune Response to Periodontal Pathogens, and Systemic Inflammation Associate With Incident Cardiovascular Disease Events. *Arter. Thromb. Vasc. Biol.* **2007**, *27*, 1433–1439. [CrossRef] [PubMed]
26. Pussinen, P.J.; Havulinna, A.S.; Lehto, M.; Sundvall, J.; Salomaa, V. Endotoxemia Is Associated With an Increased Risk of Incident Diabetes. *Diabetes Care* **2011**, *34*, 392–397. [CrossRef]
27. Lin, H.; Zhang, H.; Yan, Y.; Liu, D.; Zhang, R.; Liu, Y.; Chen, P.; Zhang, J.; Xuan, D. Knowledge, awareness, and behaviors of endocrinologists and dentists for the relationship between diabetes and periodontitis. *Diabetes Res. Clin. Pr.* **2014**, *106*, 428–434. [CrossRef]
28. World Health Organization. Available online: https://www.who.int/news-room/fact-sheets/detail/diabetes (accessed on 22 February 2020).

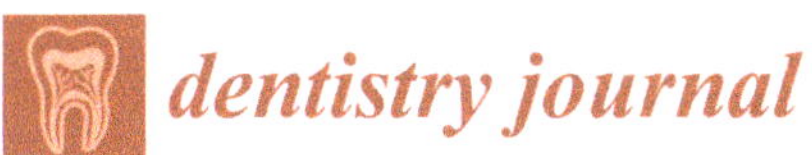 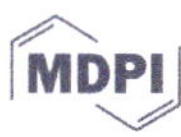

Communication

VIRDENTOPSY: Virtual Dental Autopsy and Remote Forensic Odontology Evaluation

Emilio Nuzzolese

Human Identification Laboratory, Section of Legal Medicine, University of Turin, 10124 Torino, Italy; emilio.nuzzolese@unito.it; Tel.: +39-011-6705969

Abstract: The identification of human remains relies on the comparison of post-mortem data, collected during the autopsy, with the ante-mortem data gathered from the missing persons' reports. DNA, fingerprints, and dental data are considered primary identifiers and are usually collected during any human identification process. Post-mortem dental data should be collected and analyzed by forensic odontologists, as a dental autopsy must not be confused with a dental examination. The virdentopsy project was inaugurated in 2020, during the COVID-19 pandemic, to allow the correct process of human remains by collecting dental data from teeth and jaws, which was then transmitted to forensic odontologists remotely for an expert opinion to achieve a generic profile of the unidentified human remains. The post-mortem dental biography is paramount to narrow the search for compatible missing persons but requires knowledge and experience of forensic odontologists. The virdentopsy process uses radiographic imaging (periapical X-rays, CT scans, panoramics), 2D/3D photos and video recording, photogrammetry documentation, 3D scanning, and live streaming where possible. This registered term was created by merging the terms "virtual" and "dental autopsy" but with no commercial benefits. The proposed process combines research topics under the field of the human rights of the dead and humanitarian forensic odontology services. It should enhance and accelerate the human identification process of the deceased, age estimation of the living, analysis of panoramic X-ray images, and be an educational tool for remote live training in forensic odontology and anatomy of skulls. This paper presents an overview of the virdentopsy process in the field of forensic odontology as a remote consultation as well as an educational tool for undergraduates and postgraduates.

Keywords: virdentopsy; virtual dental autopsy; autopsy imaging; human identification; dental autopsy; humanitarian forensic odontology; forensic odontology

Citation: Nuzzolese, E. VIRDENTOPSY: Virtual Dental Autopsy and Remote Forensic Odontology Evaluation. *Dent. J.* 2021, 9, 102. https://doi.org/10.3390/dj9090102

Academic Editor: Rod Moore

Received: 11 July 2021
Accepted: 2 September 2021
Published: 5 September 2021

1. Introduction

The identification of the deceased requires the involvement of several forensic experts, depending on the status of the remains. There are several methods to evaluate the evidence used to identify human remains: visual recognition; fingerprints; DNA; dental data [1]; and physical evidence (e.g., tattoos, scars, and surgical implants) [2]. The visual method is not recommended because of subjective factors and the high risk of misidentification. It can, however, lead to a single-case presumptive identification when combined with other evidence, such as personal belongings or eye-witness reports [3]. Nevertheless, it is internationally accepted that the most reliable method for identification is the collection of primary identifiers: friction ridge analysis, forensic odontology, and DNA [4].

The positive identification allows surviving family members to start the grieving process, and the death certificate following identification allows them to set insurance, legal, business, and personal affairs in order. Giving a name and an identity to unidentified human remains is also fundamental for the respect of the human rights of the dead and a dignified disposition of human remains [5,6].

The collection and analysis of dental data for the human identification process is paramount in comparing the data from the unidentified remains to the reported missing persons list and achieving a preliminary list of compatible profiles.

During the dental autopsy, forensic odontologists collect all dental and radiological evidence from teeth and jaws, as well as 3D scanning on soft tissue of the face when possible, and by analyzing this data, they estimate a generic biological profile, which is used to search for missing persons compatible with the unidentified human remains.

This assessment includes sex, geographical origin, dental age, cheiloscopy [7,8], and other biological markers, such as oral hygiene and dietary habits, and will possibly achieve a positive identification confirming a match with ante-mortem dental data of the missing persons. The principle in the human identification process is the comparison of ante-mortem with post-mortem evidence and findings among primary identifiers: fingerprints, DNA, and dental data. The correct collection and interpretation of dental information requires experienced dentists with forensic backgrounds and knowledge in disaster victim identification (DVI). Although forensic odontology is taught in most countries through postgraduate training courses for dentists, forensic odontologists are not always available or recruited systematically in the human identification process. Furthermore, the COVID-19 pandemic has raised several safety concerns when dealing with human remains of unknown medical history [9], in caseworks as well as in hands-on forensic training courses. A possible solution is the use of teledentistry [10] in forensic odontology for remote consultation of dental autopsies, as well as a supplementary means of education and hands-on training to develop skills in odontology and learn the anatomy of the skull.

2. Virtual Autopsy and Teledentistry in Forensic Odontology

The idea of using non-invasive imaging methods to perform a virtual autopsy was presented in 2003 as a tool in forensic pathology [11] to document and analyze forensic findings in dead persons [12]. It consists of whole-body volume documentation using CT, MRI, and radiology, combined with a 3D body documentation using photogrammetry and optical scanning [13], which allows an alternative and non-invasive approach to examining dead bodies and to evaluate the cause and manner of death and any other relevant forensic findings. Applications of teledentistry in a virtual autopsy have been presented by several authors [14–16] but without any humanitarian goal or applications in the identification of dead migrants. Virtual autopsy has also been proposed for odontological cases [17,18] and for the identification process [19]. As mentioned above, the major concern in the identification process is the collection of primary identifiers, including dental data through a complete dental autopsy performed by one or more odontologists who are experts in forensic odontology and disaster victim identification [20]. To be effective in the identification purpose, post-mortem dental data collected during the dental autopsy should receive a proper analysis and evaluation by forensic odontologists. If they are not available onsite, it is conceivable to split the post-mortem dental data collection, performed by dentists onsite, and the forensic odontology evaluation of data collected, performed remotely by forensic odontologists. Furthermore, when the nationality of the deceased is unknown or for challenging cases, a second expert opinion could be advisable. Finally, the involvement of remote forensic odontologists available pro bono could be a supplementary means in humanitarian forensic odontology and missing and unidentified persons as well as unidentified dead migrants.

3. The Virtual Dental Autopsy Project (VIRDENTOPSY)

The Human Identification Laboratory and the medico-legal section of the University of Turin started a research project in 2020 based on the hypothesis that the identification process of unidentified human remains must always comply with best practices in human identification, which should always include a complete dental autopsy even when no forensic odontologists are available onsite. Furthermore, teleconsultation in medicine and dentistry, especially after the COVID-19 pandemic [21] and potential risk of infection [22], can be applied also in forensics, and specifically in the human identification process. This allows forensic pathologists to perform the autopsy without compromising on the technical inputs of forensic odontologists.

At present, there are few institutions worldwide that have recognized the feasibility of remote dental autopsy [5,23] but none are currently offering teleconsultations in forensic odontology for the purpose of human identification or considering offering this service on a humanitarian basis. The project combines research topics such as pathology, odontology, anthropology, and archeology under the umbrella of human rights of the dead and humanitarian forensic odontology [24–26]. The term VIRDENTOPSY merges the terms "virtual" and "dental autopsy". It is a registered brand (Figure 1) with a dedicated website [27] in order to offer a remote forensic odontological assessment of post-mortem dental data of unidentified human remains.

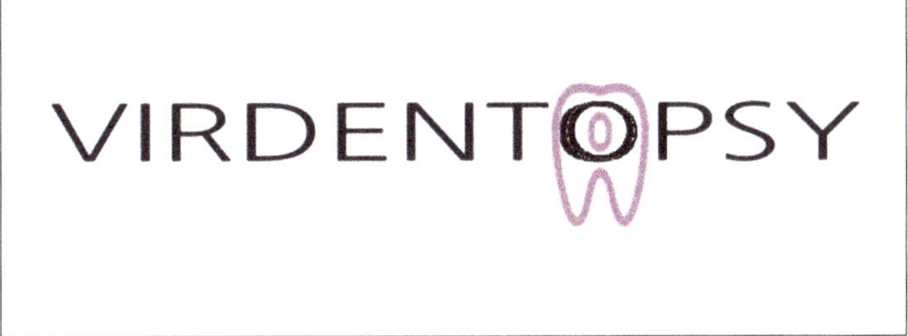

Figure 1. Virdentopsy™ registered brand (Class 44).

Virdentopsy makes provisions for the systematic collection of post-mortem dental data performed by forensic pathologists, dentists with no forensic background, dental hygienists with a forensic background, or other forensic operators authorized in the mortuary. These operators perform the dental and intraoral collection of postmortem dental data (also in livestreaming), following what is usually performed by forensic odontologists in the preliminary dental examination of human remains, which is one of the stages of a traditional dental autopsy [28]. Data can be transmitted to the human identification laboratory, where one or more forensic odontology consultants could evaluate the data received and provide charting and the dental autopsy report [28]. Provisions on the unidentified human remains consist of the following data collection:

a. 2D or 3D video recording of the dental arches and oral cavity, using intraoral camera or smartphones (Figure 2).
b. Photographic collection of the dental arches.
c. Photogrammetry of the dental arches using an intraoral scanner (Figure 3).
d. 3D scanning of jaws and skull.
e. Intraoral radiographic collection using digital sensors.
f. Any radiographic imaging of the skull (Panoramic images, OPG, TC scans, if available).
g. Live streaming using smartphone and smart glasses (Figure 4).

By registering on the Virdentopsy website, it will be possible to choose a type of assessment, either a single unidentified human remains, or an assessment within a DVI procedure, and decide if a primary or secondary expert opinion is required. Quality control checks would be carried out on the received data. The service is remunerated or pro-bono depending on the applicant entity.

This forensic service will also be available for age estimations of living individuals and for hands-on training sessions of forensic odontology courses.

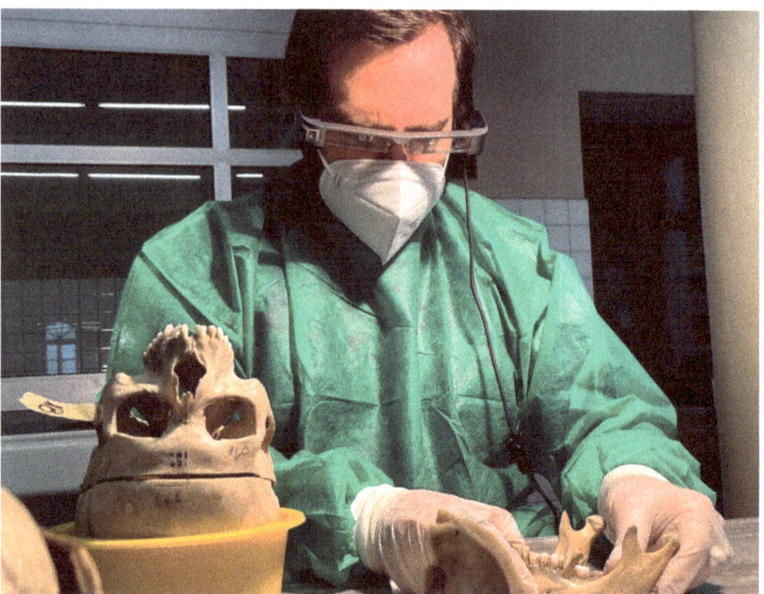

Figure 2. Operator using smart glasses to observe and record dental features on the mandible.

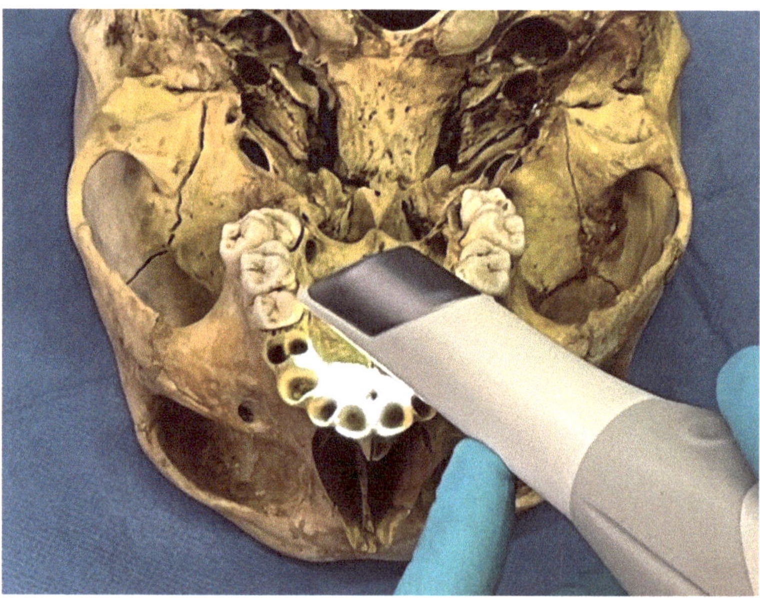

Figure 3. Post-mortem photogrammetry collection of upper dental arch using an intraoral scanner.

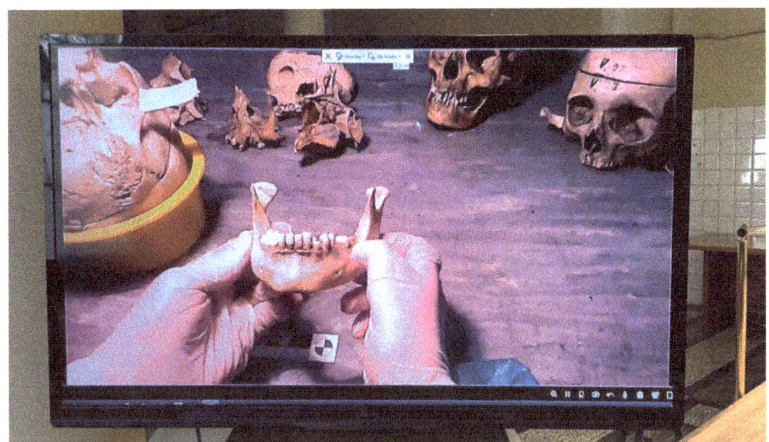

Figure 4. Live streaming images observed remotely from a forensic odontologist.

4. Discussion

The identification process of any unidentified human remains must respect best standards in forensics and should always include the collection of all identifying post-mortem data. The process requires the comparison with ante-mortem data of compatible reported missing persons and a final reconciliation of data collected. In this regard, a complete dental autopsy and further peer-review evaluation by forensic odontologists of all dental findings are crucial to achieving a generic biological profile and investigation. The simple dental examination or the collection of dental data without any evaluation performed by experts in forensic odontology and disaster victim identification does not offer any concrete contribution to the process of achieving a timely and effective personal identification. When considering the migration phenomena, there is a need for a wider collection and analysis of postmortem data [28]. In Italy, the "Missing Migrants Project" estimates that there have been 17,124 migrant deaths and disappearances since 2014, and over 60% of these victims are unidentified [29,30], while the forensic dental evaluation seems limited to a dental examination without the routine involvement of experienced forensic odontologists [31].

Virtual autopsy applications in forensic odontology involve the collection of dental data and comparison between ante-mortem and post-mortem orthopantomograms [30]. The virdentopsy process is not only the integration of a virtual autopsy in forensic odontology practice [32,33] aEs it does not rely only on radiographic imaging and CT scanning but also on 2D and 3D video, photos, and photogrammetry documentation. Virtual autopsy allows the examination of jaws and teeth by odontologists without the need to perform a traditional dental autopsy [7]. Virdentopsy broadens the horizon of this virtual approach, involving remote odontologists from various countries without the need to be physically onsite, and could become a standard of each unidentified dead body recovered.

The proposed procedure is a possible solution in the following scenarios:

- Forensic odontologists are not available on the mass disaster site or on the area of the recovery (single unidentified body of unknown nationality);
- Forensic odontologists cannot be recruited or afforded in the temporary morgue after a mass disaster;
- Forensic odontologists of the same nationalities as the victims involved in the disaster can offer remotely useful hints related to dental treatments and dental data interpretation;
- A second expert opinion on all post-mortem dental data collected could widen or confirm dental findings such as age, habits, and dental treatments, thus reducing bias;

- Archeological and paleopathological findings on ancient human remains could benefit from a complementary analysis by forensic odontologists, completing the evaluation study of jaws and teeth that are available;
- Reduce infectious risks, such as those faced during the COVID-19 pandemic, by reducing the number of experts involved in the autopsy room for the post-mortem data collection;
- Hands-on training in forensic odontology courses through live streaming using smart glasses and augmented reality.

The virdentopsy screening can reduce technical consultancy costs, as forensic odontologists do not need to be onsite; however, more importantly, it can speed up the process of human forensic identification and respect forensic human identification protocols through the complete collection and evaluation of all dental evidence, optimizing the use of human resources involved in a mass disaster scenario or a single unidentified human remains. The technology required is already incorporated in the latest generation's smartphones, making this process immediately applicable and a revolutionary humanitarian forensic odontology tool in all identification processes.

5. Conclusions

Best practices in human identification suggest the collection of primary and secondary identifiers, including post-mortem dental data. To achieve this goal, a complete dental autopsy should always be performed by one or more odontologists who are experts in forensic odontology and disaster victim identification. The virdentopsy procedure can enhance the identification autopsy through the supplementary assessment of remote forensic odontologists, providing a dental biography and generic biological profile of the unidentified human remains. Virdentopsy allows best practices in human identification when odontologists are not available onsite or when a second expert opinion is advised and can be considered a valuable humanitarian forensic odontology tool for the missing and unidentified human remains of unknown nationality, as well as an educational resource for hands-on training in forensic odontology.

Funding: This research received no external funding.

Institutional Review Board Statement: Not applicable.

Informed Consent Statement: Not applicable.

Conflicts of Interest: The author declares no conflict of interest.

References

1. Nuzzolese, E.; Di Vella, G. Future project concerning mass disaster management: A forensic odontology prospectus. *Int. Dent. J.* **2007**, *57*, 261–266. [CrossRef]
2. Disaster Victim Identification. Interpol Protocols. Available online: https://www.interpol.int/How-we-work/Forensics/Disaster-Victim-Identification-DVI (accessed on 4 July 2021).
3. International Committee of the Red Cross. Missing People, DNA Analysis and Identification of Human Remains. November 2009. Available online: https://www.icrc.org/en/doc/assets/files/other/icrc_002_4010.pdf (accessed on 4 July 2021).
4. Annexure 12: Methods of Identification. Interpol. Available online: https://www.interpol.int/content/download/5759/file/E%20DVI_Guide2018_Annexure12.pdf?inLanguage=eng-GB (accessed on 4 July 2021).
5. Nuzzolese, E. Missing People, Migrants, Identification and Human Rights. *J. Forensic Odontostomatol.* **2012**, *30* (Suppl. 1), 47–59. Available online: http://www.iofos.eu/Journals/JFOS%20sup1_Nov12/IDEALS%206-96.pdf (accessed on 11 July 2021).
6. Finegan, O.; Abboud, D.; Fonseca, S.; Malgrati, I.; Morcillo Mendez, M.D.; Burri, J.M.; Guyomarc'h, P. International Committee of the Red Cross (ICRC): Cemetery planning, preparation and management during COVID-19: A quick guide to proper documentation and disposition of the dead. *Forensic Sci. Int.* **2020**, *316*, 110436. [CrossRef] [PubMed]
7. Karim, B.; Gupta, D. Cheiloscopy and blood groups: Aid in forensic identification. *Saudi Dent. J.* **2014**, *26*, 176–180. [CrossRef] [PubMed]
8. Bernardi, S.; Bianchi, S.; Continenza, M.A.; Pinchi, V.; Macchiarelli, G. Morphological study of the labial grooves' pattern in an Italian population. *Aust. J. Forensic Sci.* **2020**, *52*, 490–499. [CrossRef]
9. Nuzzolese, E.; Pandey, H.; Lupariello, F. Dental autopsy recommendations in SARS-CoV-2 infected cases. *Forensic Sci. Int. Synerg.* **2020**, *2*, 154–156. [CrossRef]

10. Jampani, N.D.; Nutalapati, R.; Dontula, B.; Boyaoati, R. Applications of teledentistry: A Literature review and update. *J. Int. Soc. Prev. Communit. Dent.* **2011**, *1*, 37–44. Available online: https://www.jispcd.org/text.asp?2011/1/2/37/97695 (accessed on 11 July 2021).
11. Thali, M.J.; Yen, K.; Schweitzer, W.; Vock, P.; Boesch, C.; Ozdoba, C.; Schroth, G.; Ith, M.; Sonnenschein, M.; Doernhoefer, T.; et al. Virtopsy, a new imaging horizon in forensic pathology: Virtual autopsy by postmortem multislice computed tomography (MSCT) and magnetic resonance imaging (MRI)—A feasibility study. *J. Forensic Sci.* **2003**, *48*, 386–403. [CrossRef]
12. Thali, M.J.; Jackowski, C.; Oesterhelweg, L.; Ross, S.G.; Dirnhofer, R. VIRTOPSY—The Swiss virtual autopsy approach. *Leg. Med.* **2007**, *9*, 100–104. [CrossRef]
13. Perju-Dumbravă, D.; Aniþan, S.; Siserman, C.; Fulga, I.; Opincaru, I. Virtopsy—An alternative to the conventional autopsy. *Rom. J. Leg. Med.* **2010**, *1*, 75–78. [CrossRef]
14. Vadivel, J.K. Virtual autopsy. *Int. J. Forensic Odontol.* **2016**, *1*, 14–16. Available online: https://www.ijofo.org/text.asp?2016/1/1/14/185694 (accessed on 11 July 2021). [CrossRef]
15. Franco do Rosário Junior, A.; Couto Souza, P.H.; Coudyzer, W.; Thevissen, P.; Willems, G.; Jacobs, R. Virtual autopsy in forensic sciences and its applications in the forensic odontology. *Rev. Odonto Ciênc.* **2012**, *27*, 5–9. [CrossRef]
16. Tejaswi, K.B.; Aarte Hari Periya, E. Virtopsy (virtual autopsy): A new phase in forensic investigation. *J. Forensic Dent. Sci.* **2013**, *5*, 146–148.
17. Oesterhelweg, L.; Bolliger, S.A.; Thali, M.J.; Ross, S. Postmortem imaging of laryngeal foreign bodies. *Arch. Pathol. Lab. Med.* **2010**, *133*, 806–810. [CrossRef] [PubMed]
18. Aquila, I.; Falcone, C.; Di Nunzio, C.; Tamburrini, O.; Boca, D.; Ricci, P. Virtopsy versus autopsy in unusual case of asphyxia: Case report. *Forensic Sci. Int.* **2013**, *229*, e1–e5. [CrossRef]
19. Dirnhofer, R.; Jackowski, C.; Vock, P.; Potter, K.; Thali, M.J. Virtopsy—Minimally invasive, imaging guided virtual autopsy. *Radio Graph.* **2006**, *26*, 1305–1333. [CrossRef] [PubMed]
20. Berketa, J.W.; James, H.; Lake, A.W. Forensic odontology involvement in disaster victim identification. *Forensic Sci. Med. Pathol.* **2012**, *8*, 148–156. [CrossRef] [PubMed]
21. Song, X.; Liu, X.; Wang, C. The role of telemedicine during the COVID-19 epidemic in China-experience from Shandong province. *Crit. Care* **2020**, *24*, 178. [CrossRef]
22. Franco, A.; Thevissen, P.; Coudyzer, W.; Develter, W.; Van de Voorde, W.; Oyen, R.; Vandermeulen, D.; Jacobs, R.; Willems, G. Feasibility and validation of virtual autopsy for dental identification using the Interpol dental codes. *J. Forensic Leg. Med.* **2013**, *20*, 248–254. [CrossRef] [PubMed]
23. Rutty, G.N.; Biggs, M.J.P.; Brough, A.; Morgan, B.; Webster, P.; Heathcote, A.; Dolan, J.; Robinson, C. Remote post-mortem radiology reporting in disaster victim identification: Experience gained in the 2017 Grenfell Tower disaster. *Int. J. Leg. Med.* **2020**, *134*, 637–643. [CrossRef]
24. Nuzzolese, E.; Lupariello, F.; Ricci, P. Human identification and human rights through humanitarian forensic odontology. *Int. J. Forensic Odontol.* **2020**, *5*, 38–42. Available online: https://www.ijofo.org/text.asp?2020/5/1/38/288166 (accessed on 11 July 2021).
25. Yogish, P.; Yogish, A. Virtopsy: New phase in forensic odontology. *Int. J. Dent. Health Sci.* **2015**, *2*, 1548–1555.
26. Virdentopsy. Available online: https://www.virdentopsy.it (accessed on 22 June 2021).
27. Silver, E.W.; Souviron, R.R. Postmortem records. The dental autopsy. In *Dental Autopsy*; Silver, E.W., Souviron, R.R., Eds.; CRC Press: Boca Raton, FL, USA, 2009; pp. 89–112.
28. Simon, R. *Analysis of Best Practices on the Identification of Missing Migrants: Implications for the Central Mediterranean*; Central Mediterranean Route Thematic Report Series; International Organization for Migration: Geneva, Switzerland, 2019. Available online: https://publications.iom.int/system/files/pdf/identification_of_missing_migrants.pdf (accessed on 22 June 2021).
29. Olivieri, L.; Mazzarelli, D.; Bertoglio, B.; De Angelis, D.; Previderè, C.; Grignani, P.; Cappella, A.; Presciuttini, S.; Bertuglia, C.; Di Simone, P.; et al. Challenges in the identification of dead migrants in the Mediterranean: The case study of the Lampedusa shipwreck of October 3rd 2013. *Forensic Sci. Int.* **2018**, *285*, 121–128. [CrossRef]
30. Ampuero Villagran, O. *Identifying Migrant Bodies in the Mediterranean*; United Nations University Institute on Globalization, Culture and Mobility: Barcelona, Spain, 2018. Available online: https://i.unu.edu/media/gcm.unu.edu/publication/4375/Identifying-Migrant-Bodies-in-the-Mediterranean_0502.pdf (accessed on 11 July 2021).
31. Nuzzolese, E. Integration of dentistry and forensic odontology for a structured identification system and border control. *Forensic Sci. Res.* **2021**. [CrossRef]
32. Vidhya, A.; Doggalli, N.; Patil, K.; Narayan, K.; Thiruselvakumar, D.; Abirami, A. Virtual autopsy: An imaging technological integration in forensic odontology. *Int. J. Forensic Odontol.* **2019**, *4*, 2–6. Available online: https://www.ijofo.org/text.asp?2019/4/1/2/259273 (accessed on 11 July 2021). [CrossRef]
33. Rupsa, D.; Jen, S. Virtopsy in Forensic Odontology: The no Touch Autopsy. *Indian J. Forensic Med. Toxicol.* **2019**, *13*, 1883–1886.

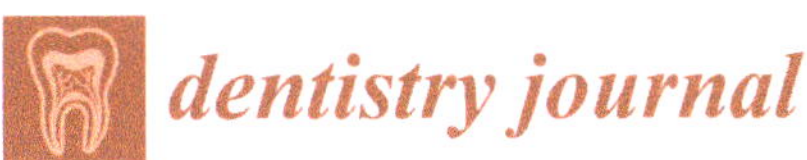

MDPI

Article

A Hands-On Exercise on Caries Diagnostics among Dental Students—A Qualitative Study

Heidi Kangas [1,†], Saujanya Karki [1,†], Tarja Tanner [1], Anne Laajala [1,2], Helvi Kyngäs [2,3] and Vuokko Anttonen [1,2,*]

1 Research Unit of Oral Health Sciences, University of Oulu, P.O. Box 5281, 90014 Oulu, Finland; heidi.kangas@student.oulu.fi (H.K.); saujanya.karki@oulu.fi (S.K.); tarja.tanner@oulu.fi (T.T.); anne.laajala@oulu.fi (A.L.)

2 Medical Research Center, Oulu University Hospital, University of Oulu, P.O. Box 21, 90029 Oulu, Finland; helvi.kyngas@oulu.fi

3 Research Unit of Nursing Sciences and Health Management, University of Oulu, P.O. Box 5281, 90014 Oulu, Finland

* Correspondence: Vuokko.anttonen@oulu.fi

† The input of the two authors was equal.

Abstract: According to current care practices, the aim is to prevent the onset of caries lesions and to stop the progression of incipient lesions. A visual lesion assessment system, International Caries Detection and Assessment System (ICDAS), has been developed to promote reliability and repeatability of assessment of different stage caries lesions. The aims of this study were to evaluate the experiences of a hands-on exercise with authentic teeth as an adjunct to lecturing among third-year dental students and to evaluate the learning process during the hands-on exercise measured by qualitative (inductive content) analysis of the given feedback. In 2018, 51 third-year dental students at the University of Oulu, Finland, participated in a hands-on exercise on caries detection, where they assessed the depth and activity of lesions in extracted teeth using the ICDAS classification. After the lecture, students evaluated the exercise, giving feedback according to five given topics, three of which were analyzed using inductive content analysis. The exercise was considered useful and necessary but, overall, also challenging. The diverse activities and materials, as well as observational methods, promoted learning. The classification of lesions, the diagnostic methods, and the fact that there was not enough time to adopt things during the exercise were found to be challenging. For developing the exercise, the students suggested that more time should be scheduled for it and there should be more individual teaching. This qualitative study showed that, despite the challenge in caries diagnostics, dental students perceive the hands-on exercise as both a communal and individual learning experience.

Keywords: dental caries; dental education; dental students; diagnosis

Citation: Kangas, H.; Karki, S.; Tanner, T.; Laajala, A.; Kyngäs, H.; Anttonen, V. A Hands-On Exercise on Caries Diagnostics among Dental Students—A Qualitative Study. *Dent. J.* **2021**, *9*, 113. https://doi.org/10.3390/dj9100113

Academic Editors: Jelena Dumancic and Božana Lončar Brzak

Received: 25 August 2021
Accepted: 24 September 2021
Published: 28 September 2021

Publisher's Note: MDPI stays neutral with regard to jurisdictional claims in published maps and institutional affiliations.

1. Introduction

Dental caries is one of the most common noncommunicable disease. On the other hand, caries is unevenly distributed in the population, i.e., it is polarized, especially in the developed countries [1]. According to the Health 2011 survey, one in five Finns in northern and southern Finland needed operative care for dental caries [2]. In the Conscripts' Oral Health Research in 2011, almost half of the conscripts were in need of operative caries treatment [3]. Caries is also common among children [4]. According to current caries care guidelines, it is important to control caries, i.e., to prevent occurrence of caries lesions and to stop the progression of incipient lesions [5]. This treatment protocol emphasizes the importance of identifying the individual risk factors of caries and detecting all lesions, including the incipient ones, and their activity as early as possible. The synthesis comprises means to influence the causes for the condition and to arrest the progression of incipient lesions or treat operatively the lesions which cannot be arrested [5].

Methods of detecting caries lesions are introduced to dental students as advised by Sculte and colleagues [6]. Lectures are the most common form of teaching in the University of Oulu, Finland, including the classifications of visual–tactile examinations, in adjunct with, e.g., fiber optic transillumination (FOTI) and radiography. Clinically, the biggest challenge for students is to detect initial caries lesions before invasive treatment is needed [7]. Visual examination usually has low sensitivity, and consequently, many lesions may go unnoticed. To improve the quality of visual examination, the ICDAS (International Caries Detection and Assessment System) classification has been developed based on which clinical signs can be used to assess the depth of lesions as well as their activity [8]. Studies have shown that the ICDAS improves distinctly the detection of caries lesions on the occlusal surfaces [9]. Similarly, the ability of dental students to assess the depth of caries lesions in extracted teeth according to ICDAS criteria after the lecture and hands-on exercise was found to be good (sensitivity 78%, specificity 87%) [7].

The aim of this study was to evaluate the experiences of a hands-on exercise with authentic teeth as an adjunct to lecturing among third-year dental students. Another aim was to evaluate the learning process during the hands-on exercise measured by qualitative (inductive content) analysis of the given feedback.

2. Materials and Methods

In the autumn of 2018, third-year dental students at the University of Oulu, Finland, were taught caries diagnostics through lectures followed by a hands-on exercise. Prior to the exercise, the lecture was summarized, covering the signs for estimating the depth and activity of different stages of caries lesions using the ICDAS criteria. In the hands-on exercise, there were 51 extracted premolar and molar teeth boiled in water and preserved in alcohol, each with at least one clinically visible enamel or dentinal lesion. A clinical digital photograph and an X-ray of each tooth had been taken before the exercise.

All the students examined the same 51 teeth with different stage caries lesions individually. At first, the students independently assessed the depth and activity of all the lesions in clinical photographs. After that, each student independently assessed the depth and activity of caries lesions of all 51 extracted teeth using visual–tactile examination and ICDAS criteria (0–6) and activity +/−. Students had the opportunity to use FOTI during the inspection. Simultaneously, they also evaluated the depth of the lesions on X-rays (mid-enamel/dento–enamel junction or outer/mid/deep dentin).

After everyone had evaluated all the teeth, each student split one tooth into two halves so that the caries lesion was visible. Each student introduced the clinically observed and radiographic findings of the tooth and evaluated the actual depth and activity of the lesion on the split tooth. They shared the clinical photographs and X-rays findings of each tooth to each other one by one using a data projector and also displayed the finding of the split tooth using the endo microscope (Leica M320 Dental Microscope, Leica Microsystems, Wetzlar, Germany). When one student was sharing the findings, the other students followed the presentations on large screens. The student also suggested a treatment plan (preventive or operative) for the lesion. The professor of cariology acted as a gold standard and gave her own opinion at the end of each student's presentation. During the exercise, the split teeth were photographed again using the endo microscope, and all material was available to the students after the teaching session.

At the end of the day, students provided feedback on the hands-on exercise on the Socrative answer platform. They were asked: 1. What helped you to learn about caries diagnostics according to the ICDAS criteria (free comments), 2. What was difficult in the exercise (free comments), 3. Was the diagnostic exercise necessary in addition to the lectures (y/n, free comments), 4. Should the exercise be developed, how (y/n, free comments) 5. What did you think about the exercise (free comments). An analysis was conducted on the contents of the answers related to questions 1, 2, and 4.

Student feedback was analyzed using inductive content analysis [10], assessing saturation for each question. Open codes were generated from open responses. Open codes indicated the core content of an open answer. The contents of the open codes were compared with each other, and the codes with similar content were combined into subcategories, which were given a name descriptive of the contents. By the same principle, the subcategories were combined into main categories. From the open-ended answers to questions 1, 2, and 4, three main categories were formed. In addition to the qualitative analysis, the subcategories were quantified by calculating how many of the subjects expressed the issue mentioned in each subcategory.

3. Results

The response rate to the survey was excellent (96%), with 49 out of 51 students responding to the feedback form on the caries diagnostics exercise. Inductive content analysis was performed on the answers to questions 1, 2, and 4. To question 3, 44 students answered that the exercise was useful in addition to the lectures, 3 did not answer and 1 thought that the lecture and/or the exercise alone would have been sufficient. In question 5, the response was an adjective (one word). A total of 42 of the responses were considered positive and 7 negative. For questions 3 and 5, no further analysis was necessary.

Figures 1–3 present the subcategories based on the feedback. The exercise offered a communal learning experience and additionally diverse working methods, materials, and detection methods. Learning caries detection was promoted by topics shown in Figure 1 using various radiographic and clinical photographs, versatile and independent working methods, and demonstration of caries lesions by splitting the extracted teeth. Interaction between the students and teachers was reported to be beneficial, too. Authenticity and the number of teeth allowing repetition were also perceived as promoting learning (Figure 1).

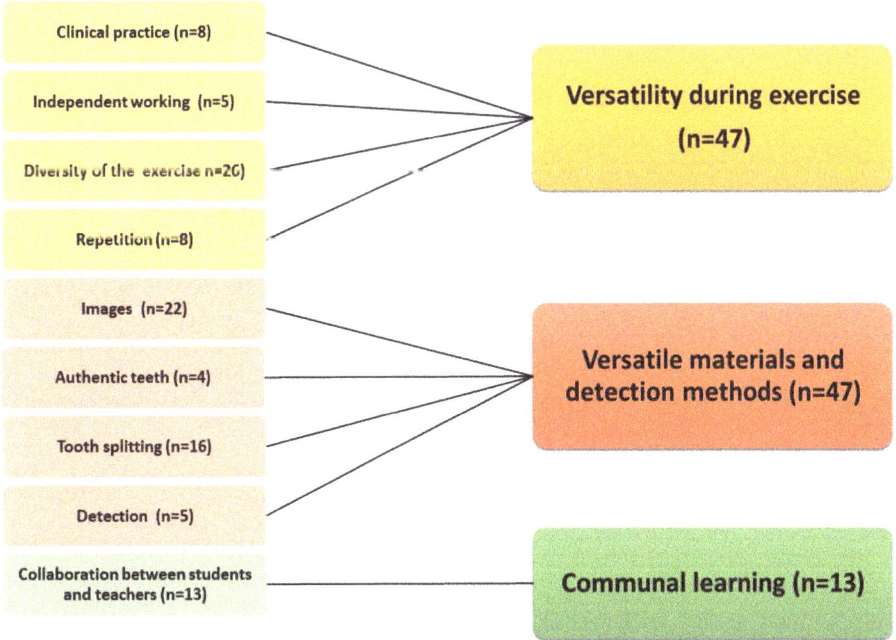

Figure 1. The topics that helped third-year dental students to learn ICDAS caries diagnostics criteria in the hands-on exercise.

The most challenging parts of the exercise were the diagnostics itself, the methods, and the learning situation. The situation was considered taxing with many repetitions. Due to the long duration of the exercise, it was difficult for some students to maintain concentration. It was also difficult to identify and distinguish between ICDAS classes, i.e., to assess both activity and depth. Interpretation and evaluation of clinical and radiographic photographs was not considered easy, nor was the use of FOTI (Figure 2).

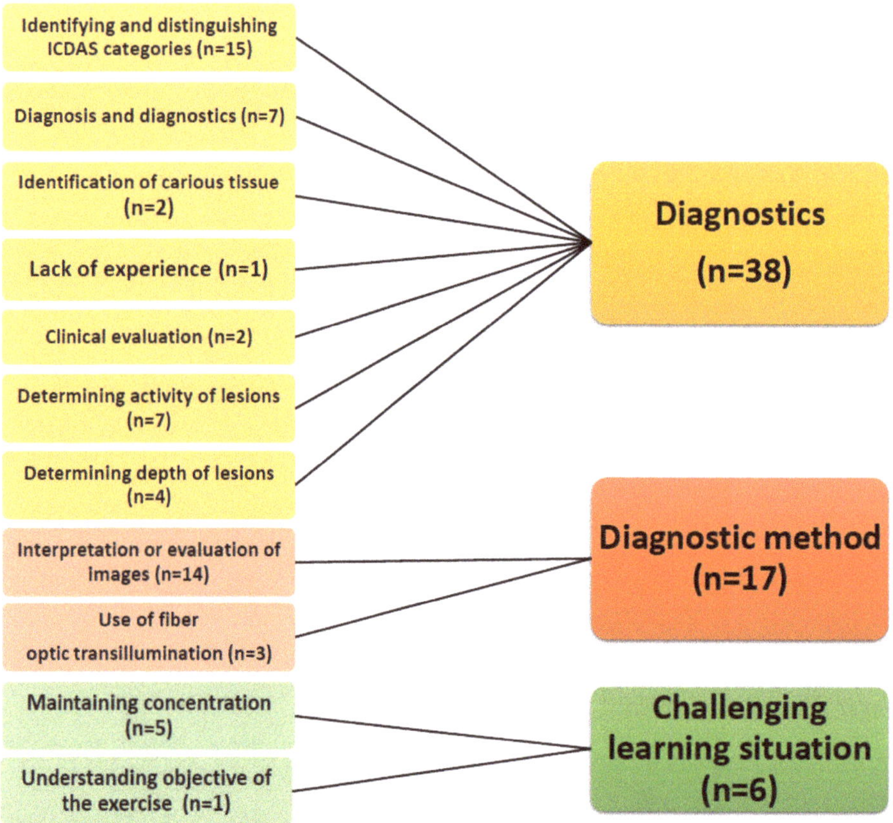

Figure 2. The most challenging issues in the hands-on exercise to introduce third-year dental students to caries diagnostics.

The fewest answers were given to the question regarding suggestions for improving and developing the exercise (n = 38). However, the students provided some developmental suggestions, i.e., teaching different diagnostic methods individually by hand (FOTI, instruments). Another suggestion was to include various sample teeth, for example, to learn to use different methods, i.e., FOTI. In particular, the students would have liked more time to complete the exercise (Figure 3).

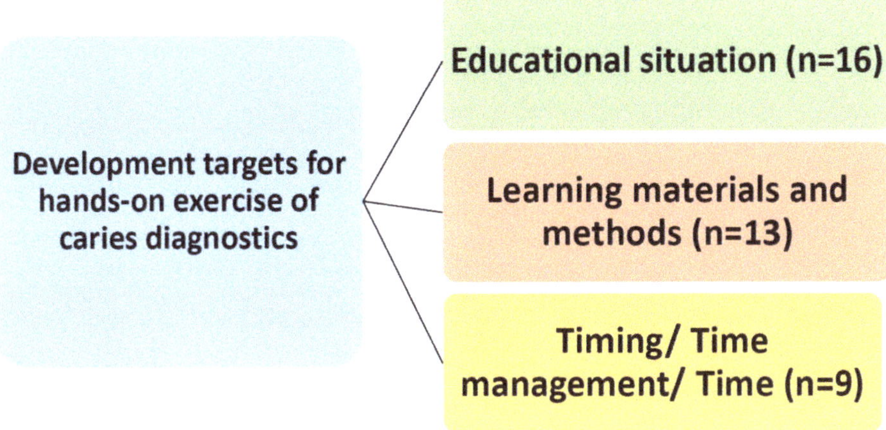

Figure 3. The topics to be developed in the hands-on exercise for third-year dental students in learning caries diagnostics.

4. Discussion

This qualitative study showed that dental students perceive the hands-on exercise on caries diagnostics as both a communal and individual learning experience. Almost everyone found practical exercise with the authentic, extracted teeth useful and necessary. The diverse methods used in the exercise complemented each other well, demonstrating various degrees of caries lesions. A benefit of such exercise was the number of repetitions. On the other hand, the exercise was considered taxing, and the exercise did not allow everyone to absorb all information during the session.

This study utilized inductive qualitative analysis developed to analyze previously uninvestigated phenomena consisting of several different components [10]. The method offered a new perspective to the teaching situation, allowing a meaningful categorization of the information obtained from feedback. Qualitative analysis thus provided important information not possible to achieve in any other way that can be utilized in the development of the teaching method in the future. To the best of our knowledge, this is the first qualitative analysis on teaching caries diagnostics to dental students. Instead, the method has been used in the past in analyses of medical education to find ways to support young teachers as they develop medical education [11].

Previous studies have quantitatively assessed the learning experience on the topic by, for example, investigating how well introduced criteria for detection of caries lesions in dental teaching have been adopted by the students [7]. This was not studied here. On the other hand, based on the research results of Zandona and colleagues [12], previous clinical experience has little relevance in learning new criteria. In their study, after lectures and hands-on exercise, there was no significant difference in the diagnostic outcomes of dental students and teachers and graduate dentists. However, it has been reported that it is difficult for both dental students and newly graduated dentists to find incipient rather than advanced lesions [7,13]. It is equally important to keep in mind that dental education is the combination of theoretical knowledge, hands-on trainings, and practices. Implication of these strategies significantly improves learning performance [14]. Learning to identify different stages of caries lesions was one of the main aims in this exercise, which, however, was not included in the analyses.

Detection of incipient lesions is important, as caries treatment increasingly focuses on controlling caries [5]. The classification of lesions has only become more common in the 2010s, which is why previously graduated dentists have no or only little knowledge of the classifications and have to learn it through postgraduate training. However, experienced dentists have the knowledge that the work brings to assess a patient's level of caries risk and estimate the lesions. Zandona and colleagues [12] report that dentists with more experience do not end up with restorative treatment in their treatment plan as often as their newly graduated counterparts. Classification of lesions according to ICDAS criteria facilitates decision-making for students and recent graduates, but most likely also benefits experienced dentists.

Almost all the students found the depth and activity exercise of caries lesions, both with photographs and authentic teeth and different additional measures, good as an adjunct to the lectures. The exercise was perceived as useful, instructive, and necessary. Thus, the aim to combine theory and practice to promote learning was achieved. The research findings are in line with the conclusions of El-Damanhoury and colleagues [13], when they reported that comprehensive caries diagnostics education requires both theoretical and practical learning supporting each other. The place of this teaching session in the curriculum or dividing it into several courses should be considered. A refresher course at the end of dental studies might be helpful. This kind of teaching could also be used to introduce caries risk assessment, treatment planning, and deciding about recall intervals [14].

Interestingly, the exercise combined individual and communal learning. The materials and methods were appreciated. Most likely, the exercise will enable learning for different kinds of learners. Having a chance to work independently and to do things with "their own hands" was also emphasized in the students' feedback, which means that doing practical implementation of theoretical knowledge promotes the learning process. The results encourage the continuance of this kind of exercise with authentic teeth in the future. At present, Finnish law allows this, as mentioned in the ethical section [15].

Regarding the learning situation, the reports emphasized the difficulty to remain focused throughout the exercise. It is possible to address this by giving enough time and opportunity for reflection on learning. In addition to people's learning differences, prior background knowledge also influences the acquisition of new knowledge. McGleenon and Morison [16] also highlighted that students are the most confident with skills in which they have prior experience. Despite a brief lecture before the exercise summarizing the main topics, it was not enough for all, and some did find the exercise difficult. The most challenging aspect of caries diagnostics was related to identifying and distinguishing between the ICDAS categories. In the future, it is worth thinking about ways to support those with poor basic knowledge in the exercise. For example, it could be useful for students to review caries diagnostic lectures independently, followed by peer-based collaborative learning and finally reviewing the exercise. Hands-on exercises on dental caries diagnosis for dental students are important for understanding and differentiating the most suitable treatment options (invasive or noninvasive) and progression (active or arrested).

The fewest answers were given to the question regarding suggestions for improving the teaching situation (n = 38). The students hoped that various diagnostic methods should be taught in even more detail, e.g., FOTI and probe. Regarding photographs, more attention should be paid to their good quality. It is important that all photographs are available even after the exercise for rehearsing. Students also wanted more time to complete the exercise, as, for example, some students did not have time to go through all the diagnostic methods properly. More time is needed, especially if new caries diagnostic methods are introduced. Teaching in smaller groups or collaborative learning could be useful, as well.

The strength of the study is that, although the study population was small, the sample size was sufficient for qualitative analysis, because the size of qualitative research data is sufficient when saturation is achieved [10]. Furthermore, students examined premolar and molar teeth during the hands-on exercise. In this study, saturation was achieved for all questions, i.e., the content of the answers began to repeat the same things that had already come up in previous answers. In addition, the material was of good quality. It described the experiences of the students in various ways. The topic of the study is important because, to our knowledge, no similar qualitative studies have been conducted before. The timing for the exercise was good, just before the start of clinical patient work, when students are motivated to learn practical things like caries diagnostics.

A practical exercise is one option for improving the learning experience of dental students in caries diagnostics in addition to lecturing. In the future, we must strive to consider the diversity of students as learners in dental education as well as aim for deeper understanding. An exercise introducing new criteria can also increase the knowledge of previously graduated dentists in the future by using an online exercise based on photographs, which were found useful. In this way, a practical exercise would provide didactically important information for pre- and postgraduate dental teaching.

5. Conclusions

In conclusion, this qualitative study showed that, despite the challenge in caries diagnostics, dental students perceive the hands-on exercise as both a communal and individual learning experience.

Author Contributions: Conceptualization, T.T., A.L. and V.A.; methodology, T.T., A.L. and V.A.; formal analysis, H.K. (Heidi Kangas), H.K. (Helvi Kyngäs) and V.A.; writing—original draft preparation, H.K. (Heidi Kangas) and S.K.; writing—review and editing, H.K. (Heidi Kangas), S.K., T.T., A.L. and H.K. (Helvi Kyngäs); supervision, V.A. All authors have read and agreed to the published version of the manuscript.

Funding: This research received no external funding.

Institutional Review Board Statement: Not applicable. As per the Finnish legislation, ethical permission is not required for the survey.

Informed Consent Statement: Finnish law on the medical use of organs, human tissues, and cells declares that samples taken for detecting or treating a disease or for detection of the cause of death may be donated for use in medical research, for the development of new methods, in quality control, and for teaching. The consent of the unit responsible for the sample must be achieved. No personal identifications can be made. The teeth in this study had been extracted from patients in the City of Oulu, Finland, to treat dental caries, periodontitis, or pericoronitis. After extraction, the teeth were donated to the University of Oulu for research and education. The identity of patients cannot be tracked in any case.

Data Availability Statement: Data are available upon request.

Acknowledgments: The authors would like to thank Päivi Haataja her help in the preparation of materials for this study. We are also grateful to all the students for their participation in this study.

Conflicts of Interest: The authors declare no conflict of interest.

References

1. Bernabe, E.; Marcenes, W.; Hernandez, C.R.; Bailey, J.; Abreu, L.G.; Alipour, V.; Amini, S.; Arabloo, J.; Arefi, Z.; Arora, A.; et al. Global, Regional, and National Levels and Trends in Burden of Oral Conditions from 1990 to 2017: A Systematic Analysis for the Global Burden of Disease 2017 Study. *J. Dent. Res.* **2020**, *99*, 362–373. [PubMed]
2. Suominen, A.L.; Varsio, S.; Helminen, S.; Nordblad, A.; Lahti, S.; Knuuttila, M. Dental and periodontal health in Finnish adults in 2000 and 2011. *Acta Odontol. Scand.* **2018**, *76*, 305–313. [CrossRef] [PubMed]
3. Tanner, T.; Kämppi, A.; Päkkilä, J.; Patinen, P.; Rosberg, J.; Karjalainen, K.; Järvelin, M.-R.; Tjäderhane, L.; Anttonen, V. Prevalence and polarization of dental caries among young, healthy adults: Cross-sectional epidemiological study. *Acta Odontol. Scand.* **2013**, *71*, 1436–1442. [CrossRef] [PubMed]
4. Pitts, N.B.; Carter, N.L.; Tsakos, G. The Brussels Statement on the Future Needs for Caries Epidemiology and Surveillance in Europe. *Community Dent. Health* **2018**, *35*, 66. [PubMed]
5. Pitts, N.; Ismail, A.; Martignon, S.; Ekstrand, K.; Douglas, G.; Longbottom, C. ICCMS™ Guide for Practitioners and Educators. 2014. Available online: https://www.iccms-web.com/uploads/asset/592845add7ac8756944059.pdf (accessed on 20 August 2020).
6. Schulte, A.G.; Pitts, N.B.; Huysmans, M.C.; Splieth, C.; Buchalla, W. European Core Curriculum in Cariology for undergraduate dental students. *Eur. J. Dent. Educ.* **2011**, *15* (Suppl. 1), 9–17. [CrossRef] [PubMed]
7. Parviainen, H.; Vähänikkilä, H.; Laitala, M.-L.; Tjäderhane, L.; Anttonen, V. Evaluating performance of dental caries detection methods among third-year dental students. *BMC Oral Health* **2013**, *13*, 70. [CrossRef] [PubMed]
8. Pitts, N.B.; Ekstrand, K.R. ICDAS Foundation. International Caries Detection and Assessment System (ICDAS) and its International Caries Classification and Management System (ICCMS)—Methods for staging of the caries process and enabling dentists to manage caries. *Community Dent. Oral Epidemiol.* **2013**, *41*, e41–e52. [CrossRef] [PubMed]

9. Diniz, M.B.; Lima, L.M.; Santos-Pinto, L.; Eckert, G.J.; Zandoná, A.G.F.; Cordeiro, R.D.C.L. Influence of the ICDAS E-Learning Program for Occlusal Caries Detection on Dental Students. *J. Dent. Educ.* **2010**, *74*, 862–8688. [CrossRef] [PubMed]
10. Elo, S.; Kyngäs, H. The qualitative content analysis process. *J. Adv. Nurs.* **2008**, *62*, 107–115. [CrossRef] [PubMed]
11. Browne, J.; Webb, K.; Bullock, A. Making the leap to medical education: A qualitative study of medical educators' experiences. *Med. Educ.* **2018**, *52*, 216–226. [CrossRef] [PubMed]
12. Zandona, A.G.; Al-Shiha, S.; Eggertsson, H.; Eckert, G. Student versus faculty performance using a new visual criteria for the detection of caries on occlusal surfaces: An in vitro examination with histological validation. *Oper. Dent.* **2009**, *34*, 598–604. [CrossRef] [PubMed]
13. El-Damanhoury, H.M.; Fakhruddin, K.S.; Awad, M.A. Effectiveness of teaching International Caries Detection and Assessment System II and its e-learning program to freshman dental students on occlusal caries detection. *Eur. J. Dent.* **2014**, *8*, 493–497. [CrossRef] [PubMed]
14. Varvara, G.; Bernardi, S.; Bianchi, S.; Sinjari, B.; Piattelli, M. Dental Education Challenges during the COVID-19 Pandemic Period in Italy: Undergraduate Student Feedback, Future Perspectives, and the Needs of Teaching Strategies for Professional Development. *Healthcare* **2021**, *9*, 454. [CrossRef] [PubMed]
15. Finlex, Laki Lääketieteellisestä Tutkimusesta. Available online: http://www.finlex.fi/fi/laki/ajantasa/1999/19990488 (accessed on 20 November 2020).
16. McGleenon, E.L.; Morison, S. Preparing dental students for independent practice: A scoping review of methods and trends in undergraduate clinical skills teaching in the UK and Ireland. *Br. Dent. J.* **2021**, *230*, 39–45. [CrossRef] [PubMed]

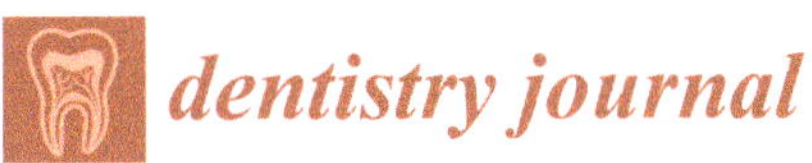

MDPI

Article

The Impact of the COVID-19 Pandemic on Dental Education: An Online Survey of Students' Perceptions and Attitudes

Ana Badovinac [1], Matej Par [2], Laura Plančak [3], Marcela Daria Balić [4], Domagoj Vražić [1], Darko Božić [1] and Larisa Musić [1,*]

1 Department of Periodontology, School of Dental Medicine, University of Zagreb, HR-10000 Zagreb, Croatia; badovinac@sfzg.hr (A.B.); vrazic@sfzg.hr (D.V.); bozic@sfzg.hr (D.B.)

2 Department of Endodontics and Restorative Dentistry, School of Dental Medicine, University of Zagreb, HR-10000 Zagreb, Croatia; mpar@sfzg.hr

3 School of Dental Medicine, University of Zagreb, HR-10000 Zagreb, Croatia; lplancak@sfzg.hr

4 Private Dental Practice, HR-10000 Zagreb, Croatia; balic.marcela@gmail.com

* Correspondence: lmusic@sfzg.hr; Tel.: +385-1480-2219

Abstract: Purpose: Dental education institutions worldwide experienced disruptive changes amid the COVID-19 pandemic, with a rapid switch to the online learning format. Thus, this study aimed to assess the impact of the COVID-19 pandemic on dental education and evaluates the perceptions and attitudes of students towards the introduction of online learning in the School of Dental Medicine in Zagreb, Croatia. Methods: A survey was conducted on a population of undergraduate students. It was comprised of perceptions and attitudes of students on the impact of the COVID-19 pandemic on their psychoemotional status, changes introduced in the educational system, and online learning in particular. Results: Of the 352 students that completed the survey, 66.2% of students reported being psychoemotionally affected by the lockdown. The most significant impact of the switch from in-person to online learning was observed in terms of missing contact with lecturers (60.3%) and peers (90.3%) and loss of practical courses, regarding which 65% of students agreed that they could not be compensated. While only 36.1% reported that online teaching fully met their expectations, the majority of the students (61.9%) agreed that online lectures were as valuable as in-person lectures and that the theoretical courses could be carried out online in the future as well (69.9%). Conclusions: Students reported relative satisfaction with changes in the learning format and a positive attitude towards online learning; however, several challenges and obstacles were identified.

Keywords: dental education; dental students; online learning; COVID-19; surveys and questionnaires

Citation: Badovinac, A.; Par, M.; Plančak, L.; Balić, M.D.; Vražić, D.; Božić, D.; Music, L. The Impact of the COVID-19 Pandemic on Dental Education: An Online Survey of Students' Perceptions and Attitudes. *Dent. J.* **2021**, *9*, 116. https://doi.org/10.3390/dj9100116

Academic Editor: Hans S. Malmstrom

Received: 31 July 2021
Accepted: 28 September 2021
Published: 9 October 2021

1. Introduction

After less than three months of the first official report on the identification of the novel coronavirus in China, now known as SARS-CoV-2, the World Health Organisation declared a global pandemic in mid-March 2020 due to its unprecedented spread rate [1–3]. Exposure to infectious respiratory fluids was defined as the main mode of viral transmission, mostly in a non-contact manner through droplets and aerosols [4–7]. A series of behavioural and social measures, among which physical distancing, was recommended and introduced to prevent and reduce viral transmission [8,9].

Educational institutions worldwide responded by cessation of education onsite and introduction of remote learning. United Nations Educational, Scientific and Cultural Organization (UNESCO) reported that at the peak of the crisis in March and April 2020, more than 1.6 billion learners of 190 countries were affected by school closures, and some still remain affected [10]. In Croatia, all onsite university-level classes were suspended on 13 March 2020 and transferred to online learning until the end of the academic semester.

Given that the dental curriculum features theoretical education and practical training, switching to online learning, which is generally applicable to the theoretical content, greatly affected dental faculties worldwide. Early released position papers addressed the challenges dental education faced in the wake of the pandemic: the infrastructure, no access to preclinical and clinical training, and meeting the examination and graduation requirements [11–14].

Online learning is certainly not a novelty. In fact, higher education institutions initially started with online courses as early as the beginning- and mid-1990s [15]. With the development of technology, online learning has become more accessible and diverse. Synchronous online learning runs similar to traditional classes, as the lecturer and students are present in the same interactive online environment at different physical locations. Examples of this mode of online learning are online lectures/webinars, virtual congresses, or real-time chats. Asynchronous learning modes allow the students to interact with the educational material and the teacher on their own flexible schedule. Examples of asynchronous learning are pre-recorded video lessons, lectures and viewing demonstrations, reading sources and even virtual libraries, and research projects. Both modes may use features such as audio, video, text, or even interactive apps and blackboards [16].

The undergraduate study programme at the School of Dental Medicine University of Zagreb spans over 12 semesters; the first to sixth semesters include basic medical and theoretical dental and preclinical courses, while clinical courses are introduced from the seventh semester onwards. Before the COVID-19 pandemic, the teaching of all course forms was primarily delivered in person. However, the digitalisation of teaching and examination has long been introduced through a remote learning system Merlin, provided by the Croatian Academic and Research Network (CARNet). With the cessation of in-person teaching in March 2020, synchronous (Zoom Cloud Meetings, Google Meet, Skype) and asynchronous (Merlin) formats were exclusively used to deliver online lessons until the end of the academic semester. The examination and assessment of knowledge were also conducted remotely, using synchronous formats. As the epidemiological situation improved, certain examinations were conducted in person under particular conditions (use of personal protective equipment (PPE), maintenance of physical distance, maximum 2 students).

In 2021 we are witnessing a gradual return of in-person educational activities. However, due to the unpredictability of the contagion and subsequent public health policies, the development of flexible curricula inclusive of online learning is adamant. Wagner et al. [17] highlighted that the success of online learning lies in the rate to which it meets the needs and addresses the concerns of the key stakeholders. Students, in fact, represent one of the stakeholder groups as they are the direct consumers of online learning. Creating an effective framework for it requires identifying barriers and enablers/solutions [18,19].

The aim of this study was to assess the impact of the COVID-19 pandemic on dental education and evaluate the perceptions and attitudes of students towards the introduced online learning in the School of Dental Medicine in Zagreb, Croatia.

2. Materials and Methods

2.1. Study Design

This is a cross-sectional observational study that was conducted using an electronically distributed survey on a population of undergraduate students enrolled in the academic year 2019/2020.

2.2. Ethical Considerations

The study was approved by the Ethics Committee of the School of Dental Medicine (No: 05-PA-30-XIX-9/2020). Participant information and a consent form were provided in written form before the beginning of the survey. Participation was voluntary and anonymous, and the participants could withdraw at any point.

2.3. Survey

A survey was developed for the purpose of this study. It was prepared in Google Forms and sent via e-mail to all of the undergraduate students enrolled in the academic year 2019/2020. The survey was conducted in September 2020, after the official end of the summer exam session. It was open for a total of two weeks, and a reminder was sent after four and ten days. As it was stated in the participant information, the statements referred to the period of the switch from in-person to remote learning during Croatia's lockdown and until the end of the academic semester and exam session.

The survey was created de novo for the purpose of this study by a group of four researchers with previous experience in dental education research, one postgraduate student, and one undergraduate student. The development commenced with a focus group discussion. Next, a pool of preliminary statements was made based on the main research question. The questions were further refined, divided into thematic sections, and the final number was reached upon mutual agreement. The first section on sociodemographic data included information regarding gender, age, year of study, place of residence, and living circumstances during the "lockdown" period. The second section of three statements focused on the self-perceived psychological impact of the SARS-CoV-2 contagion and the introduction of strict public health policies and measures. The third section consisted of 15 statements on attitudes and opinions about changes introduced to learning and teaching during the pandemic and loss of clinical practice in the summer semester 2019/20. Finally, the fourth part was assessed through 15 statements attitudes and perceptions of online learning and teaching. Participants evaluated their agreement with the statements on a five-point Likert type scale, ranging from 1 (strongly disagree) to 5 (strongly agree).

2.4. Data Analysis

Responses "completely disagree" and "disagree" were regarded as disagreement with the statement, while "agree" and "completely agree" as an agreement. The statement "neither agree nor disagree" was regarded as a neutral response. Categorical data were reported as frequencies and percentages, whereas the data for the Likert type scale were represented by mean $\pm$ SD. Differences in responses to statements S1–S33 between genders, as well as between the groups of preclinical and clinical students, were tested using a two-tailed t-test for independent observations and homogeneous variance [20]. An explanatory factor analysis using principal component analysis with varimax rotation was performed to investigate underlying factors explaining students' responses to S1–S33 [21].

The statistical analysis was performed using SPSS (version 25, IBM, Armonk, NY, USA) at an overall level of significance of $\alpha = 0.05$.

3. Results

3.1. Demographic Data

The demographic characteristics of the participating students are presented in Table 1. Of the 568 students enrolled in the academic year 2019/20 at the School of Dental Medicine University of Zagreb, 352 (62.0%) participated and completed the survey. The mean age was 22.5 $\pm$ 2.0 years, and 83.5% of the participants were female. According to their year of study, the proportion of respondents (%) was not equally distributed; however, relatively similar, with most respondents in their fifth year (20.2%) and least in the first year (13.1%) of study. Three hundred and eleven (88.4%) students lived with their families and 323 (91.7%) in their place of residence during the lockdown. Twenty-seven (7.7%) students were tested for SARS-CoV-2, of which six (1.7%) tested positive. Five out of six students who tested positive reported experiencing prejudice due to SARS-CoV-2 infection.

Table 1. Sociodemographic characteristics of participants (N = 352).

Characteristic	N (%)
Age	22.5 ± 2.0
Gender	
Female	294 (83.5%)
Male	58 (16.5%)
Year of study	
First	46 (13.1%)
Second	67 (19.0%)
Third	53 (15.1%)
Fourth	63 (17.9%)
Fifth	71 (20.2%)
Sixth	52 (14.8%)
Place of residence during lockdown	
In the place of residence	323 (91.7%)
In Zagreb, which isn't my place of residence	21 (6.0%)
Other	8 (2.3%)
Living with during lockdown	
Alone	12 (3.4%)
Family	311 (88.4%)
Partner	23 (6.5%)
Other	6 (1.7%)
Tested on SARS-CoV-2	
Yes, I was negative	21 (6.0%)
Yes, I was positive	6 (1.7%)
(I've experienced prejudice)	(5 (83.3%)
No, I haven't been tested	325 (92.3%)

3.2. *The Self-Perceived Psychoemotional Impact of the COVID-19 Pandemic*

Data on the psychoemotional impact of the COVID-19 pandemic is shown in Table 2. Students reported different perceptions of the viral emergence and subsequent possibility of infection versus an introduction of a radical public health measure, i.e., lockdown. Around one-third (31.3%) of students reported feeling worried and insecure about the emergence of the SARS-CoV-2, while 26.4% expressed fear about the possible infection. However, two-thirds of the students (66.2%) reported that the lockdown was the cause of feelings of anxiety and insecurity. No differences between preclinical and clinical students were observed. Female students, however, expressed more significant concern and insecurity with regards to the introduction of lockdown ($p = 0.043$).

3.3. *The Self-Perceived Educational Impact of the COVID-19 Pandemic*

Data on the impact of the COVID-19 pandemic on education and educational changes are presented in Table 3. The majority of the students (62.8%) expressed concern about the outcome of the academic year 2019/20, female students significantly more so ($p < 0.001$). In general, it seems that the COVID-19 pandemic did not necessarily influence students' perception of the academic year as more stressful, their motivation for studying, and their perception of studying as more difficult; however, significant differences in the responses could be observed among female students and preclinical students. Female students had significantly more agreed ($p < 0.001$) that the semester was more stressful than the previous ones, and both females and preclinical students agreed more that they were not equally motivated to study ($p = 0.038$ and $p = 0.014$, respectively) and that studying was more challenging during the COVID-19 pandemic ($p = 0.005$ and $p = 0.002$, respectively). Almost half of the respondents (47.1%) agreed that they had more time to study, which they have used well and have benefited from.

Table 2. The self-perceived psychoemotional impact of the COVID-19 pandemic.

	Statement	Level of Agreement with the Statement 1	2	3	4	5	Mean ± SD		p-Value Gender	p-Value Pre/Clinical
S1	The emergence of the SARS-CoV-2 made me feel concerned and insecure.	13.1%	24.1%	31.5%	22.2%	9.1%	Total	2.9 ± 1.2	0.205	0.819
							Female	2.9 ± 1.2		
							Male	2.7 ± 1.1		
							Preclinical	2.9 ± 1.2		
							Clinical	2.9 ± 1.2		
S2	The introduction of a strict public health measure, i.e., lockdown, in Croatia made me feel concerned and insecure.	2.0%	10.8%	21.0%	45.7%	20.5%	Total	3.7 ± 1.0	**0.043** *	0.490
							Female	3.8 ± 1.0		
							Male	3.5 ± 1.0		
							Preclinical	3.7 ± 1.0		
							Clinical	3.8 ± 1.0		
S3	I feel fear and concern about the possibility of SARS-CoV-2 contagion.	11.4%	28.7%	33.5%	21.9%	4.5%	Total	2.8 ± 1.1	0.128	0.688
							Female	2.8 ± 1.1		
							Male	2.6 ± 1.0		
							Preclinical	2.8 ± 1.1		
							Clinical	2.8 ± 1.0		

* Differences between genders and between preclinical and clinical students were tested using a two-tailed *t*-test. Significant difference ($p < 0.05$); 1—completely disagree, 2—disagree, 3—neither agree, nor disagree, 4—agree, 5—completely agree.

Table 3. The self-perceived educational impact of the COVID-19 pandemic.

	Statement	Level of Agreement with the Statement 1	2	3	4	5	Mean ± SD		p-Value Gender	p-Value Pre/Clinical
S4	I was concerned about the outcome of the academic year 2019/20.	7.7%	14.5%	15.1%	32.7%	30.1%	Total	3.6 ± 1.3	**<0.001** *	0.780
							Female	3.8 ± 1.2		
							Male	2.9 ± 1.3		
							Preclinical	3.7 ± 1.3		
							Clinical	3.6 ± 1.2		
S5	The summer semester of the academic year 2019/20 was more stressful than the previous ones.	13.4%	24.1%	23.6%	18.8%	20.2%	Total	3.1 ± 1.3	**<0.001** *	0.323
							Female	3.2 ± 1.3		
							Male	2.4 ± 1.1		
							Preclinical	3.2 ± 1.3		
							Clinical	3.0 ± 1.4		
S6	Due to the uncertainty caused by the COVID-19 pandemic, I was not equally motivated to study.	17.3%	22.7%	22.2%	18.5%	19.3%	Total	3.0 ± 1.4	**0.038** *	**0.014** *
							Female	3.1 ± 1.4		
							Male	2.7 ± 1.3		
							Preclinical	3.2 ± 1.4		
							Clinical	2.8 ± 1.4		
S7	During the period of strict public health measures (i.e., lockdown) studying was more difficult than usual.	19.0%	21.9%	16.8%	24.4%	17.9%	Total	3.0 ± 1.4	**0.005** *	**0.002** *
							Female	3.1 ± 1.4		
							Male	2.5 ± 1.3		
							Preclinical	3.2 ± 1.3		
							Clinical	2.8 ± 1.4		
S8	During the period of strict public health measures (i.e., lockdown) I had more time for studying, which I've used well and have benefited from.	8.2%	21.0%	23.6%	28.1%	19.0%	Total	3.3 ± 1.2	0.055	0.355
							Female	3.2 ± 1.2		
							Male	3.6 ± 1.2		
							Preclinical	3.2 ± 1.3		
							Clinical	3.3 ± 1.2		

Table 3. *Cont.*

	Statement	Level of Agreement with the Statement					Mean ± SD		p-Value Gender	p-Value Pre/Clinical
		1	2	3	4	5				
S9	I missed social contact with teachers.	5.7%	9.4%	24.7%	31.0%	29.3%	Total Female Male Preclinical Clinical	3.7 ± 1.2 3.7 ± 1.1 3.4 ± 1.3 3.9 ± 1.1 3.5 ± 1.2	0.064	**0.010** *
S10	I missed social contact with colleagues.	2.8%	2.8%	4.0%	24.1%	66.2%	Total Female Male Preclinical Clinical	4.5 ± 1.0 4.5 ± 0.9 4.4 ± 1.0 4.6 ± 0.8 4.4 ± 1.0	0.548	0.058
S11	Adaptation in knowledge assessment/examination (online exams) was a source of stress for me.	18.8%	24.4%	19.0%	24.7%	13.1%	Total Female Male Preclinical Clinical	2.9 ± 1.3 3.0 ± 1.3 2.6 ± 1.3 3.0 ± 1.2 2.8 ± 1.4	**0.034** *	0.071
S12	Adaptation in knowledge assessment/examination (oral exams in-person, with PPE—gloves and face masks) was a source of stress for me.	21.9%	29.5%	23.9%	16.2%	8.5%	Total Female Male Preclinical Clinical	2.6 ± 1.2 2.7 ± 1.3 2.3 ± 1.1 2.7 ± 1.2 2.6 ± 1.3	0.050	0.462
S13	The teachers were as available for contact and communication as usual.	5.4%	17.0%	27.6%	34.1%	15.9%	Total Female Male Preclinical Clinical	3.4 ± 1.1 3.4 ± 1.1 3.5 ± 1.0 3.3 ± 1.2 3.4 ± 1.0	0.523	0.326
S14	The suspension and loss of practical courses in the summer semester of the academic year 2019/20 can be fully compensated.	36.6%	28.4%	18.5%	8.8%	7.7%	Total Female Male Preclinical Clinical	2.2 ± 1.3 2.2 ± 1.3 2.3 ±1.2 2.5 ± 1.2 2.0 ± 1.2	0.490	**<0.001** *
S15	The suspension and loss of practical courses affected my knowledge during knowledge assessments (exams).	7.7%	18.5%	28.1%	26.4%	19.3%	Total Female Male Preclinical Clinical	3.3 ± 1.2 3.4 ± 1.2 3.1 ± 1.1 3.2 ± 1.2 3.4 ± 1.2	0.146	0.185
S16	Due to the suspension and loss of practical courses, it was more difficult to understand and adopt the study materials needed for the knowledge assessments (exams).	7.7%	19.0%	26.1%	26.4%	20.7%	Total Female Male Preclinical Clinical	3.3 ± 1.2 3.4 ± 1.2 3.2 ± 1.1 3.3 ± 1.2 3.4 ± 1.2	0.266	0.684
S17	If there was an opportunity to compensate for the lost practical courses during the summer and/or winter holidays, I would agree to that.	7.4%	11.9%	21.9%	29.5%	29.3%	Total Female Male Preclinical Clinical	3.6 ± 1.2 3.6 ± 1.2 3.5 ± 1.2 3.3 ± 1.2 3.9 ± 1.2	0.514	**<0.001** *
S18	If there was an opportunity to compensate for the lost practical courses by extending my graduate studies, I would agree to that.	35.2%	19.6%	19.6%	12.2%	13.4%	Total Female Male Preclinical Clinical	2.5 ± 1.4 2.5 ± 1.5 2.3 ± 1.2 2.1 ± 1.1 2.8 ± 1.5	0.250	**<0.001** *

* Differences between genders and between preclinical and clinical students were tested using a two-tailed t-test. Significant difference ($p < 0.05$); 1—completely disagree, 2—disagree, 3—neither agree, nor disagree, 4—agree, 5—completely agree.

As many as 90.3% of the students agreed that they had missed the social contact with colleagues. A total of 60.3% of the students missed the social contact with teachers, and preclinical students were more likely to agree ($p = 0.001$). Half of the participants reported that the teachers were available for contact and communication as usual.

The students did not seem to be particularly negatively affected by the adaptation in knowledge assessments. However, online exams and exams in presence with the use of

PPE seemed to have been a more significant source of stress for female students ($p = 0.034$ and $p = 0.05$, respectively).

Students expressed significant concerns about the loss of practical courses. A total of 65.0% of students disagreed that the lost practical courses can be fully compensated. Clinical students were significantly more likely to disagree with that statement ($p < 0.001$). Furthermore, almost half of the students, 47.1%, reported that due to this loss, it was more challenging to adopt the learning material needed for the knowledge assessments, and has, thus, affected their knowledge during the examination (45.7%).

When students were asked about the opportunities to compensate for the lost practical courses during summer and/or winter holidays, 58.8% of students agreed with this possibility, with clinical students agreeing significantly more ($p < 0.001$). On the contrary, if they were offered to compensate for the suspended practical courses by extending their study programme, only 25.6% of the students would agree to it. Preclinical students were significantly more likely to disagree with that opportunity ($p < 0.001$).

3.4. Students' Attitudes and Perception of Online Learning during the COVID-19 Pandemic

Data on the perception and attitudes towards online learning is presented in Table 4. The majority of the students (91.8%) agreed that they had all the prerequisites to follow online classes. However, 37.5% reported that they had encountered technical issues that made it impossible to follow online classes. More than half of the students (58.5%) agreed that the teaching faculty managed to organise online classes well in the short time frame, and 61.3% stated that the quality of online classes improved over time. High levels of agreement were recorded in the statements that the quality of online classes differed among subjects and among the members of the teaching faculty, 88.9% and 95.5%, respectively.

Table 4. Students' attitudes and perception of online learning.

	Statement	Level of Agreement with the Statement					Mean ± SD		p-Value Gender	p-Value Pre/Clinical
		1	2	3	4	5				
S19	I had all the prerequisites enabling me to follow online classes	0.6%	3.1%	4.5%	23.6%	68.2%	Total	4.4 ± 0.9	0.382	0.244
							Female	4.5 ± 0.8		
							Male	4.6 ± 0.6		
							Preclinical	4.5 ± 0.8		
							Clinical	4.6 ± 0.7		
S20	I encountered technical issues that sometimes made it impossible to follow online classes.	26.4%	21.6%	14.5%	26.4%	11.1%	Total	2.8 ± 1.4	0.407	0.251
							Female	2.8 ± 1.4		
							Male	2.6 ± 1.3		
							Preclinical	2.8 ± 1.4		
							Clinical	2.7 ± 1.4		
S21	During online classes, I received the same amount of information as did the previous student generations in the same period.	15.9%	23.3%	25.6%	23.9%	11.4%	Total	2.9 ± 1.3	**0.039** *	0.450
							Female	2.9 ± 1.3		
							Male	3.2 ± 1.2		
							Preclinical	2.9 ± 1.2		
							Clinical	3.0 ± 1.3		
S22	Online lectures are as valuable as onsite lectures.	9.4%	13.6%	15.1%	22.4%	39.5%	Total	3.7 ± 1.4	0.600	**<0.001** *
							Female	3.7 ± 1.4		
							Male	3.8 ± 1.3		
							Preclinical	3.4 ± 1.4		
							Clinical	3.9 ± 1.3		
S23	I was able to be more focused during online lectures than I would during onsite lectures.	12.8%	11.1%	18.5%	20.2%	37.5%	Total	3.6 ± 1.4	0.680	**0.008** *
							Female	3.6 ± 1.4		
							Male	3.7 ± 1.2		
							Preclinical	3.4 ± 1.4		
							Clinical	3.8 ± 1.4		

Table 4. *Cont.*

	Statement	Level of Agreement with the Statement					Mean ± SD		p-Value Gender	p-Value Pre/Clinical
		1	2	3	4	5				
S24	I would master the curriculum more successfully if in person/direct contact with the teacher.	10.5%	21.0%	34.1%	17.6%	16.7%	Total Female Male Preclinical Clinical	3.1 ± 1.2 3.1 ± 1.2 3.2 ± 1.3 3.3 ± 1.1 3.0 ± 1.3	0.571	**0.022** *
S25	Lectures and theoretical courses could be carried out online (virtually) in the future as well.	6.8%	8.8%	14.8%	19.0%	50.6%	Total Female Male Preclinical Clinical	4.0 ± 1.3 3.9 ± 1.3 4.1 ± 1.2 3.9 ± 1.2 4.0 ± 1.3	0.294	0.268
S26	The use of online education platforms prepared me well for further education and improvement.	5.1%	14.2%	36.4%	25.6%	18.8%	Total Female Male Preclinical Clinical	3.4 ± 1.1 3.4 ± 1.1 3.4 ± 0.9 3.3 ± 1.1 3.5 ± 1.1	0.639	**0.040** *
S27	The teaching faculty managed to organise online classes well in the short time frame.	6.3%	11.6%	23.6%	35.2%	23.3%	Total Female Male Preclinical Clinical	3.6 ± 1.2 3.6 ± 1.2 3.6 ± 1.0 3.7 ± 1.2 3.5 ± 1.1	0.750	0.186
S28	The quality of online classes differed among subjects.	0.6%	2.0%	6.8%	26.4%	64.2%	Total Female Male Preclinical Clinical	4.5 ± 0.8 4.5 ± 0.8 4.4 ± 0.7 4.4 ± 0.8 4.6 ± 0.7	0.089	0.071
S29	The quality of online classes differed among the members of the teaching faculty.	0.6%	1.1%	2.8%	26.7%	68.8%	Total Female Male Preclinical Clinical	4.6 ± 0.7 4.6 ± 0.6 4.5 ± 0.7 4.5 ± 0.7 4.7 ± 0.6	0.083	**0.004** *
S30	The quality of online classes improved over time (over the course of the semester).	4.3%	6.5%	27.8%	40.3%	21.0%	Total Female Male Preclinical Clinical	3.7 ± 1.1 3.7 ± 1.1 3.7 ± 0.8 3.7 ± 1.0 3.7 ± 1.0	0.677	0.734
S31	Online teaching influenced the amount of the acquired knowledge.	2.0%	6.0%	27.6%	38.6%	25.9%	Total Female Male Preclinical Clinical	3.8 ± 1.0 3.8 ± 1.0 3.6 ± 0.9 3.8 ± 0.9 3.8 ± 1.0	0.148	0.472
S32	Online teaching influenced the results of the exams I sat.	4.0%	16.5%	27.0%	31.0%	21.6%	Total Female Male Preclinical Clinical	3.5 ± 1.1 3.5 ± 1.1 3.3 ± 1.1 3.6 ± 1.0 3.4 ± 1.2	0.076	0.199
S33	Online teaching fully met my expectations.	10.8%	16.5%	36.6%	25.0%	11.1%	Total Female Male Preclinical Clinical	3.1 ± 1.1 3.0 ± 1.2 3.3 ± 1.0 3.1 ± 1.2 3.1 ± 1.1	0.062	0.918

* Differences between genders and between preclinical and clinical students were tested using a two-tailed *t*-test. Significant difference ($p < 0.05$); 1—completely disagree, 2—disagree, 3—neither agree, nor disagree, 4—agree, 5—completely agree.

Around one-third (35.3%) of the students agreed that they had received the same amount of information during online classes as did the previous generations in the same period. Female students had a significantly higher level of disagreement with that statement ($p = 0.039$). Nearly two-thirds (64.5%) reported that online teaching influenced the amount of the acquired knowledge, while more than half of the respondents (52.6%) believed that online teaching influenced the results of the exams they sat.

The majority of the students (61.9%) agreed that online lectures were as valuable as in-person lectures, while 69.9% of the students agreed that lectures and theoretical courses could be carried out online in the future as well. A total of 34.3% agreed that they would master the curriculum more successfully if in-person. More than half of the students (57.7%) stated that they were able to focus more during online lectures than they would during onsite lectures.

Finally, around one-third of the respondents (36.1%) agreed that online teaching fully met their expectations, while 44.4% agreed that the use of online education platforms prepared them well for further education and professional improvement.

3.5. Attitudes toward SARS-CoV-2, Teaching and Online Teaching during COVID-19 Pandemic Grouped in Dimensions by Explanatory Factor Analysis

The factor analysis identified nine principal components with eigenvalues ≥1. Of these, the first four principal components were selected as the main factors that explained the responses to S1–S33. These four principal components explained cumulatively 43.9% of the total variance. The variance percentages explained by individual principal components (1st–4th) amounted to 20.9, 9.6, 7.1, and 6.3, respectively.

The loadings of statements S1–S33 with regards to their respective principal components are presented in Table 5. The interpretation of factors and the number of statements grouped within each factor (principal component) is as follows:

1. Modality of teaching—seven statements related to various aspects of offline and online schooling;
2. Impact of distress—five statements related to learning abilities in the period of the pandemic;
3. Satisfaction with online teaching—five statements related to online teaching;
4. Response to the pandemic—four statements related to the impact of the pandemic.

Table 5. Perceptions and attitudes toward SARS-CoV-2, teaching, and online teaching during COVID-19 pandemic grouped in dimensions by explanatory factor analysis.

Factor		Statements	Loading
1. Modality of teaching	S25	Lectures and theoretical courses could be carried out online (virtually) in the future as well.	0.794
	S23	I was able to be more focused during online lectures than I would during onsite lectures.	0.776
	S24	**I would master the curriculum more successfully if in person/direct contact with the teacher.**	**−0.763**
	S22	Online lectures are as valuable as onsite lectures.	0.732
	S26	The use of online education platforms prepared me well for further education and improvement.	0.625
	S9	**I missed social contact with teachers.**	**−0.556**
	S10	**I missed social contact with colleagues.**	**−0.434**

Table 5. *Cont.*

Factor		Statements	Loading
2. Impact of distress	S7	During the period of strict public health measures (i.e., lockdown), studying was more difficult than usual.	0.862
	S6	Due to the uncertainty caused by the COVID-19 pandemic, I was not equally motivated to study.	0.827
	S8	**During the period of strict public health measures, I had more time for studying, which I've used well and have benefited from.**	**−0.685**
	S5	The summer semester of the academic year 2019/20 was more stressful than the previous ones.	0.522
	S16	Due to the suspension and loss of practical courses, it was more difficult to understand and adopt the study materials needed for the exams.	0.449
3. Satisfaction with online teaching	S27	The teaching faculty managed to organise online classes well in the short time frame.	0.814
	S13	The teachers were as available for contact and communication as usual.	0.698
	S33	Online teaching fully met my expectations.	0.656
	S30	The quality of online classes improved over time (over the course of the semester).	0.630
	S21	During online classes, I received the same amount of information as did the previous generations in the same period.	0.457
4. Response to the pandemic	S3	I was and am feeling fear and concern about the possibility of becoming infected with SARS–CoV–2.	0.752
	S2	The introduction of a strict public health measure, i.e., lockdown, in Croatia made me feel concerned and insecure.	0.748
	S1	The emergence of the SARS-CoV-2 made me feel concerned and insecure.	0.743
	S4	I was feeling concerned about the outcome of the academic year 2019/20.	0.422

Positive correlation coefficients, **negative correlation coefficients**.

4. Discussion

The present study evaluated the self-perceived impact of the COVID-19 pandemic on dental education and students' perspectives and attitudes towards online learning. The obtained data suggest a generally positive perception of online learning and its continued use in the future; however, several obstacles to a better satisfaction rate were identified.

Several published studies evaluated the psychological impact of COVID-19 on the population of students. An Italian survey of 501 university students from Rome reported that the COVID-19 pandemic put the student population at risk for psychological distress, and one of the factors associated with the increase of anxiety was the female gender [22]. A large study on 2534 university students in the United States highlighted that the majority of the respondents, 45%, experienced a high psychological impact from COVID-19 [23]. Furthermore, a Turkish study on a population of dental students reported higher anxiety scores in females and clinical students [24]. The data obtained with this present study, while limited, suggests that the most significant source of feelings of fear and insecurity in students was the introduction of a very radical public health policy/measure, i.e., the lockdown. The emergence of the novel virus and contagion with it caused distress to a lesser extent. While there is no clear explanation for this finding, it could be speculated that the lockdown represents a novel situation that is characterised by what can be evaluated as potential stressors: coping with fears and insecurity and isolation [25–27].

Interestingly, one of the identified factors ("Response to the pandemic") suggests that the students who most frequently reported feelings of insecurity due to the virus emergence, fear of contagion, and worriedness due to the lockdown also reported worry about the academic year outcome. Another of the identified factors ("Impact of distress") pointed to changes in studying activities during the pandemic period. Students who found studying during the pandemic more difficult were also less motivated to study, did not use the extra time well, found the semester more stressful than previous ones, and had more difficulties adopting theoretical material for the exams due to the loss of practical courses. Hung et al. were among the first to report on the significant impact of the pandemic on difficulties with learning, particularly focusing on school work and difficulties in finding the motivation to study [28].

Students negatively appreciated the loss of practical courses, which is in concordance with the results of Iosif et al. and Hattar et al. [29,30]. Only around 16% of our students felt that the lost practical courses could be fully compensated, and clinical students were less likely to agree with that statement. While preclinical practical courses (i.e., practicals on manikins) are undoubtedly important in dental education for developing and training manual skills, the loss of clinical hours and practice on patients can hardly be replaced during dental education. Interestingly, in the present study, almost two-thirds of students reported that they would be willing to compensate for the lost clinical hours during their winter and summer holidays. However, only one-quarter would be willing to extend their studies, with preclinical students less willing to do so. Comparatively, Hung et al. reported a significantly higher reluctance to make up for the lost educational time and clinical experience, only up to 11% of the participants, in a population of undergraduate students and orthodontic residents through reduction of winter vacation, cancelling travel plans and the extension of working hours or the working week [28].

The impact of the suspension of clinical activities on long-term students' professional competencies is not yet clear. Students themselves reported anticipating a decrease in their clinical professional skills, as highlighted in the studies by Loch et al. and Agius et al. [31,32]. Whether this may affect the quality of provided care can only be speculated.

The switch to distance learning could also be observed in terms of its social impact. A significant number of students reported missing the usual contact with the teachers and colleagues, 60% and 80%, respectively. Interestingly, one of the identified factors ("Modality of teaching") suggests that students that were less likely to report to miss social contact with their teachers and peers, suggesting less need for social interaction, also appreciated various aspects of online learning more. With the rise of distance learning, a growing number of studies are looking to identify students' personality traits and behaviours influencing their preferences for different modalities of education [33–37]. The data could be considered instrumental in structuring effective teaching and learning systems, accommodating different student learning styles.

It is important to highlight that e-learning has been used to various extents already employed in our school before the pandemic. Around 60% of students considered that the teaching faculty switched promptly to remote learning and organised the classes well in a short amount of time, and an even greater proportion agreed that the quality of classes improved over time. In another study by Puljak et al. conducted on a Croatian population of health science (non-dental) university students, the authors reported a similar percentage of agreement, 68%, with the efforts of their institutions to organise and adapt to online learning [38]. An important finding from our study in terms of possible improvements of online learning in the future is that over 90% of our students reported that the quality of classes differed significantly among different lecturers and different subjects. This may be an indicator of the need for further education of the teaching staff in the use of online tools.

A trend was also noticed concerning a factor related to "Satisfaction with online teaching". Satisfied students rated the organisation of online classes and availability of lecturers for communication positively and also reported that online teaching improved over time, met their expectations, and gave them the same amount of information as they would expect to get in regular conditions.

Some of the frequently reported challenges of remote learning in the published literature are the technical problems and difficulties with access to technology [18,19,39–41].

This presents as another disparity between the developed and developing countries. For example, while almost all of our students had all the prerequisites to follow online classes, 37.5% of them encountered technical problems that made it impossible for them to follow classes at times. Due to the unprecedented increase in traffic, CARNet, provider of the online learning platform Merlin, faced difficulties in the first period upon switching to online learning. Shrivastava et al. reported that the most common problem encountered among dental students across India was internet connectivity [39]; conversely only 5% of students encountered this problem among the population of students in Giessen, Germany, as highlighted by Schlenz et al. [42].

This study presents some limitations. As it was conducted at only one dental school, the generalisation of the results is limited. Furthermore, at the inception of the study, no validated questionnaire was available; thus, we have created a new one. The full list of statements can be found in the tables accompanying this article.

Despite the gradual return of students to classrooms, we are witnessing a change in educational systems. A complete switch back to education exclusively in presence can hardly be expected. Thus, we believe that the data obtained by studies such as ours can improve students' educational experience. As highlighted by our result, much of the responsibility for the quality and students' appreciation of delivered online courses were directly related to lecturers. Thus, we have identified the need for further education of the faculty staff in the use of synchronous and asynchronous teaching tools. As practical classes are an integral part of the dental curriculum, their omission in the long perspective is unacceptable. As practical classes are re-assumed, a high level of protective measurements must be maintained to ensure safety, particularly for clinical practices. Overcrowding should be addressed by reorganising practical classes with smaller groups of students, in a manner and to the extent that institutional scheduling allows.

5. Conclusions

The COVID-19 pandemic affected a significant proportion of our student population negatively. While the students at our school reported relative satisfaction with changes implemented to their education due to the COVID-19 pandemic and introduction of online learning, this study has identified several challenges and obstacles that need to be addressed in the future. The results of this and similar studies may be used to implement changes in the existing online learning model, tailoring it better to students' needs.

Author Contributions: Conceptualisation, A.B. and L.M.; methodology, A.B., L.M., D.V. and D.B.; software and statistical analysis, M.P.; investigation, M.D.B. and L.P.; writing—original draft preparation, A.B., L.M., D.V. and D.B.; writing—review and editing, A.B. and L.M.; Visualisation, L.M. and A.B. All authors have read and agreed to the published version of the manuscript.

Funding: This research received no external funding.

Institutional Review Board Statement: The study was approved by the Ethics Committee of the School of Dental Medicine University of Zagreb (No: 05-PA-30-XIX-9/2020).

Informed Consent Statement: Participant information was provided in written form before students moved forward with the survey. They were informed about the type and the purpose of the survey and the ability to withdraw at any point in time.

Data Availability Statement: Not applicable.

Acknowledgments: The authors would like to thank the undergraduate students of the School of Dental Medicine University of Zagreb for participation in this study.

Conflicts of Interest: The authors declare no conflict of interest.

References

1. World Health Organization. WHO Director-General's Opening Remarks at the Media Briefing on COVID-19. 11 March 2020. Available online: https://www.who.int/director-general/speeches/detail/who-director-general-s-opening-remarks-at-the-media-briefing-on-covid-19---11-march-2020 (accessed on 20 December 2020).
2. Gorbalenya, A.E.; Baker, S.C.; Baric, R.S.; de Groot, R.J.; Drosten, C.; Gulyaeva, A.A.; Haagmans, B.L.; Lauber, C.; Leontovich, A.M.; Neuman, B.W.; et al. The species Severe acute respiratory syndrome-related coronavirus: Classifying 2019-nCoV and naming it SARS-CoV-2. *Nat. Microbiol.* **2020**, *5*, 536–544. [CrossRef]
3. Lu, R.; Zhao, X.; Li, J.; Niu, P.; Yang, B.; Wu, H.; Wang, W.; Song, H.; Huang, B.; Zhu, N.; et al. Genomic characterisation and epidemiology of 2019 novel coronavirus: Implications for virus origins and receptor binding. *Lancet* **2020**, *395*, 565–574. [CrossRef]
4. Meyerowitz, E.A.; Richterman, A.; Gandhi, R.T.; Sax, P.E. Transmission of SARS-CoV-2: A Review of Viral, Host, and Environmental Factors. *Ann. Intern. Med.* **2021**, *174*, 69–79. [CrossRef] [PubMed]
5. Klompas, M.; Baker, M.A.; Rhee, C. Airborne Transmission of SARS-CoV-2: Theoretical Considerations and Available Evidence. *JAMA* **2020**, *324*, 441–442. [CrossRef] [PubMed]
6. Patel, K.P.; Vunnam, S.R.; Patel, P.A.; Krill, K.L.; Korbitz, P.M.; Gallagher, J.P.; Suh, J.E.; Vunnam, R.R. Transmission of SARS-CoV-2: An update of current literature. *Eur. J. Clin. Microbiol. Infect. Di.s* **2020**, *39*, 2005–2011. [CrossRef]
7. Morawska, L.; Cao, J. Airborne transmission of SARS-CoV-2: The world should face the reality. *Environ. Int.* **2020**, *139*, 105730. [CrossRef]
8. World Health Organization. Advice for the public on COVID-19—World Health Organization. Available online: https://www.who.int/emergencies/diseases/novel-coronavirus-2019/advice-for-public (accessed on 20 December 2020).
9. Barabari, P.; Moharamzadeh, K. Novel Coronavirus (COVID-19) and Dentistry—A Comprehensive Review of Literature. *Dent. J.* **2020**, *8*, 53. [CrossRef]
10. United Nations Educational, Scientific and Cultural Organization (UNESCO). One year into COVID-19 education disruption: Where do we stand? Available online: https://en.unesco.org/news/one-year-covid-19-education-disruption-where-do-we-stand (accessed on 21 July 2021).
11. Emami, E. COVID-19: Perspective of a Dean of Dentistry. *JDR Clin. Trans. Res.* **2020**, *5*, 211–213. [CrossRef]
12. Iyer, P.; Aziz, K.; Ojcius, D.M. Impact of COVID-19 on dental education in the United States. *J. Dent. Educ.* **2020**, *84*, 718–722. [CrossRef]
13. Machado, R.A.; Bonan, P.R.F.; Perez, D.E.d.C.; Martelli Júnior, H. COVID-19 pandemic and the impact on dental education: Discussing current and future perspectives. *Braz. Oral Res.* **2020**, *34*, e083. [CrossRef]
14. Deery, C. The COVID-19 pandemic: Implications for dental education. *Evid. Based Dent.* **2020**, *21*, 46–47. [CrossRef]
15. Kentnor, H. Distance Education and the Evolution of Online Learning in the United States. *Curric. Teach. Dialogue* **2015**, *17*, 21–34.
16. Martin, F.; Parker, M.A. Use of Synchronous Virtual Classrooms: Why, Who, and How? *J. Online Learn. Teach.* **2014**, *10*, 192–210.
17. Wagner, N.; Hassanein, K.; Head, M. Who is responsible for E-Learning Success in Higher Education? A Stakeholders' Analysis. *J. Educ. Technol. Soc.* **2008**, *11*, 26–36.
18. Regmi, K.; Jones, L. A systematic review of the factors—Enablers and barriers—Affecting e-learning in health sciences education. *BMC Med. Educ* **2020**, *20*, 91. [CrossRef]
19. O'Doherty, D.; Dromey, M.; Lougheed, J.; Hannigan, A.; Last, J.; McGrath, D. Barriers and solutions to online learning in medical education—An integrative review. *BMC Med. Educ.* **2018**, *18*, 130. [CrossRef]
20. Mircioiu, C.; Atkinson, J. A Comparison of Parametric and Non-Parametric Methods Applied to a Likert Scale. *Pharmacy* **2017**, *5*, 26. [CrossRef] [PubMed]
21. Jordan, A.; Badovinac, A.; Špalj, S.; Par, M.; Šlaj, M.; Plančak, D. Factors influencing intensive care nurses' knowledge and attitudes regarding ventilator-associated pneumonia and oral care practice in intubated patients in Croatia. *Am. J. Infect. Control.* **2014**, *42*, 1115–1117. [CrossRef] [PubMed]
22. Villani, L.; Pastorino, R.; Molinari, E.; Anelli, F.; Ricciardi, W.; Graffigna, G.; Boccia, S. Impact of the COVID-19 pandemic on psychological well-being of students in an Italian university: A web-based cross-sectional survey. *Glob. Health* **2021**, *17*, 39. [CrossRef] [PubMed]
23. Browning, M.H.E.M.; Larson, L.R.; Sharaievska, I.; Rigolon, A.; McAnirlin, O.; Mullenbach, L.; Cloutier, S.; Vu, T.M.; Thomsen, J.; Reigner, N.; et al. Psychological impacts from COVID-19 among university students: Risk factors across seven states in the United States. *PLoS ONE* **2021**, *16*, e0245327. [CrossRef]
24. Yildirim, T.T.; Atas, O. The evaluation of psychological state of dental students during the COVID-19 pandemic. *Braz. Oral Res.* **2021**, *35*, e069. [CrossRef] [PubMed]
25. Büssing, A.; Recchia, D.R.; Hein, R.; Dienberg, T. Perceived changes of specific attitudes, perceptions and behaviors during the Corona pandemic and their relation to wellbeing. *Health Qual. Life Outcomes* **2020**, *18*, 374. [CrossRef]
26. Marelli, S.; Castelnuovo, A.; Somma, A.; Castronovo, V.; Mombelli, S.; Bottoni, D.; Leitner, C.; Fossati, A.; Ferini-Strambi, L. Impact of COVID-19 lockdown on sleep quality in university students and administration staff. *J. Neurol.* **2021**, *268*, 8–15. [CrossRef] [PubMed]
27. Adam, M.; Urbančič-Rak, T.; Crnić, T. Dental Students' Discomfort and Anxiety During the First and the Second Lockdown Due to COVID-19 Pandemic at the School of Dental Medicine, University of Zagreb. *Acta Stomatol. Croat.* **2021**, *55*, 186–197. [CrossRef] [PubMed]

28. Hung, M.; Licari, F.W.; Hon, E.S.; Lauren, E.; Su, S.; Birmingham, W.C.; Wadsworth, L.L.; Lassetter, J.H.; Graff, T.C.; Harman, W.; et al. In an era of uncertainty: Impact of COVID-19 on dental education. *J. Dent. Educ.* **2021**, *85*, 148–156. [CrossRef]
29. Iosif, L.; Ţâncu, A.M.C.; Didilescu, A.C.; Imre, M.; Gălbinașu, B.M.; Ilinca, R. Self-Perceived Impact of COVID-19 Pandemic by Dental Students in Bucharest. *Int. J. Environ. Res. Public. Health* **2021**, *18*, 5249. [CrossRef] [PubMed]
30. Hattar, S.; AlHadidi, A.; Sawair, F.A.; Alraheam, I.A.; El-Ma'aita, A.; Wahab, F.K. Impact of COVID-19 pandemic on dental education: Online experience and practice expectations among dental students at the University of Jordan. *BMC Med. Educ.* **2021**, *21*, 151. [CrossRef]
31. Loch, C.; Kuan, I.B.J.; Elsalem, L.; Schwass, D.; Brunton, P.A.; Jum'ah, A. COVID-19 and dental clinical practice: Students and clinical staff perceptions of health risks and educational impact. *J. Dent. Educ.* **2021**, *85*, 44–52. [CrossRef]
32. Agius, A.-M.; Gatt, G.; Zahra, E.V.; Busuttil, A.; Gainza-Cirauqui, M.L.; Cortes, A.; Attard, N.J. Self-reported dental student stressors and experiences during the COVID-19 pandemic. *J. Dent. Educ.* **2021**, *85*, 208–215. [CrossRef]
33. Batra, K.; Urankar, Y.; Batra, R.; Gomes, A.F.; S, M.; Kaurani, P. Knowledge, Protective Behaviors and Risk Perception of COVID-19 among Dental Students in India: A Cross-Sectional Analysis. *Healthcare* **2021**, *9*, 574. [CrossRef]
34. Gherheș, V.; Stoian, C.E.; Fărcașiu, M.A.; Stanici, M. E-Learning vs. Face-To-Face Learning: Analyzing Students' Preferences and Behaviors. *Sustainability* **2021**, *13*, 4381. [CrossRef]
35. Goolsby, S.; Stilianoudakis, S.; Carrico, C. A pilot survey of personality traits of dental students in the United States. *Br. Dent. J.* **2020**, *229*, 377–382. [CrossRef]
36. Batra, M.; Malčić, A.I.; Shah, A.F.; Sagtani, R.; Mikić, I.M.; Knežević, P.T.; Krmek, S.J.; Illeš, D. Self Assessment of Dental students' Perception of Learning Environment in Croatia, India and Nepal. *Acta Stomatol. Croat.* **2018**, *52*, 275–285. [CrossRef]
37. Kellesarian, S.V. Flipping the Dental Anatomy Classroom. *Dent. J.* **2018**, *6*, 23. [CrossRef]
38. Puljak, L.; Čivljak, M.; Haramina, A.; Mališa, S.; Čavić, D.; Klinec, D.; Aranza, D.; Mesarić, J.; Skitarelić, N.; Zoranić, S.; et al. Attitudes and concerns of undergraduate university health sciences students in Croatia regarding complete switch to e-learning during COVID-19 pandemic: A survey. *BMC Med. Educ.* **2020**, *20*, 416. [CrossRef] [PubMed]
39. Shrivastava, K.J.; Nahar, R.; Parlani, S.; Murthy, V.J. A cross-sectional virtual survey to evaluate the outcome of online dental education system among undergraduate dental students across India amid COVID-19 pandemic. *Eur. J. Dent. Educ.* **2021**, 12679. [CrossRef]
40. Barrot, J.S.; Llenares, I.I.; Del Rosario, L.S. Students' online learning challenges during the pandemic and how they cope with them: The case of the Philippines. *Educ. Inf. Technol.* **2021**, 1–18. [CrossRef]
41. Singal, A.; Bansal, A.; Chaudhary, P.; Singh, H.; Patra, A. Anatomy education of medical and dental students during COVID-19 pandemic: A reality check. *Surg. Radiol. Anat.* **2021**, *43*, 515–521. [CrossRef]
42. Schlenz, M.A.; Schmidt, A.; Wöstmann, B.; Krämer, N.; Schulz-Weidner, N. Students' and lecturers' perspective on the implementation of online learning in dental education due to SARS-CoV-2 (COVID-19): A cross-sectional study. *BMC Med. Educ.* **2020**, *20*, 354. [CrossRef] [PubMed]

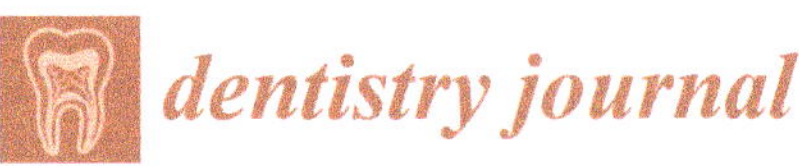

MDPI

Article

A Contemporary Evaluation on Posterior Direct Restoration Teaching among Undergraduates in Dental Schools in Malaysia

Muhammad Syafiq Alauddin [1,*], Norazlina Mohammad [1], Azlan Jaafar [2], Faizah Abdul Fatah [1] and Aimi Amalina Ahmad [1]

[1] Department of Conservative Dentistry and Prosthodontics, Universiti Sains Islam Malaysia, Kuala Lumpur 55100, Malaysia; norazlina79@usim.edu.my (N.M.); drfaizah@usim.edu.my (F.A.F.); aimiamalina@usim.edu.my (A.A.A.)

[2] Department of Periodontology and Community Oral Health, Universiti Sains Islam Malaysia, Kuala Lumpur 55100, Malaysia; drazlan_jaafar@usim.edu.my

* Correspondence: syafiq.alauddin@usim.edu.my

Abstract: There is a current trend to restore posterior teeth with composite resin due to increasing demands on natural tooth colour restoration and increased concern about the safety of amalgam restorations. The objective was to evaluate the current teaching of posterior direct restoration among restorative dental lecturers in Malaysia compared to available international literature. An online questionnaire, which sought information on the teaching of posterior restoration was developed and distributed to 13 dental schools in Malaysia. The response rate for the questionnaire was 53.8%. The most popular posterior restoration teaching methods among the respondents were lecture (95.7%), demonstration (87.0%) and problem-based learning (PBL) (73.9%), while continuous assessment and a practical competency test (82.6%) were the most popular assessment methods. Placing a hard setting calcium hydroxide and GIC base for deep cavity restored by composite restoration was taught in 79.2% of cases. The standard protocols for posterior composite restoration were incremental filling in deep cavity (87.5%), using circumferential metal bands with wooden wedge (91.7%), with a total etch system (95.8%), using a light emitting diode (LED) light curing unit (91.7%), finishing using water cooling (80%) and finishing with a disc (87.5%). Graduates from dental schools in Malaysia received similar theoretical, preclinical and clinical teaching on posterior restoration techniques, although there were variations in the delivery methods, techniques and assessments, pointing to a need for uniformity and consensus.

Keywords: dental education; composite restoration; conservative dentistry; operative dentistry; undergraduate dental student; dentin bonding

Citation: Alauddin, M.S.; Mohammad, N.; Jaafar, A.; Abdul Fatah, F.; Ahmad, A.A. A Contemporary Evaluation on Posterior Direct Restoration Teaching among Undergraduates in Dental Schools in Malaysia. *Dent. J.* **2021**, *9*, 123. https://doi.org/10.3390/dj9100123

Academic Editors: Rod Moore and Luca Testarelli

Received: 1 September 2021
Accepted: 8 October 2021
Published: 19 October 2021

1. Introduction

Composite resin restoration is one of the dental practitioner choices besides traditional amalgam restoration. Rapid advances in the adhesive technology of the resin composites have resulted in them becoming the main choice to restore carious and traumatic posterior teeth [1,2]. After all, dental amalgams are a well-proven material with durability, excellence in maintaining structural integrity of the tooth-restoration complex in the long-term, as well as less technique sensitive steps being required for it. Nevertheless, due to its metallic greyish appearance and non-aesthetical optical properties, there is a current trend for metal free restorations. Moreover, there is a continuous issue with regards to its inability to bond to the tooth structure, marginal leakage and the high occurrence of secondary caries [3,4]. Evidence shows that a well restored composite resin restoration is able to provide a high survival and success rate of the posterior restoration [3,5,6]. It is also more aesthetically pleasing compared to the traditional amalgam restoration. With growing research and improvements in modern adhesive technology and science, contemporary resin composites are able to bond properly to the remaining tooth structure and reduce common risks associated with the resin composite restorations, such as polymerization shrinkage, marginal discolouration, bulk fracture, chipping of the restoration and microleakage [7–10], There is also a current trend worldwide in reducing use of mercury in dental practices. Amalgam restorations are known to emit mercury vapour during daily activities such as drinking hot water and eating, with potential, unfavourable toxicity side effects [11]. Furthermore, the current concept of a minimal invasive approach, which focuses more on collaborative work for conservative techniques, and treatment being introduced and advocated worldwide, means resin composites is seen as a more appropriate method. This is because dental amalgam restoration technically requires the removal of unnecessary, yet sound, tooth structure to provide more mechanical resistance and retention features. Thus, it is considered less conservative than resin composite restoration [12,13].

A plethora of components on competency-based pedagogy have been introduced during undergraduate clinical years, including training on posterior teeth restorations. Arguably the competency of undergraduate students in dental schools will predict the future outcome of these graduates in clinical practice after graduation, even though the competency of dental practitioners is commonly associated with experience and years of practice [14]. Therefore, it is of utmost importance that the faculty members and teaching staff constantly evaluate contemporary theoretical and clinical teaching methods, particularly in a routine dental procedure such as restoration of the posterior teeth. Undergraduate dental students should possess and exhibit acceptable competence in this field, particularly in biomaterial science and the use of modern contemporary materials, and use appropriate techniques to perform this procedure under the guidance of faculty members.

Several nationwide and regional surveys have been conducted over the past decades to evaluate the teaching of posterior restorations, especially for composite resin, and these have shown widely varying and notable differences in teaching programmes within and among the countries where the research had been conducted [15–23]. Apart from in Japan and Malaysia, these surveys provided limited data on the teaching of posterior composite resin restorations in Asian regions [24,25]. Taking into consideration the growing interest in metal free restorations and the need to homogenize and form coherency in the teaching of posterior restoration, the rationale of this study was to assess the current standard and approach for the teaching of posterior direct restorations on posterior teeth. The aim was to evaluate the trends, extent, nature and practice of contemporary teaching of posterior restoration to undergraduate dental students in Malaysia.

2. Materials and Methods

Ethical approval for this study was granted by the local institutional ethical committee [USIM/FPg-MEC/2016/No. (45)] for a cross-sectional and quantitative methodological approach conducted from January 2019 to May 2020.

A survey questionnaire was adopted, developed and then underwent minor modifications based on previous studies [20,25,26] (see Supplementary Figure S1). The questionnaire was then administered and distributed as an online survey via Google Form with the corresponding link being sent primarily via e-mail and then via WhatsApp to the heads and lecturers of the Operative/Conservative/Restorative Dentistry Department in all 13 dental schools in Malaysia that conduct dental degree programmes. The questionnaire was made up of 36 questions with a combination of open and closed questions. The majority were multiple choice questions with predefined answers that enabled the respondents to select more than one answer. The targeted respondents, who were Heads of Department Operative/Conservative/Restorative Dentistry and senior lecturers with 5 years or more experience in teaching posterior restoration to undergraduates, were initially given 12 weeks to complete the questionnaire. A second and third e-mail reminder was sent to participants who had not responded. They were informed that their participation in this research would remain anonymous and that the results would be confidential in that no individual and dental school would be identified in any preliminary findings, reports or publications.

The information sought from the respondents comprised of (a) the teaching technique and methodology of posterior restoration, including types of assessments, (b) the practice, nature and extent of the preclinical teaching, (c) the practice, nature and extent of the clinical teaching including relevant assessment techniques and (d) the contemporary restorative protocol taught and practiced for posterior teeth restoration with composite resins. Information derived from the questionnaires were entered into a Microsoft (R) Excel spreadsheet and descriptive data analysis was then performed to express results in terms of mean, range and total percentage in order to provide coherency of the reporting style associated with previous studies.

3. Result

3.1. Response Rate

From a total of 13 dental schools invited to collaborate in this study, seven schools responded to the questionnaire, a response rate of 53.8%. The findings stated are the responses given by the participating teachers from the dental schools, with responses to all or the majority of the questions.

3.2. Contemporary Teaching Methodology and Strategies

The theoretical pedagogical components including the mode of delivery, teaching aids and materials used to supplement the delivery of the core components and contemporary assessment methods involved in the teaching of posterior restoration in Malaysia are detailed in Table 1. According to the responses received, the most favourable teaching approaches for posterior tooth restoration were formal lectures (95.7%), followed by preclinical and clinical demonstrations (87%), problem-based learning (PBL) (73.9%), tutorials (69.6%) and seminars (47.8%). As for the teaching materials used to enhance learning activities, the majority of the respondents (65.2%) favoured the use of demonstrations through teeth models as compared to the distribution of validated instruction manuals which included clinical pro forma (43.5%). When it came to assessment methods to evaluate a student's knowledge on posterior restoration throughout the undergraduate pro-gramme, a large number of the respondents (82.6%) preferred to conduct continuous assessments and clinical competency tests rather than written examinations (69.6%).

Table 1. Teaching strategies for posterior restoration (n = 23).

Teaching Strategies	N (%)
Mode of Delivery (Core)	
Formal lecture	22 (95.7)
Demonstration	20 (87.0)
Problem-based learning (PBL)	17 (73.9)
Tutorial	16 (69.6)
Seminar	11 (47.8)
Material (Supplementary)	
Instruction manual	19 (82.6)
Models	15 (65.2)
Projection slides	8 (34.8)
Video tape	5 (21.7)
Overhead projector	1 (4.3)
Assessment methods	
Continuous assessment	19 (82.6)
Practical competency test	19 (82.6)
Written paper	16 (69.6)
Self-assessment	10 (43.5)
Peer assessment	8 (34.8)
Objective structural practical exam	7 (30.4)
Objective Structured Clinical Examination (OSCEs)	1 (4.3)

3.2.1. Preclinical Simulation Laboratory/Phantom Head Teaching Programme

According to the results of this study, all the respondents agreed that the preclinical simulation laboratory practice should be a compulsory prerequisite for the students prior to treating patients during the clinical years (23 = (95.8%)). When asked about the types of posterior materials taught in the preclinical year, composite resin (*n* = 22 (95.7%)) was the most popular, then amalgam (*n* = 20 (87%)), followed by glass ionomer cement (GIC) (*n* = 8 (34.8%)) and resin modified GIC (*n* = 3 (13%)). The undergraduate students at most of the dental schools were provided with comprehensive manuals and instructions (*n* = 20 (81%)) on what was taught in class to aid them in the practice of preclinical simulation in the laboratory for posterior restorations, which mostly used both extracted natural teeth and artificial teeth (*n* = 12 (52.2%)). The schools unanimously agreed that students were required to complete a proximal amalgam and composite restoration as a prerequisite to start their clinical session. The average amount of preclinical time devoted to teaching composite resin placement during preclinical years was more than 24 h (*n* = 7 (30.4%)), followed by between 4 to 8 h (*n* = 7 (30.4%)), 12 to 16 h (*n* = 6 (26.1%)) and 20 to 24 h (*n* = 3 (13%)). During this time, the mean number of teeth required for the undergraduate to undergo training suggested by the respondents for preclinical simulation is shown in Table 2.

Table 2. The mean number of teeth needed for preclinical simulation laboratory practice (*n* = 23).

Type of Cavity	Type of Restoration							
	Amalgam				Composite			
	Range	Premolar Mean (±SD)	Range	Molar Mean (±SD)	Range	Premolar Mean (±SD)	Range	Molar Mean (±SD)
Shallow cavity	0–3	1.09 (±0.85)	0–4	1.43 (±0.93)	0–3	1.26 (±0.81)	0–3	1.29 (±0.78)
Moderate cavity	1–4	1.70 (±0.77)	-	-	1–3	1.52 (±0.67)	1–3	1.48 (±0.68)
Deep cavity	0–4	1.52 (±0.95)	1–4	1.67 (±0.86)	0–3	1.48 (±0.79)	1–3	1.43 (±0.60)

3.2.2. Clinical Teaching Programme

The majority of the respondents stated that the teaching of amalgam restorations as a choice for posterior tooth restorative material was still relevant (*n* = 20 (83.4%)) except for 16.7% (*n* = 4) of respondents who responded otherwise. In this regard, the undergraduate students were required to complete amalgam restorations (*n* = 21 (87.5%)) and composite restorations (*n* = 22 (97.1%)), respectively, as part of their prerequisite requirement prior to the final examination during the 5th year of their undergraduate study.

Several assessment methods were used to evaluate the clinical competency of the undergraduate students. Among them were a clinical competency examination (*n* = 21 (87.5%)), followed by an objective structural clinical examination (OSCE) (*n* = 14 (58.3%)) and self-assessment (*n* = 10 (41.7%)). The least favoured assessments utilized by the dental schools were peer review/assessment (*n* = 5 (20.8%) (and viva voce examination (*n* = 7 (29.2%)).

3.3. *The Management of Operatively and Partially Exposed Dentine*

In the management of a moderate cavity depth restored using the amalgam restoration technique, no liner/base (45.8%) and hard setting calcium hydroxide (45.8%) and GIC base were preferred by respondents. The options selected were similar for composite resin restoration with no liner/base (50%) and hard setting calcium hydroxide (54.2%) considered as the most favourable options. In a deep cavity situation, the combination of hard setting calcium hydroxide liner and GIC base were the preferred options for both the amalgam (91.7%) and composite restoration (71.2%). As for a shallow cavity depth, none of the respondents reported teaching the use of cavity liner and/or base. The rest of the materials taught the use of liners, and the results are summarized in Table 3.

Table 3. The use of liners/base prior to the placement of restoration in Malaysia dental schools (n = 24).

Cavity Depth	Type of Restoration	
	Amalgam	Composite
	N (%)	N (%)
Moderate		
No liner/base	11 (45.8)	12 (50.0)
GIC (base)	8 (33.3)	9 (37.5)
Hard-setting calcium hydroxide (liner)	8 (33.3)	13 (54.2)
Hard-setting calcium hydroxide (liner) + GIC base	11 (45.8)	7 (29.2)
Deep		
No liner/base	4 (16.7)	4 (16.7)
GIC (base)	6 (25.0)	8 (33.3)
Hard-setting calcium hydroxide (liner)	7 (29.2)	9 (37.5)
Hard-setting calcium hydroxide (liner) + GIC base	22 (91.7)	19 (79.2)

3.4. Restorative Materials Recommendation and Placed Sites on the Posterior Teeth

Maxillary and mandibular molars were the two most recommended and commonly placed sites for amalgam restorations, while maxillary and mandibular premolars were the most recommended and commonly placed sites for composite restorations. On the other hand, there were one (4.2%) and two (8.3%) respondents who recommended using GIC as an option to restore posterior sites. Further details and distribution with regards to the recommended and commonly placed restorative materials on posterior sites are summarized in Table 4.

Table 4. Restorative materials taught for posterior tooth (n = 24).

Posterior Sites	Type of Restoration		
	Amalgam	Composite	GIC
	N (%)	N (%)	N (%)
Recommended			
Maxillary premolar	7 (29.2)	22 (91.7)	1 (4.2)
Maxillary molar	18 (75.0)	18 (75.0)	1 (4.2)
Mandibular premolar	7 (29.2)	23 (95.8)	1 (4.2)
Mandibular molar	18 (75.0)	17 (70.8)	1 (4.2)
Commonly placed			
Maxillary molar	15 (62.5)	15 (62.5)	2 (8.3)
Mandibular premolar	5 (20.8)	20 (83.3)	2 (8.3)
Mandibular molar	14 (58.3)	16 (66.7)	2 (8.3)
Maxillary premolar	5 (20.8)	20 (83.3)	2 (8.3)

3.5. Contemporary Operative Techniques Utilised in Dental Schools in Malaysia

3.5.1. Moisture Control

All the respondents from various schools were in agreement that rubber dams were mandatory for composite restorations of posterior teeth (n = 24 (100%)). They were most commonly used to isolate the operative site for the placement of a posterior amalgam (n = 16 (66.7%)) and GIC (n = 18 (75%)), respectively. Besides the use of rubber dams, cotton rolls were considered as suitable alternative isolation tools for amalgam (n = 12 (50%)) and GIC (n = 8 (33.3%)) restorations.

3.5.2. Beveling Technique

The most common technique taught to dental students was beveling the proximal box margins (n = 18 (75%)), followed by beveling the occlusal margin (n = 15 (62.5%)).

Nevertheless, about 12.5% (n = 3) of the respondents reported not teaching any beveling techniques for posterior composite restorations.

3.5.3. Adhesive

When asked about the adhesive bonding technique taught in dental schools in Malaysia, the majority of the respondents reported teaching the total etch system (n = 23 (95.8%)), whereas 45.8% (n = 11) of the respondents taught the self-etch technique for posterior composite resin restorations.

3.5.4. Interproximal Matrix and Wedging Techniques

As for the isolation and wedge technique, a circumferential metal band with a wooden wedge (n = 22 (91.7%)) was the most common taught technique, followed by the sectional matrix system (n = 12 (50%)), sectional metal band with wooden wedge (n = 11 (45.8%)) and transparent matrix band with a light-transmitting wedge (n = 9 (37.5%)).

3.5.5. Restorative Technique

According to the survey, the most common composite restoration technique taught for both deep and moderate cavity for composite restorations was incremental fill, with scores of 87.5% (n = 21) and 83.3% (n = 20), respectively. Nevertheless, 16.7% (n = 4) and 20.8% (n = 5) of the respondents reported teaching the bulk fill technique in deep and moderate cavity respectively.

3.5.6. Light Curing Technologies

The majority of the respondents taught the students using a light-emitting diode (LED) curing light (n = 22 (91.7%)), and a small number of the respondents (n = 2 (8.3%)) reported still teaching the use of a "traditional" quartz-tungsten-halogen curing light for posterior composite restorations.

3.5.7. Finishing Techniques

There was a considerable variety of finishing instruments used after completion of posterior restorations. Finishing discs and finishing strips were the most common finishing techniques taught, with scores of 87.5% and 75%, respectively. The utilization of diamond burs as one of the materials for finishing was the least taught in the dental schools (45.8%). Table 5 shows the variety of finishing technique/instruments taught for posterior restoration training in the dental schools in Malaysia.

Table 5. Taught finishing technique/materials for posterior restoration taught in Malaysia (n = 24).

Instruments/Devices	N	%
Diamond burs	11	45.8
Tungsten carbide (TC) burs	14	58.3
Finishing discs	21	87.5
Finishing strips	18	75.0
With water cooling	20	80
Without water cooling	5	20

4. Discussion

The overall participating response rate of dental schools, 53.8% (n = 7), in this study was among the lowest compared to previous surveys of a similar nature. The authors were not able to increase the response rate despite multiple attempts made to reach out to the selected dental schools. The initial part of the study focused on assessing the teaching strategies and methodology used for posterior restorations in Malaysia, as they had not been highlighted by other studies previously. The results of this study indicated that the respondents were almost in complete agreement that formal lectures and preclinical and clinical demonstrations formed a fundamental and integral part of teaching about posterior restorations. This has been reinforced in multiple studies and through surveys derived from dental students that revealed the teaching strategies used allowed comprehensive two-way interaction between the learners and the lecturers, with positive results achieved compared to other methods [27,28]. The majority (n = 19 (82.6%)) of the lecturers supplied a comprehensive instruction manual to their students. The materials were conventionally adopted from various guidelines that originated from manufacturers' guidelines, recommendations from international professional bodies and societies, and fundamental core textbooks and literature in the respective fields. In assessing students, the two most popular assessment modalities reported were continuous assessments throughout the undergraduate years of study and practical competency tests. In assessing posterior restorations, the faculty members must first determine the desired learning outcome before selecting the assessment method, as the selection should be done according to the conventional outcome-based curriculum rather than the teacher-input-orientated traditional curriculum. The assessments conducted in the dental schools in Malaysia were made up of quizzes, mini examinations, clinical assessments and competency performance assessments designed in accordance with the four levels of Miller's Pyramid of clinical competence and the affective, psychomotor and affective domains in Bloom's Taxonomy of theoretical educational framework [29–32]. In this modern technological age, digital education implementation in posterior restoration teaching, such as e-learning and internet web-based education, is more desirable due to their practicality in facilitating the overall learning experience between students, lecturers, and faculty members. However, the findings for this are not reported in this study [33].

Prior to assessing dental students, the training carried out for them in various undergraduate dentistry programmes plays a major role at every step of the way. These students acquire the necessary theoretical knowledge at different stages of their studies and are assessed from time to time before they are finally ready for a clinical training placement mimicking the future roles as professional healthcare providers in a work setting. The fundamental challenge during this educational journey is to bridge these two training stages through gradual preclinical training. This integral training equips the undergraduates with the necessary skills to apply and integrate during theoretical and clinical practice prior to their clinical placement [34,35]. In this survey, the respondents unanimously agreed (100%) that the undergraduate dental students must complete preclinical training, as well as the restoration of proximal amalgam and composite, prior to any clinical training placements. Amalgam and composite resin restoration trainings had almost the same distribution in terms of the number of teeth (preclinical exercise) required to be completed during preclinical training, despite the prediction, based on previous studies, that amalgam restoration training might undergo marked reduction in the near future [16]. A clear majority of the restorative lecturers concluded that amalgam is still relevant to be taught in the dental curricular (83.4%). Apart from findings in Japan, the findings in this study were consistent with previous surveys which concluded that preclinical and clinical training of amalgam restoration is still relevant and considered as common practice in the UK, Germany, Austria and Switzerland [15,16,24–26,36]. Nevertheless, the Malaysia National Oral Health Survey (NOHSA) is on board to follow the call set by the global trend on phasing out amalgam, and it is perhaps beneficial to note that possible reduction on the preclinical training of amalgam restoration by using other suitable alternative materials will be implemented in the near future in the dental schools in Malaysia. However, other technical aspects, such as didactic training on repairing and maintaining existing restored amalgam of dental patients in Malaysia, should not be neglected [37,38]. It is regrettable that the authors were not able to compare the differences on preclinical training time dedicated between amalgam and composite resin restoration due to the inconsistent answers provided and the limited replies given for this section, as opposed to reports obtained from other studies [19,39].

It is noteworthy that one of the findings of this study indicated that the conventional teaching of placing a liner underneath an amalgam and composite restoration was considered not unusual in the dental schools in Malaysia. This is in contrast to the findings of other surveys of the same nature [15,18]. The routine practice of placing a liner underneath a composite restoration in a deep cavity is somehow controversial, and is considered an unnecessary step in moderately deep cavities [40]. The addition of a liner occupies part of the space for a composite resin bonding area, thus reducing the efficacy and effectiveness of the dentin bonding capability of the adhesive system. On another note, almost all the participating dental schools unanimously agreed to practicing the total etch system (95.8%), which, theoretically, is able to increase the sealing of dentine after effective selective etching [41,42]. The total etch system is able to ensure the effective removal of the smear layer after cavity preparation, which then promotes the ability of the adhesive resin system to permeate and seal the dentine. This prevents the need for lining materials to be used as additional protection [43]. Another finding in the study showed that the setting of calcium hydroxide, Ca(OH)2, was routinely taught as the only liner material, or to be used in combination with GIC. The biomechanical properties of Ca(OH)2 include its brittle nature and high solubility [41,42]. This has a negative impact upon polymerisation shrinkage of the composite resin, as it leaves the residual Ca(OH)2 exposed to undesired physical changes. When this happens, microleakage might follow, which then allows localised bacterial migration that might lead to recurrent caries. Anecdotal evidence that indicates a lining placement is able to inhibit hybrid layer degradation, and function as an antibacterial layer, has been refuted by previous evidence [44,45]. Rather, the traditional thought is that linings are placed in deep cavities for amalgam restorations to provide thermal insulation to the vital dentine and also for planned deep carious dentine remineralisation [41,43].

In this survey, the results indicated that the participants were more inclined towards teaching that the composite resin should be routinely placed on the premolar site while amalgam restorations should be mostly performed at the molar site. This is in line with previous studies that showed that amalgam has a high survival rate, with the majority of studies reporting more than 85% survival rate in an extensive cavities [46–48]. Moreover, composite resin restoration also has a low failure rate, with the majority of studies reporting an annual failure rate of less than 5%, thus making it a desirable material of choice for posterior teeth [1]. To ensure predictable and successful longevity of a posterior resin restoration, multiple studies concluded that there was a necessity to introduce caries preventive measures, or at least good caries control methods [3,5]. Nonetheless, despite the abundance of evidence showing the longevity of an amalgam restoration, necessary steps and plans are required by the operative dentistry community worldwide to support the global call to reduce the usage of amalgam as a restorative material.

Another finding from this study is in relation to the matrix and wedge technique used, with almost all respondents (91.7%) agreeing that the circumferential metal band with wooden wedge was commonly taught and practised in undergraduate dentistry programmes. This finding is consistent with surveys from other studies, which proves that the utilisation of this technique provided a more reliable posterior restoration outcome especially with Class II composite resin restorations [15,16,18,49–51]. Transparent matrices and stiff wedges, such as light-transmitting wedges, are nonrigid and are pliable in nature. This may cause possible mechanical deformation during clinical application especially during a composite resin restoration. Unlike amalgam, composite resin is unable to exert adequate physical force to hold the matrix system. This further complicates the conformity of the restoration in achieving proximal contact tightness with the adjacent teeth, which then results in a proximal overhang, open proximal contact and inappropriate contour [49]. Another point to note from this survey is that all the respondents from various backgrounds and schools agreed that rubber dams were considered mandatory for composite resin restorations. This finding was heavily reflected in this survey, and comparable to others of similar nature [15,16,18,20]. According to this survey, apart from cotton roll isolation, rubber dams were extensively used for amalgam and GIC posterior restorations as a precautionary measure. Composite resin restoration is a hydrophobic material and involves a technique-sensitive procedure. If it exposed to moisture intraorally, this might complicate successful bonding to the tooth structure. As such, common clinical conditions and situations, such as the presence of a deep subgingival margin, or the patient's inability to tolerate rubber dams might be the most common contraindication for the application of rubber dams [18].

Some studies noted that confusion over additional beveling of the occlusal and proximal box margin in posterior restorations was influenced by the construction of beveling in anterior composite resin restorations [52]. Additional beveling in those locations can result in a number of disadvantages including improper marginal adaptation of the restoration at the tooth-restoration-matrix system area, the removal of unnecessary enamel structure that is paramount for effective bonding, thin composite resin residue at the beveling location of the cavosurface margin resulting in the possibility of a composite resin fracture or chipped restorations under physiological masticatory load in the future, and difficulties for the operators to identify between tooth tissues and composite resin restoration in future operative repair work. Regrettably, only 12.5% of the respondents thought that beveling in the proximal and occlusal margin was unnecessary, unlike those from the Spanish dental schools survey [16,18,23,24].

The majority of the restorative dentistry lecturers taught students to use a conventional light emitting diode (LED) curing light (97.1%). This finding represents one of the highest scores for this survey criterion as compared to the Japanese and Spanish dental school surveys [18,24]. Contemporary LED light curing units are, allegedly, able to provide more depth of cure, generate less heat, and have exceptional power and light intensity with less light exposure time, and are comparable, if not more effective, than traditional quartz tungsten halogen light curing units [53,54]. This survey also found that 37.5% of the respondents taught the bulk-fill composite resin technique in undergraduate dentistry programmes when compared to previous surveys of a similar nature [15]. Even though numerous studies showed that bulk fill composite resins are more controversial in their physical and biomechanical properties compared to other types and techniques of composite resin restorations, their feasibility and their major advantage of being able to reduce the chairside time makes them very attractive in dental practices [55–58].

In a recent publication by Sidhu, P. et al., in 2021, the study was similar in nature to the current study [59]. The respondents in the study included all the Heads of Conservative/Operative Dentistry Department, while in our study the questionnaire was sent to heads and lecturers who had a minimum of 5 years of teaching posterior restoration experience to undergraduates within the Operative/Conservative/Restorative Dentistry Department in all 13 dental schools in Malaysia. In the management of operatively and partially exposed dentine, both studies concluded that there should be no liners used in shallow cavities. According to this study, the combination of Ca(OH)2 and GIC was commonly taught and utilised as a lining material for amalgam (n = 22 (91.7%)) and resin composite (n = 19 (79.2%)) in deep cavities, while the study conducted by Sidhu, P. et al. 2021 received a score of 85% (n = 11). In the same study, the majority of the respondents selected rubber dams as mandatory tools for moisture control prior to resin composite placement (n = 11 (85%)) with the alternative tool being a cotton roll (n = 12 (92%)). This is similar to our findings [59]. Almost all respondents in both studies taught and utilized a conventional light emitting diode (LED) curing light and finishing techniques such as finishing discs and strips in the restoration of resin composites involving occlusal-proximal cavities. There was a slight notable discrepancy between the studies though. In our study, it was reported that the bulk fill technique was taught by 20.8% (n = 5) of the respondents, while there were no schools which practiced bulk fill teaching in the study carried out by Sidhu, P. et al. 2021 [59]. The specific teaching and learning activities in which the bulk fill technique was taught are not reported in our study.

Sidhu, P. et al. 2021 also reported on the contraindication of composite restoration placement at the posterior cavity, the contemporary composite materials and bonding systems used in dental schools, the fees charged by the dental schools for the restoration of a posterior cavity done by the students, and the teaching of indirect posterior composite resin restoration [59]. These were not included in our study The additional information obtained through the above-mentioned study is very much needed as it encourages a shift in the use of composite resins as a step towards a more modern way of dentistry, such as minimal intervention dentistry [59]. Nonetheless, this study was conducted with the aim of identifying the theoretical, didactic and clinical teaching used in the teaching and learning process, and covered the theoretical pedagogical component, teaching materials and common assessment types performed by dental schools in Malaysia. Findings on preclinical simulation programmes, and common types of assessment to evaluate clinical competency of the dental students, were also included. With both studies being conducted in Malaysia, it shows that there is a pressing need to address the harmonization of the teaching of posterior restoration as part of a global collaborative approach in phasing out the use of amalgam in this part of the world.

5. Conclusions

There are notable variations and diversities in the teaching of posterior restoration which shows a lack of consensus and agreement among dental schools. Therefore, there is a pressing need for uniformity, harmonization and consistency in the approaches used in primary dental qualification curricular. This action demands a collaborative effort by the dental schools in Malaysia. This study can be considered as an initial initiative in acquiring comprehensive information with regarding the operative dentistry teaching curriculum in dental schools in Malaysia. The global approach in phasing out the use of dental amalgam should not be ignored.

Supplementary Materials: The following are available online at https://www.mdpi.com/article/10.3390/dj9100123/s1, Figure S1: Teaching of Posterior Composite Resin Restorations in Undergraduate Dental Schools in Malaysia.

Author Contributions: Conceptualization, N.M., M.S.A., F.A.F. and A.A.A.; data curation, A.J. and M.S.A.; formal analysis, A.J. and M.S.A.; funding acquisition, N.M. and A.A.A.; methodology, N.M., A.A.A., F.A.F. and A.J.; writing—original draft, M.S.A.; writing—review and editing, M.S.A., N.M., F.A.F. and A.J. All authors have read and agreed to the published version of the manuscript.

Funding: This research was funded by Universiti Sains Islam Malaysia (USIM) Research Grant [Grant number: PPPI/FPG/0217/051000/11918].

Institutional Review Board Statement: The study was conducted according to the guidelines of the Declaration of Helsinki, and approved by the Ethics Committee of USIM [USIM/FPg-MEC/2016/No. (45).

Informed Consent Statement: Informed consent was obtained from all subjects involved in the study.

Conflicts of Interest: The authors declare no conflict of interest.

References

1. Demarco, F.F.; Corrêa, M.B.; Cenci, M.S.; Moraes, R.R.; Opdam, N.J. Longevity of posterior composite restorations: Not only a matter of materials. *Dent. Mater.* **2012**, *28*, 87–101. [CrossRef] [PubMed]
2. Gilmour, A.S.; Evans, P.; Addy, L.D. Attitudes of general dental practitioners in the UK to the use of composite materials in posterior teeth. *Br. Dent. J.* **2007**, *202*, E32. [CrossRef] [PubMed]
3. Opdam, N.J.; Bronkhorst, E.M.; Loomans, B.A.; Huysmans, M.C. 12-year survival of composite vs. amalgam restorations. *J. Dent. Res.* **2010**, *89*, 1063–1067. [CrossRef] [PubMed]
4. Agnihotry, A.; Fedorowicz, Z.; Nasser, M. Adhesively bonded versus non-bonded amalgam restorations for dental caries. *Cochrane Database Syst. Rev.* **2016**, *3*, CD007517. [CrossRef]
5. Opdam, N.J.; Van De Sande, F.H.; Bronkhorst, E.; Cenci, M.S.; Bottenberg, P.; Pallesen, U.; Gaengler, P.; Lindberg, A.; Huysmans, M.C.; Van Dijken, J.W. Longevity of posterior composite restorations: A systematic review and meta-analysis. *J. Dent. Res.* **2014**, *93*, 943–949. [CrossRef]
6. Alcaraz, M.G.; Veitz-Keenan, A.; Sahrmann, P.; Schmidlin, P.R.; Davis, D.; Iheozor-Ejiofor, Z. Direct composite resin fillings versus amalgam fillings for permanent or adult posterior teeth. *Cochrane Database Syst. Rev.* **2014**, *3*, CD005620. [CrossRef]
7. Pires, P.M.; de Almeida Neves, A.; Makeeva, I.M.; Schwendicke, F.; Faus-Matoses, V.; Yoshihara, K.; Banerjee, A.; Sauro, S. Contemporary restorative ion-releasing materials: Current status, interfacial properties and operative approaches. *Br. Dent. J.* **2020**, *229*, 450–458. [CrossRef]

8. Zhou, X.; Huang, X.; Li, M.; Peng, X.; Wang, S.; Zhou, X.; Cheng, L. Development and status of resin composite as dental restorative materials. *J. Appl. Polym. Sci.* **2019**, *136*, 48180. [CrossRef]
9. Nedeljkovic, I.; De Munck, J.; Vanloy, A.; Declerck, D.; Lambrechts, P.; Peumans, M.; Teughels, W.; Van Meerbeek, B.; Van Landuyt, K.L. Secondary caries: Prevalence, characteristics, and approach. *Clin. Oral Investig.* **2020**, *24*, 683–691. [CrossRef]
10. Ferracane, J.L. Resin composite—State of the art. *Dent. Mater.* **2011**, *27*, 29–38. [CrossRef]
11. Svare, C.W.; Peterson, L.C.; Reinhardt, J.W.; Boyer, D.B.; Frank, C.W.; Gay, D.D.; Cox, R.D. The effect of dental amalgams on mercury levels in expired air. *J. Dent. Res.* **1981**, *60*, 1668–1671. [CrossRef]
12. Pitts, N.B.; Ismail, A.I.; Martignon, S.; Ekstrand, K.; Douglas, G.V.; Longbottom, C. *ICCMS™ Guide for Practitioners and Educators*; King's College London: London, UK, 2014.
13. McCracken, M.S.; Gordan, V.V.; Litaker, M.S.; Funkhouser, E.; Fellows, J.L.; Shamp, D.G.; Qvist, V.; Meral, J.S.; Gilbert, G.H. A 24-month evaluation of amalgam and resin-based composite restorations: Findings from The National Dental Practice-Based Research Network. *J. Am. Dent. Assoc.* **2013**, *144*, 583–593. [CrossRef]
14. Mocny-Pachońska, K.; Doniec, R.J.; Wójcik, S.; Sieciński, S.; Piaseczna, N.J.; Duraj, K.M.; Tkacz, E.J. Evaluation of the Most Stressful Dental Treatment Procedures of Conservative Dentistry among Polish Dental Students. *Int. J. Environ. Res. Public Health* **2021**, *18*, 4448. [CrossRef]
15. Kanzow, P.; Büttcher, A.F.; Wilson, N.H.; Lynch, C.D.; Blum, I.R. Contemporary teaching of posterior composites at dental schools in Austria, Germany, and Switzerland. *J. Dent.* **2020**, *96*, 103321. [CrossRef]
16. Loch, C.; Liaw, Y.; Metussin, A.P.; Lynch, C.D.; Wilson, N.; Blum, I.R.; Brunton, P.A. The teaching of posterior composites: A survey of dental schools in Oceania. *J. Dent.* **2019**, *84*, 36–43. [CrossRef]
17. Kanzow, P.; Wiegand, A.; Wilson, N.H.; Lynch, C.D.; Blum, I.R. Contemporary teaching of restoration repair at dental schools in Germany–Close to universality and consistency. *J. Dent.* **2018**, *75*, 121–124. [CrossRef]
18. Castillo-de Oyagüe, R.; Lynch, C.; McConnell, R.; Wilson, N. Teaching the placement of posterior resin-based composite restorations in Spanish dental schools. *Med. Oral Patol. Oral Cirugía Bucal.* **2012**, *17*, e661. [CrossRef]
19. Lynch, C.D.; Frazier, K.B.; McConnell, R.J.; Blum, I.R.; Wilson, N.H. Minimally invasive management of dental caries: Contemporary teaching of posterior resin-based composite placement in US and Canadian dental schools. *J. Am. Dent. Assoc.* **2011**, *142*, 612–620. [CrossRef]
20. Lynch, C.D.; Frazier, K.B.; McConnell, R.J.; Blum, I.R.; Wilson, N.H. State-of-the-art techniques in operative dentistry: Contemporary teaching of posterior composites in UK and Irish dental schools. *Br. Dent. J.* **2010**, *209*, 129–136. [CrossRef]
21. Sadeghi, M.; Lynch, C.D.; Wilson, N.H. Trends in Dental Education in the Persian Gulf—An Example From Iran: Contemporary Placement of Posterior Composites. *Eur. J. Prosthodont. Restor. Dent.* **2009**, *17*, 182.
22. Gordan, V.V.; Mjör, I.A.; Ritter, A.V. Teaching of posterior resin-based composite restorations in Brazilian dental schools. *Quintessence Int.* **2000**, *31*, 10.
23. Awad, M.M.; Salem, W.S.; Almuhaizaa, M.; Aljeaidi, Z. Contemporary teaching of direct posterior composite restorations in Saudi dental schools. *Saudi J. Dent. Res.* **2017**, *8*, 42–51. [CrossRef]
24. Hayashi, M.; Seow, L.L.; Lynch, C.D.; Wilson, N.H. Teaching of posterior composites in dental schools in Japan. *J. Oral Rehabil.* **2009**, *36*, 292–298. [CrossRef]
25. Hayashi, M.; Yamada, T.; Lynch, C.D.; Wilson, N.H. Teaching of posterior composites in dental schools in Japan–30 years and beyond. *J. Dent.* **2018**, *76*, 19–23. [CrossRef]
26. Lynch, C.D.; McConnell, R.J.; Wilson, N.H. Teaching of posterior composite resin restorations in undergraduate dental schools in Ireland and the United Kingdom. *Eur. J. Dent. Educ.* **2006**, *10*, 38–43. [CrossRef]
27. Shqaidef, A.J.; Abu-Baker, D.; Al-Bitar, Z.B.; Badran, S.; Hamdan, A.M. Academic performance of dental students: A randomized trial comparing live, audio recorded, and video recorded lectures. *Eur. J. Dent. Educ.* **2021**, *25*, 377–384. [CrossRef]
28. Ramlogan, S.; Raman, V.; Sweet, J. A comparison of two forms of teaching instruction: Video vs. live lecture for education in clinical periodontology. *Eur. J. Dent. Educ.* **2014**, *18*, 31–38. [CrossRef]
29. Patel, U.S.; Tonni, I.; Gadbury-Amyot, C.; Van der Vleuten, C.P.; Escudier, M. Assessment in a global context: An international perspective on dental education. *Eur. J. Dent. Educ.* **2018**, *22*, 21–27. [CrossRef]
30. Miller, G.E. The assessment of clinical skills/competence/performance. *Acad. Med.* **1990**, *65*, S63–S67. [CrossRef]
31. Bloom, B.S.; Krathwohl, D.R.; Masia, B.B. *Bloom Taxonomy of Educational Objectives*; Allyn and Bacon, Pearson Education: New York, NY, USA, 1984.
32. Othman, N.I.; Ismail, H.U.; Mohammad, N.; Ghazali, N.; Alauddin, M.S. An Evaluation on Deep Caries Removal Method and Management Performed by Undergraduate Dental Students: A Malaysia Experience. *Eur. J. Dent.* **2021**, *15*, 281–289.
33. Alauddin, M.S.; Baharuddin, A.S.; Mohd Ghazali, M.I. The Modern and Digital Transformation of Oral Health Care: A Mini Review. *Healthcare* **2021**, *9*, 118. [CrossRef] [PubMed]
34. Serrano, C.M.; Botelho, M.G.; Wesselink, P.R.; Vervoorn, J.M. Challenges in the transition to clinical training in dentistry: An ADEE special interest group initial report. *Eur. J. Dent. Educ.* **2018**, *22*, e451–e457. [CrossRef] [PubMed]
35. Schwibbe, A.; Kothe, C.; Hampe, W.; Konradt, U. Acquisition of dental skills in preclinical technique courses: Influence of spatial and manual abilities. *Adv. Health Sci. Educ.* **2016**, *21*, 841–857. [CrossRef] [PubMed]

36. Lynch, C.D.; Blum, I.R.; McConnell, R.J.; Frazier, K.B.; Brunton, P.A.; Wilson, N.H. Teaching posterior resin composites in UK and Ireland dental schools: Do current teaching programmes match the expectation of clinical practice arrangements? *Br. Dent. J.* **2018**, *224*, 967–972. [CrossRef]
37. Oral Health Division Malaysia. *National Oral Health Survey of Adults 2010 (NOHSA 2010)*; Government Printers: Putrajaya, Malaysia, 2013.
38. WHO. *Promoting the Phase Down of Dental Amalgam in Developing Countries*; United Nations Enviroment Programme, World Health Organization: Geneva, Switzerland, 2014.
39. Ottenga, M.E.; Mjör, I.A. Amalgam and composite posterior restorations: Curriculum versus practice in operative dentistry at a US dental school. *Oper. Dent.* **2007**, *32*, 524–528. [CrossRef]
40. Schenkel, A.B.; Veitz-Keenan, A. Dental cavity liners for Class I and Class II resin-based composite restorations. *Cochrane Database Syst. Rev.* **2019**, *3*, CD010526. [CrossRef]
41. Hume, W.R. *Pulp Protection During and After Tooth Restoration. Preservation and Restoration of Tooth Structure*, 2nd ed.; Knowledge Books and Software: Brisbane, Australia, 2005; pp. 289–298.
42. Ritter, A.V. *Sturdevant's Art & Science of Operative Dentistry-e-Book*; Elsevier Health Sciences: Amsterdam, The Netherlands, 2017.
43. Lynch, C.D.; Mcconnell, R.J.; Wilson, N.H. Posterior composites: The future for restoring posterior teeth? *Prim. Dent. J.* **2014**, *3*, 49–53. [CrossRef]
44. Schwendicke, F.; Kniess, J.L.; Paris, S.; Blunck, U. Margin integrity and secondary caries of lined or non-lined composite and glass hybrid restorations after selective excavation in vitro. *Oper. Dent.* **2017**, *42*, 155–164. [CrossRef]
45. Göstemeyer, G.; Schwendicke, F. Inhibition of hybrid layer degradation by cavity pretreatment: Meta-and trial sequential analysis. *J. Dent.* **2016**, *49*, 14–21. [CrossRef]
46. Plasmans, P.J.; Creugers, N.H.; Mulder, J. Long-term survival of extensive amalgam restorations. *J. Dent. Res.* **1998**, *77*, 453–460. [CrossRef]
47. Bernardo, M.; Luis, H.; Martin, M.D.; Leroux, B.G.; Rue, T.; Leitão, J.; DeRouen, T.A. Survival and reasons for failure of amalgam versus composite posterior restorations placed in a randomized clinical trial. *J. Am. Dent. Assoc.* **2007**, *138*, 775–783. [CrossRef]
48. Dutra, T.T.; Tapety, Z.I.; Mendes, R.F.; Moita Neto, J.M.; Prado Júnior, R.R. Survival time of direct dental restorations in adults. *Rev. Odontol. UNESP* **2015**, *44*, 213–217. [CrossRef]
49. Müllejans, R.; Badawi, M.O.; Raab, W.H.; Lang, H. An in vitro comparison of metal and transparent matrices used for bonded Class II resin composite restorations. *Oper. Dent.* **2003**, *28*, 122–126.
50. Kampouropoulos, D.; Paximada, C.; Loukidis, M.; Kakaboura, A. The influence of matrix type on the proximal contact in Class II resin composite restorations. *Oper. Dent.* **2010**, *35*, 454–462. [CrossRef]
51. Wirsching, E.; Loomans, B.A.; Klaiber, B.; Dörfer, C.E. Influence of matrix systems on proximal contact tightness of 2-and 3-surface posterior composite restorations in vivo. *J. Dent.* **2011**, *39*, 386–390. [CrossRef]
52. Lynch, C.D.; Opdam, N.J.; Hickel, R.; Brunton, P.A.; Gurgan, S.; Kakaboura, A.; Shearer, A.C.; Vanherle, G.; Wilson, N.H. Guidance on posterior resin composites: Academy of operative dentistry-European section. *J. Dent.* **2014**, *42*, 377–383. [CrossRef]
53. Neeraj Malhotra, M.D.; Kundabala Mala, M.D. Light-curing considerations for resin-based composite materials: A review. Part, I. *Compendium* **2010**, *31*, 498–505.
54. Kramer, N.; Lohbauer, U.; Garcia-Godoy, F.; Frankenberger, R. Light curing of resin-based composites in the LED era. *Am. J. Dent.* **2008**, *21*, 135.
55. Leprince, J.G.; Palin, W.M.; Vanacker, J.; Sabbagh, J.; Devaux, J.; Leloup, G. Physico-mechanical characteristics of commercially available bulk-fill composites. *J. Dent.* **2014**, *42*, 993–1000. [CrossRef]
56. Ilie, N.; Bucuta, S.; Draenert, M. Bulk-fill resin-based composites: An in vitro assessment of their mechanical performance. *Oper. Dent.* **2013**, *38*, 618–625. [CrossRef]
57. Rosatto, C.M.; Bicalho, A.A.; Veríssimo, C.; Bragança, G.F.; Rodrigues, M.P.; Tantbirojn, D.; Versluis, A.; Soares, C.J. Mechanical properties, shrinkage stress, cuspal strain and fracture resistance of molars restored with bulk-fill composites and incremental filling technique. *J. Dent.* **2015**, *43*, 1519–1528. [CrossRef]
58. Van Ende, A.; De Munck, J.; Lise, D.P.; Van Meerbeek, B. Bulk-fill composites: A review of the current literature. *J. Adhes. Dent.* **2017**, *19*, 95–109.
59. Sidhu, P.; Sultan, O.S.; Math, S.Y.; Ab Malik, N.; Wilson, N.H.; Lynch, C.D.; Blum, I.R.; Daood, U. Current and future trends in the teaching of direct posterior resin composites in Malaysian dental schools: A cross-sectional study. *J. Dent.* **2021**, *110*, 103683. [CrossRef]

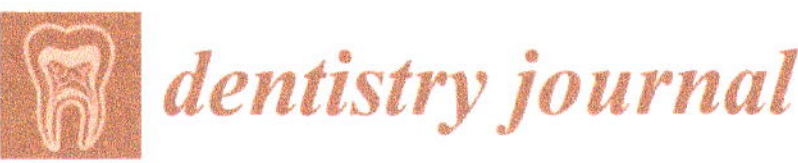

Communication

Use of Computer Simulation in Dental Training with Special Reference to Simodont

Angie Lok-Sze Leung, Conson Yeung, Samantha Chu, Amy Wai-Yee Wong, Ollie Yiru Yu and Chun-Hung Chu *

Faculty of Dentistry, The University of Hong Kong, Prince Philip Dental Hospital, 34 Hospital Road, Sai Ying Pun, Hong Kong, China; angie667@connect.hku.hk (A.L.-S.L.); conson@hku.hk (C.Y.); chus@connect.hku.hk (S.C.); drawong@hku.hk (A.W.-Y.W.); ollieyu@hku.hk (O.Y.Y.)
* Correspondence: chchu@hku.hk

Abstract: Simulation-based dental education has been increasingly implemented in dental training. Virtual reality simulators are being explored as an adjunct to dental education. Simulation-based dental education could serve as a powerful aid to preclinical instruction. This article provides an overview of how dental simulators can be used in dental instruction and manual dexterity training, utilizing the Simodont dental trainer as a reference. The Simodont dental trainer provides a platform for students to hone their manual dexterity skills and practice repeatedly prior to conventional clinical simulations. Additionally, it can reduce resource wastage. However, the financial cost of setting up and maintaining the system can be high. The high cost would ultimately limit the number of devices each individual school could afford, as a potential drawback to meeting the training needs of many dental students at one time. The machine's force-feedback mechanism provides trainees with the tactile experience of drilling into various tissues. Students are empowered via self-learning and assessment, with guidance provided for diagnosis and treatment. From training students on basic operative skills to providing basic aptitude tests for entrance examinations, the Simodont dental trainer's functions and potential for further development may make it a valuable tool in the field of simulation-based dental education.

Keywords: virtual reality; haptics; simulation; education; Simodont

Citation: Leung, A.L.-S.; Yeung, C.; Chu, S.; Wong, A.W.-Y.; Yu, O.Y.; Chu, C.-H. Use of Computer Simulation in Dental Training with Special Reference to Simodont. *Dent. J.* **2021**, 9, 125. https://doi.org/10.3390/dj9110125

Academic Editors: Jelena Dumancic, Rod Moore and Božana Lončar Brzak

Received: 13 September 2021
Accepted: 19 October 2021
Published: 21 October 2021

1. Introduction

With the advancement of technology, simulation and virtual reality have facilitated teaching, learning and professional training in dentistry [1]. In disciplines such as dentistry involving unpredictable situations and requiring a certain level of manual dexterity, much attention has been paid to simulation and virtual reality as possible tools with which to provide a realistic training environment for students to practice high-risk procedures. In medicine, medical technologies have already been developed for surgical training, including endoscopy, laparoscopic and neurosurgery simulators. A report on sigmoidoscopy simulator training found that it improved examination times and hand-to-eye skill measures [2].

The acquisition of psychomotor skills makes up a substantial part of the dental curriculum. As dentists perform detailed work on a small scale, hand–eye coordination is crucial for carrying out operative procedures. Restorative dentistry students should gain sufficient hands-on practice in a simulation environment to prevent mishaps caused by human error before they enter the clinical setting [3]. Therefore, simulation-based dental education is being explored as a clinical environment simulator in which preclinical training can be carried out safely.

Conventional preclinical training involves mannequin heads mounted on a metal rod. These phantom heads contain a set of plastic maxillary and mandibular teeth. Dental simulation systems are a newer practice method. Example of these include PerioSim, the Simodont dental trainer and DentSim. These simulators utilize computer-assisted simulation, which connects computer learning software to a simulator. The simulator generates 3D images for students to operate on using dental handpieces. The results are sent to the computer for evaluation and feedback [4]. Students can practice on these devices before practicing on phantom heads and, eventually, on real patients. The Simodont dental trainer (MOOG, Nieuw Vennep, The Netherlands) is one such simulator. The Simodont brand is developed by Nissin Dental Products Europe BV (Nieuw-Vennep, The Netherlands). The various components of Simodont Dental Trainer are shown in Figure 1.

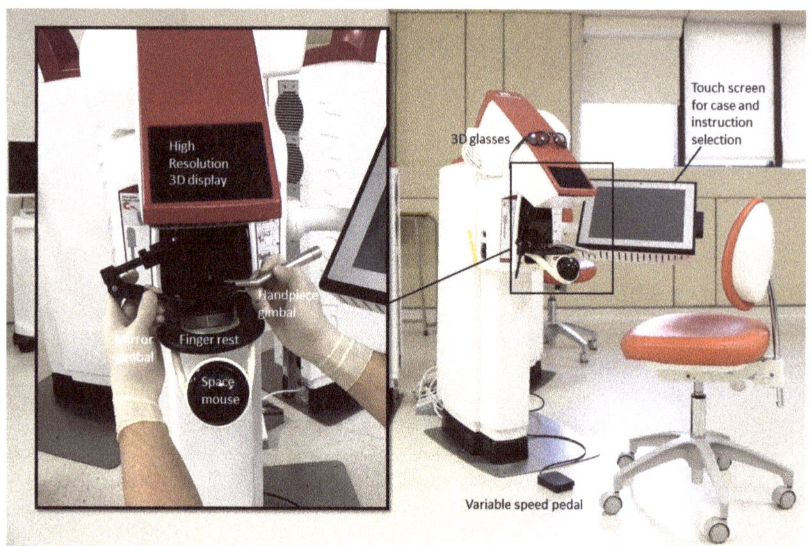

Figure 1. Components of Simodont.

Simodont provides a 3D display of the instrument and tooth on-screen in true size [5]. The gimbals on either side of the machine appear in full size on-screen, and one of them functions as a handpiece with which to work on the selected model. The required instruments are selected before starting. A force-feedback mechanism is applied so that the tactile sensation of drilling into the tooth is transmitted when the handpiece touches the model. Auditory and visual effects also are provided for realism [5]. Afterward, the computer evaluates the operation and displays the results on the PC interface as completion percentages for each assessment criterion. A variety of cases are housed in an online library, and real clinical cases can be uploaded for sharing [6]. How Simodont can serve as a valuable adjunct to traditional preclinical teaching will now be discussed.

2. Attributes of Simodont in Preclinical Training

2.1. Haptics

Different dental tissues possess different resistance to cutting by the handpiece. Hence, the user experiencing the tactile sensation of drilling into these tissues is important. As dentists may not always be able to see the work area clearly, they sometimes rely on their sense of touch for navigation [7]. With force feedback, the Simodont dental trainer mimics the touch sensation when drilling, preparing cavities, removing caries and delivering other restorative procedures. The tactile feeling is transmitted through the gimbal, and it differs according to each tooth tissue's hardness level [7]. This improves the resemblance of the cutting resistance of enamel, dentine and pulp, in comparison to the plastic teeth used in conventional simulation. Simodont can also imitate the softness of caries to acquaint students with the feeling of drilling carious lesions [6]. Homogeneous plastic teeth cannot replicate this function. In addition, the trainer detects and records the pressure applied by the trainee's hand at specific locations [7]. This may help students to gain better control over the force they use and adjust it accordingly to obtain better results.

Typodont teeth are available with different cutting characteristics for enamel, dentine, pulpal tissue and carious tooth structures. These typodont teeth include RTX Caries Teeth (Acadental, Overland Park, KS, USA) and Candent (Candent, Mississauga, ON, Canada). However, no manufacturers have explained how they created typodont teeth that reproduce the cutting characteristics of sound and carious dental tissues. In Simodont, the amount of opposing force that is generated against the handpiece is a function of three determinants [7,8]: (1) the hardness of the virtual material, (2) the drill's speed and (3) the push force. The hardness of the material is determined according to the grey value of the tooth scan. In addition to issues related to how well the typodont teeth reproduce the cutting characteristics of sound and carious dental tissues, typodont teeth with caries and pulp space are expensive [9,10].

2.2. Personnel Cost

As most dental schools do not have adequate dental teachers, generally only a few instructors are available for teaching dental students. The students usually are grouped together and assigned to one teacher, who is responsible for evaluating their work and offering guidance. This teaching model presents a number of challenges. The teacher must provide feedback and address the questions of many students, so students waste time waiting [8]. This reduces the quantity and sometimes quality of the advice they receive. The evaluation system in Simodont provides instantaneous feedback by displaying the completion percentage for each criterion. Students can receive basic evaluation before instructor assessment, which can reduce the time cost. This also alleviates the waiting time for each student. In addition, Simodont allows students to restart if they damage the tooth during a procedure [11] (p. 58). This allows students to be less cautious about making mistakes, especially regarding 'cutting too much', which may contribute to faster learning.

2.3. Human and Plastic Teeth as Resources

Theoretically, extracted human teeth are the best material for practice. However, the challenges faced to collect them restrict their usage in training. As human teeth supply is unstable, the number of teeth that students can receive is limited and may even be insufficient to carry out proper practice using solely human teeth. Oftentimes, only teeth with extensive damage are extracted, while others have had work performed on them, such as restoration and root canal treatment, which renders them unsuitable for further usage. In addition, occlusal and proximal relations cannot be simulated using extracted human teeth. Furthermore, parents of patients often wish to keep the extracted primary teeth of their children [12].

Plastic models have a standardized size and morphology and an absence of defects. Virtual teeth are produced by scanning extracted teeth with the desired morphology and pathology using cone beam tomography, thus creating a more realistic appearance as compared to plastic teeth [13]. This covers the variation in human dentition more comprehensively. Resources can be pooled using a shared library, as interesting cases can be uploaded for other students to download and work on [11]. This could include cases that are rarely encountered in the clinic, which students otherwise may be unable to see even during their clinical years [6]. Encountering such cases would broaden the range of their experience and improve their understanding of tooth structure and pathology. The translucency of virtual teeth can be adjusted to show the inner structures of the tooth, thus helping students to acquire a more complete understanding of its structure and pathology [6]. The teacher can manipulate and reposition the orientation of the tooth or jaw [6], to simulate a wider range of proximal and occlusal relations. Virtual teeth in Simodont can be regenerated infinitely, which avoids the problem of supply [6]. Students can practice on the same tooth repeatedly until they reach skill competency and familiarity with the morphology, and then choose another tooth to work on. Simodont possesses an online library housing a collection of tooth models, from which a large variety of cases can be downloaded [6]. Virtual teeth usage also skirts the need for disinfection and storage, as well as eliminates the cost of collecting teeth [12].

2.4. Diagnosis and Treatment Planning

Proper diagnosis and disease identification must occur before any treatment. While plastic teeth are all standardized and pathology-free, the teeth in Simodont provide a range of healthy and diseased structures for diagnosis and treatment practice. Simodont provides an examination mode and a practice mode, which provides step-by-step guidance for defect and disease recognition [6]. A more detailed examination is possible by magnifying and viewing the model from multiple angles, which has been shown to enhance student understanding of the task at hand and improve students' confidence in their skills during training [4]. Teachers can add patient records and guiding questions to simulate different clinical situations [6]. Student knowledge is solidified by combining theory and practice. Students can construct their own treatment plans prior to preparation, which can be saved and compared with the actual preparation carried out afterwards for self-assessment.

2.5. Instructor Guidance

The dental trainers are connected to a computer, which can display the monitors of six simulators live at once [8]. Teachers then can view the students' practice through a live screen, without any obstruction from the students' hands and instruments [6]. Improper techniques and missteps can be spotted by reviewing the procedures being carried out, instead of requiring the instructors to guess the causes of the mistakes just from inspecting the final product. The procedure can also be recorded for future evaluation and comparison [11] (p. 53). The teacher then can provide more accurate corrective advice regarding the performed techniques.

2.6. Self-Learning

The Simodont dental trainer displays the completion percentages for each surface as well as over-drilled areas [14]. Continuous feedback is provided throughout the procedure. Students are informed of any mistakes they have made immediately; therefore, they can self-correct on the spot. This can also help to prevent gross over-preparation to the extent that switching to a new virtual tooth is required. The Simodont dental trainer also provides a snapshot function. If a student has difficulty with a certain part of the procedure, they can create a save point, so that they can revisit that particular point in the tooth-preparation procedure [6]. Thus, students can repeat their practice at specific points throughout the preparation sequence, instead of having to start from a new tooth each time. This greatly improves practice effectiveness. The Simodont dental trainer also provides a more flexible learning schedule [15]. Students can use it outside of school hours for review and remediation. This means that students can practice independently at their own pace. This also encourages them to take charge of their own learning.

2.7. Manual Dexterity

The Simodont dental trainer provides simple manual dexterity exercises for beginner trainees to develop the basic psychomotor skills needed for restorative work. A virtual block is generated for students to practice drilling, and the requirements of the exercise resemble the principles of cavity preparation [6]. Students then move on to practicing on virtual teeth. Apart from building confidence, students accumulating manual dexterity skills prior to conventional practice prevents them from wasting resources by accidentally causing irreversible damage on plastic teeth [12].

The gimbals on the Simodont dental trainer are designed to resemble the weight and grip of dental hand instruments. A hand rest is also provided for students to practice proper finger grip and hand positioning, which are important skills for students to possess. The position (left or right) of the handpiece gimbal and the mirror gimbal can be exchanged to accommodate people with different dominant sides. A wide range of burs are available for students to practice with [6]. The skills learnt via the dental trainer can be retained and remain transferable to real clinical settings [16]. This suggests that earlier training on a virtual cavity is effective in improving dexterity when students experience a physical model for the first time.

2.8. Self-Assessment

The Simodont dental trainer evaluates student work using a set of standard criteria [5]. For a caries-removal exercise, the computer measures the percentages of carious tissue that has been removed and of over-drilled tissue on each side of the cavity. If the amount of over-drilled tissue exceeds a certain margin, immediate failure results. This imitates caries removal in minimally invasive dentistry, in which dentists avoid damaging healthy tissue surrounding a carious lesion. Using the V4 software, the exercise analyses the under- or over-preparedness of the cavity, contour smoothness, depth of the cavity, convergence, divergence, etc., using the Site-Stage (SI/STA) Classification System [17]. This classification system designates the site (SI) and stage (STA) components of the caries lesion and provides guidance on the selection of restorative material. As teachers show the same and standardised criterion for evaluation, students are guided to assess their own outcomes, so that they may gauge the quality of their work and determine key areas for improvement. Students who can actively assess their work will have a better idea about the goal of the treatment simulation they are performing, which may give them clearer direction and bolster their confidence [14].

Self-assessment also allows students to identify potential challenges in learning. By comparing the feedback for different practice runs, students may notice salient performance gaps (for example, the student may score consistently lower for a specific assessment criterion). The students may decide to put more effort into practicing and improving their weaker areas. Variations in the feedback given by different teachers may confuse trainees at an early stage in their career development. Using a standard set of criteria for the machine to generate basic and objective feedback can improve clarity, avoid confusion and instil confidence. Students can learn alternative restorative treatment once they have mastered the basic operative skills. The students' exercise results are sent to the teaching module. Slower or weaker learners could be identified early and given timely remediation, such that they can catch up with their peers faster.

2.9. Other Issues Related to Preclinical Training

The challenge of patient management in paediatrics is that the time for carrying out restorative work is limited. It is important that dentists are able to deliver procedures efficiently, which requires a solid understanding of and familiarity with dental pathology and morphology [12]. Simodont provides pulpotomy and drilling exercises for students to hone their manual dexterity skills on primary dentition. Students can clearly feel the pulp chamber drop using Simodont when they perform simulated root canal treatment. When the students perform crown preparation, they can visualise the original tooth outline on the prepared tooth to aid with comparison and measurement. They also can observe the damage to the neighbouring teeth through the display screen of the Simodont. A summary of the main findings of studies of Simodont in dental education is given in Table 1.

Table 1. Main findings of studies of Simodont in dental education.

Authors, Year [Ref]	Main Findings
De Boer et al., 2016 [18]	Simodont enhanced student performance and appreciation of students working in a virtual learning environment.
Zafer et al., 2020 [12]	Simodont assisted pre-clinical training in restorative procedures in paediatric dentistry.

Table 1. *Cont.*

Authors, Year [Ref]	Main Findings
Murbay et al., 2020 [17]	Simodont facilitated the effectiveness of pre-clinical training in operative dentistry.
Yuan et al., 2021 [19]	Simodont improved the effectiveness in pre-clinical teaching of access and coronal cavity preparation in operative dentistry

3. Limitations of Simodont in Preclinical Training

The haptic limitation of the Simodont dental trainer in tactile sensation in different tooth structures requires improvement. In a pulpotomy exercise, "only 27% of interviewees agreed that the hardness, texture and tactile sensations of Simodont felt realistic for performing pulpotomy and stainless-steel crown exercises" [12]. Furthermore, 79% agreed that conventional simulations felt more realistic. Better simulation fidelity is also required to emulate the texture of pulpal tissues and the mechanical hardness of tooth structures. As mentioned before, another advantage of Simodont is reducing resource wastage. Students do not need to purchase plastic teeth or collect, store or disinfect human teeth for practice. However, the cost of the initial setup and maintenance can be high and will increase the cost of the curriculum. The high cost would ultimately limit the number of devices each individual dental school could afford, as a potential drawback to meeting the training needs of many dental students at one time. Furthermore, students cannot wear loupes while practicing with Simodont due to the need to wear 3D glasses. Many dental schools are training students to perform operative procedures with magnifying loupes, which is becoming an accepted norm amongst dentists and part of the training in simulation laboratory [20]. Additionally, as the trainer only simulates tooth structures, students cannot practice the management of soft tissue such as the tongue and the lips.

4. Simodont as an Assessment Tool and Its Future Perspectives

In comparison to traditional entrance examinations involving wire bending or wax carving, an aptitude test conducted using the Simodont dental trainer has a higher resemblance to performing dental restorative work. Candidates' manual dexterity can be assessed without concerns of injury and the time cost of setting up stations. The potential of the Simodont dental trainer to reduce human bias may prove useful in providing objective assessment for higher-level certification. However, a deeper investigation is warranted into the reliability and evaluation accuracy before this can be implemented [21].

There has been discussion about external accreditation for licensing. This would require (1) a highly reliable means of recording and (2) assessing candidates' performance according to the criteria set by the examiners. The current challenge lies in acquiring highly reliable data that can prove the candidates' competence [21]. There is potential for Simodont dental trainer programmes to spread into other dental fields beyond restorative dentistry. Roy et al. [8] discussed the development of a dental hygiene and periodontics programme.

5. Conclusions

In conclusion, simulation-based dental education could serve as a powerful aid to preclinical instruction. The Simodont dental trainer provides a platform for students to hone their manual dexterity skills and practice repeatedly prior to conventional preclinical simulation. However, the cost of the initial setup and maintenance can be high. The machine's force-feedback mechanism provides trainees with the tactile experience of drilling various tissues. It empowers students via self-learning and assessment, with guidance provided for diagnosis and treatment. From training students on basic operative skills to providing basic aptitude tests in entrance examinations, the Simodont dental trainer's functions and potential for further development may make it a valuable tool for simulation-based dental education.

Author Contributions: Conceptualization, C.Y., S.C., A.W.-Y.W., O.Y.Y. and C.-H.C.; investigation, A.L.-S.L., C.Y., S.C., A.W.-Y.W. and O.Y.Y.; data curation, A.L.-S.L., C.Y., S.C., A.W.-Y.W., O.Y.Y. and C.-H.C.; writing—original draft preparation, A.L.-S.L.; writing—review and editing, C.Y., S.C., A.W.-Y.W., O.Y.Y. and C.-H.C.; supervision, C.-H.C.; project administration, C.-H.C. All authors have read and agreed to the published version of the manuscript.

Funding: This research received no external funding.

Institutional Review Board Statement: Not applicable.

Informed Consent Statement: Not applicable.

Data Availability Statement: Not applicable.

Conflicts of Interest: The authors declare no conflict of interest.

References

1. Afrashtehfar, K.I.; Yang, J.W.; Al- Sammarraie, A.A.H.; Chen, H.; Saeed, M.H. Pre-clinical undergraduate students' perspectives on the adoption of virtual and augmented reality to their dental learning experience: A one-group pre- and post-test design protocol. *F1000Research* **2021**, *10*, 473. [CrossRef]
2. Tuggy, M.L. Virtual reality flexible sigmoidoscopy simulator training: Impact on resident performance. *J. Am. Board Fam. Pract.* **1998**, *11*, 426–433. [CrossRef] [PubMed]
3. Vincent, M.; Joseph, D.; Amory, C.; Paoli, N.; Ambrosini, P.; Mortier, E.; Tran, N. Contribution of haptic simulation to analogic training environment in restorative dentistry. *J. Dent. Educ.* **2020**, *84*, 367–376. [CrossRef] [PubMed]
4. Nassar, H.M.; Tekian, A. Computer simulation and virtual reality in undergraduate operative and restorative dental education: A critical review. *J. Dent. Educ.* **2020**, *84*, 812–829. [CrossRef] [PubMed]
5. Mirghani, I.; Mushtaq, F.; Allsop, M.J.; Al-Saud, L.M.; Tickhill, N.; Potter, C.; Keeling, A.; Mon-Williams, M.A.; Manogue, M. Capturing differences in dental training using a virtual reality simulator. *Eur. J. Dent. Educ.* **2018**, *22*, 67–71. [CrossRef] [PubMed]
6. Simodont®Dental Trainer. Available online: https://www.simodontdentaltrainer.com/product (accessed on 14 February 2021).
7. De Boer, I.R.; Lagerweij, M.D.; de Vries, M.W.; Wesselink, P.R.; Vervoorn, J.M. The effect of force feedback in a virtual learning environment on the performance and satisfaction of dental students. *Simul. Healthc.* **2017**, *12*, 83–90. [CrossRef] [PubMed]
8. Roy, E.; Bakr, M.M.; George, R. The need for virtual reality simulators in dental education: A review. *Saudi. Dent. J.* **2017**, *29*, 41–47. [CrossRef] [PubMed]
9. Candent Composite Resin Teeth with Caries. Available online: https://candent.ca/products/composite-resin-teeth-with-caries.html (accessed on 13 April 2021).
10. Acadental. RTX Caries Teeth. Available online: https://acadental.com/product_page.php?id=236468860-3797379 (accessed on 13 April 2021).
11. Simodont Teacher Manual. Available online: http://moocs.csmu.edu.tw/sysdata/doc/1/1314663a38aa450c/pdf.pdf (accessed on 2 October 2021).
12. Zafar, S.; Lai, Y.; Sexton, C.; Siddiqi, A. Virtual reality as a novel educational tool in pre-clinical paediatric dentistry training: Students' perceptions. *Int. J. Paediatr. Dent.* **2020**, *30*, 791–797. [CrossRef] [PubMed]
13. De Boer, I.R.; Bakker, D.R.; Serrano, C.M.; Koopman, P.; Wesselink, P.R.; Vervoorn, J.M. Innovation in dental education: The "on-the-fly" approach to simultaneous development, implementation and evidence collection. *Eur. J. Dent. Educ.* **2018**, *22*, 215–222. [CrossRef] [PubMed]
14. Aliaga, I.; Pedrera-Canal, M.; Vera, V.; Rico Martin, S.; Garcia Barbero, E.; Leal-Hernandez, O.; Moran, J.M. Preclinical assessment methodology using a dental simulator during dental students' first and third years. *J. Oral Sci.* **2020**, *62*, 119–121. [CrossRef] [PubMed]
15. Jasinevicius, T.R.; Landers, M.; Nelson, S.; Urbankova, A. An evaluation of two dental simulation systems: Virtual reality versus contemporary non-computer-assisted. *J. Dent. Educ.* **2004**, *68*, 1151–1162. [CrossRef] [PubMed]
16. Bakker, D.; Lagerweij, M.; Wesselink, P.; Vervoorn, M. Transfer of manual dexterity skills acquired in the Simodont, a dental haptic trainer with a virtual environment, to reality: A pilot study. *Bio-Algorithms Med.-Syst.* **2010**, *6*, 21–24.
17. Murbay, S.; Neelakantan, P.; Chang, J.W.W.; Yeung, S. Evaluation of the introduction of a dental virtual simulator on the performance of undergraduate dental students in the pre-clinical operative dentistry course. *Eur. J. Dent. Educ.* **2020**, *24*, 5–16. [CrossRef] [PubMed]
18. De Boer, I.R.; Wesselink, P.R.; Vervoorn, J.M. Student performance and appreciation using 3D vs. 2D vision in a virtual learning environment. *Eur. J. Dent. Educ.* **2016**, *20*, 142–147. [CrossRef] [PubMed]
19. Yuan, C.Y.; Wang, X.Y.; Dong, Y.M.; Gao, X.J. Effect of digital virtual simulation system for preclinical teaching of access and coronal cavity preparation. *Zhonghua Kou Qiang Yi Xue Za Zhi* **2021**, *56*, 479–484. [CrossRef] [PubMed]
20. James, T.; Gilmour, A.S. Magnifying loupes in modern dental practice: An update. *Dent. Update* **2010**, *37*, 633–636. [CrossRef] [PubMed]
21. McGaghie, W.C.; Issenberg, S.B.; Petrusa, E.R.; Scalese, R.J. A critical review of simulation-based medical education research: 2003–2009. *Med. Educ.* **2010**, *44*, 50–63. [CrossRef]

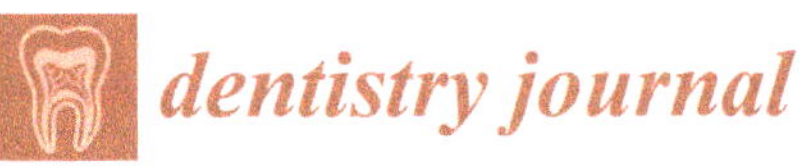

MDPI

Article

Knowledge of Dental Students from Croatia, Slovenia, and Bosnia and Herzegovina about Dental Care of Oncology Patients

Iva Pedic [1], Livia Cigic [2,3,*], Danijela Kalibovic Govorko [3,4], Katarina Vodanovic [5], Ruzica Bandic [5], Robert Glavinic [6] and Ivana Medvedec Mikic [3,7]

1 Private Dental Clinic Ceprnja, Bastijanova 2a, 10000 Zagreb, Croatia; iva.pedic@gmail.com
2 Department of Oral Medicine and Periodontology, Study Programme of Dental Medicine, School of Medicine, University of Split, Soltanska 2, 21000 Split, Croatia
3 Clinic of Dental Medicine, University Hospital of Split, 21000 Split, Croatia; dkalibovic@gmail.com (D.K.G.); imedvedecmikic@gmail.com (I.M.M.)
4 Department of Orthodontics, Study Programme of Dental Medicine, School of Medicine, University of Split, Soltanska 2, 21000 Split, Croatia
5 Study Programme of Dental Medicine, School of Medicine, University of Split, Soltanska 2, 21000 Split, Croatia; katarina.vodanovic@mefst.hr (K.V.); ruzica.bandic@mefst.hr (R.B.)
6 Clinic of Infectious Diseases, University Hospital of Split, Spinciceva 1, 21000 Split, Croatia; robert.glavinic@yahoo.com
7 Department of Endodontics and Restorative Dental Medicine, Study Programme of Dental Medicine, School of Medicine, University of Split, Soltanska 2, 21000 Split, Croatia
* Correspondence: lcigic@mefst.hr; Tel.: +385-21557874

Abstract: The central role of the dentist in the treatment of oncology patients is to care for the patient's oral cavity before, during, and after radio/chemotherapy. The aim of this research was to determine the knowledge of dental students from five universities in three neighboring countries, Croatia (Split, Rijeka, and Zagreb), Bosnia and Herzegovina (Sarajevo), and Slovenia (Ljubljana), about oncology patients' dental care. A total of 140 students in their fourth, fifth, and sixth year of dental medicine studies participated in this research. A questionnaire with 36 specific questions was designed for this research and included questions about dental care of oncologic patients before, during, and after the oncology therapy. Most students are familiar with the incidence and most common type of head and neck tumors, while knowledge about tumor treatment and the side-effects of radiation therapy and/or chemotherapy is weak. Students did not show satisfactory knowledge about osteoradionecrosis, which is the most serious side-effect of radiotherapy; therefore, the emphasis on additional education should be greatest in this area. Teaching staff should be aware of lack of student knowledge and try to offer more information and practice in providing dental care for oncology patients.

Keywords: dental students; dental care; oncology; chemotherapy; radiotherapy; osteoradionecrosis

Citation: Pedic, I.; Cigic, L.; Kalibovic Govorko, D.; Vodanovic, K.; Bandic, R.; Glavinic, R.; Medvedec Mikic, I. Knowledge of Dental Students from Croatia, Slovenia, and Bosnia and Herzegovina about Dental Care of Oncology Patients. *Dent. J.* **2021**, 9, 132. https://doi.org/10.3390/dj9110132

Academic Editor: Rod Moore

Received: 3 September 2021
Accepted: 8 November 2021
Published: 15 November 2021

1. Introduction

The central role of the dentist in the treatment of patients with head and neck cancer is to care for the patient's oral cavity before, during, and after radio/chemotherapy. Since the oncology patients have a treatment plan that consists of different doses of radio- or chemotherapy, a detailed dental assessment is needed, and the ideal time is before oncology therapy even starts. A dental assessment includes intra/extraoral clinical examination of the head and neck, radiographic imaging analysis, laboratory reports, and insight into the complete medical history of the patient including the medications that the patient was or is still using. In addition, all teeth with caries, periapical pathoses, and a damaged periodontium or broken and half-impacted teeth may need to be treated. The treatment includes removing caries, endodontic or periodontal therapy, and, if needed, extraction. The removal of retained teeth should also be considered, especially in younger patients where some complications can be expected with unerupted third molars. In the elderly population, above 60 years, retained teeth, if they are without symptoms or clinical signs, should be left in the bone because there are more post-extraction complications, as published in the study of Trybek et al. [1]. The best time for dental treatment is at least 3 weeks before the beginning of oncology therapy. In case of a period shorter than 10 days, and, if the patient is not in acute inflammation, teeth extractions are performed during the so-called "golden window period" after radiation [2]. Dental care before oncology therapy includes oral hygiene instructions, descaling, promoting a noncariogenic diet, prophylactic treatment with fluorine preparations, and removing all sources of irritation and infection [3].

During chemotherapy and radiation therapy, good oral hygiene is crucial for patients. All elective dental treatments should be delayed until the end of oncology therapy. However, in the case of an active dental infection, a dentist and an oncologist should make a decision and a plan for helping the patient [4]. Patients on chemotherapy without radiation therapy may receive dental care, routine or necessary, but only if their counts are stable (leukocytes at least 2000 cells/mm^3, neutrophils >1000 cells/mm^3, platelets >50,000 cells/mm^3). Therefore, it is necessary to do a complete blood count (CBC) and differential blood count (DBC) on the day of dental treatment [4].

The period after oncology treatment requires frequent dental check-ups so that dentists can monitor a patient's condition through clinical examinations and detect possible local recurrences, metastatic lesions in the head and neck area, or secondary malignant lesions. The interval of "recall" visits is estimated individually, according to the patient's risk, but is likely to be no less frequent than 3 months, at least in the first instance [5]. Regular check-ups are performed for prevention, early diagnosis, and treatment of late radiation complications. After radiotherapy, tooth extractions and other oral surgical procedures are avoided, and the most important goal is to establish adequate fluoridation of teeth. In case that tooth extraction or some other oral surgical procedure is needed, Trybek et al. [6] suggest the technique of applying platelet-rich fibrin to the post-extraction alveolus in order to reduce the severity of post-extraction complications.

The aim of this research was to determine the knowledge of dental students from five universities in three neighboring countries, Croatia (Split, Rijeka, and Zagreb), Bosnia and Herzegovina (Sarajevo), and Slovenia (Ljubljana), about oncology patients' dental care. Moreover, the need for additional education on this topic during the time of their study was assessed.

2. Material and Methods

A total of 140 subjects, 21 to 27 years old, participated in this research. They were all students of fourth, fifth, and sixth year of dental medicine studies at five different universities (Split, Zagreb, Rijeka, Sarajevo, and Ljubljana) from three countries. The participation of all respondents was voluntary. The research was approved by the Ethics Committee of the University of Split, School of Medicine.

The research consisted of 36 specific questions as an online Google form from January to April 2020. The questionnaire was specially designed for this research and included questions about dental care of oncologic patients before, during, and after the oncology therapy. Using the correct statement from the literature, question sentences were formed, and answers "I agree with the statement", "I am not sure", "I do not agree with the statement" were offered. Moreover, data about gender, age, and the year of study were collected. After gathering all completed questionnaires, a statistical analysis of acquired data was conducted.

For statistical data processing, the STATISTICA 11.0 software package was used. Frequency tables were calculated for each question. Kruskal–Wallis ANOVA test was used to confirm the potential difference in responses between subjects from five different faculties of dental medicine studies. A general regression model was used to determine the potential influence of predictor variables (gender, year of study, and faculty). Both correlation coefficients and their significance express the potential interdependence of dependent and predictor variables. Statistical significance in all used methods was reduced to $p < 0.05$.

3. Results

The mean values of the age of respondents for the five faculties were very similar. The youngest students were from Split (23.0 ± 1.0 years), and the oldest were from Sarajevo (24.4 ± 0.8 years).

As for the gender of participants in this study, 115 (82.1%) were women and 25 (17.9%) were men (Table 1). The final year students (sixth year) were most numerous (Table 2).

Table 1. Frequency and percentage of respondents by gender for the five selected faculties of dental medicine.

	Ljubljana		Rijeka		Split		Sarajevo		Zagreb		In total	
	N	%	N	%	N	%	N	%	N	%	N	%
Female	5	62.5	14	87.5	38	79.2	23	76.7	35	92.1	115	82.1
Male	3	37.5	2	12.5	10	20.8	7	23.3	3	7.9	25	17.9
Total	8		16		48		30		2	38	140	

N—number of respondents, %—percentage of respondents.

Table 2. Frequency and percentage of respondents according to the year of study for five selected faculties of dental medicine.

Year of Study	Ljubljana		Rijeka		Split		Sarajevo		Zagreb		In total	
	N	%	N	%	N	%	N	%	N	%	N	%
4	4	50	7	43.8	16	33.3	17	56.7	20	45.7	64	45.8
5	0	0	9	56.2	16	33.3	13	43.3	7	32.1	45	32.1
6	4	50	0	0	16	33.3	0	0	11	22.1	31	22.1

N—number of respondents, %—percentage of respondents.

Dental students already learn about the dental care of oncologic patients. To the question "Did you learn about providing dental care to oncology patients as part of your studies?", 93.8% respondents from Rijeka responded affirmatively in contrast to 50% of students from Sarajevo.

Although most respondents received some education about oncology patients, their certainty that they can provide adequate care to cancer patients was generally low. Thus, the answer to the question "Do you think you have enough knowledge to help oncology patients?" was "Yes" from only 3.3% of students from Sarajevo and 34.2% of students from Zagreb.

As for the dental medicine students' knowledge about the most frequent carcinoma in the head and neck area, students from Zagreb showed the worst results. A total of 13.2% answered incorrectly. Students from Split answered correctly in 87.5% of cases.

To the statement, "Pre-therapy assessment of an oncology patient must include a detailed clinical examination of the oral cavity and radiological imaging.", the largest percentage of respondents from Sarajevo answered "I agree" (96.7%), and the largest percentage of respondents from Ljubljana answered "I disagree" (12.5%).

Responses to the statement "Total radiation dose greater than 40 Gray (Gy) poses a risk to osteoradionecrosis (ORN)." showed that students do not have the required level of knowledge about the strength of radiation dose that poses a risk of ORN. Approximately half of the respondents from all faculties, except Ljubljana, answered "I am not sure" (Table 3).

To the question "Do you think that antibiotic prophylaxis, before tooth extraction after oncology therapy, is a safe protection of the patient from ORN?", most negative answers were offered by respondents from Split (68.8%), and most positive answers were from the students from Sarajevo (60%). A large number of students from all faculties answered "I do not know", which shows us that students do not have the required level of knowledge in this area.

Table 3. Frequency and percentage of respondents with respect to responses to the statement "Total radiation dose greater than 40 Gy poses a risk to ORN." for five selected faculties of dental studies.

	Ljubljana		Rijeka		Split		Sarajevo		Zagreb	
	N	%	*N*	%	*N*	%	*N*	%	*N*	%
I agree	5	62.5	8	50	17	35.4	15	50	17	44.7
I am not sure	2	25.0	8	50	23	57.5	15	50	19	50
I disagree	1	12.5	0	0	8	7.1	0	0	2	5.3

N—number of respondents, %—percentage of respondents.

To the statement "In case an emergency invasive dental procedure must be performed, and the platelet count is less than 50,000 cells/mm^3, a platelet transfusion is required.", most respondents answered "I agree". In general, there is a large discrepancy in responses both within and between faculties (Table 4).

Table 4. Frequency and percentage of respondents regarding the answers to the statement "In case an emergency invasive dental procedure must be performed, and the platelet count is less than 50,000 cells/mm^3, platelet transfusion is required." for five selected faculties of dental medicine.

	Ljubljana		Rijeka		Split		Sarajevo		Zagreb	
	N	%	*N*	%	*N*	%	*N*	%	*N*	%
I agree	5	62.5	8	50.1	24	50	24	**80**	30	76.4
I am not sure	2	25.0	5	31.3	19	39.6	5	16.7	7	18.4
I disagree	1	12.5	3	**18.8**	5	10.4	1	3.3	2	5.2

N—number of respondents, %—percentage of respondents.

Students also showed uncertainty in the case of responses to the statement "During chemotherapy, if the granulocyte count is less than 2000 cells/mm^3, antibiotic prophylaxis is required." (Table 5). However, it can be seen that more than half of the students, except those from Ljubljana, agreed that antibiotic prophylaxis is needed.

Table 5. Frequency and percentage of respondents regarding the answers to the statement "During chemotherapy, if the granulocyte count is less than 2000 cells/mm^3, antibiotic prophylaxis is required." for five selected faculties of dental medicine.

	Ljubljana		Rijeka		Split		Sarajevo		Zagreb	
	N	%	*N*	%	*N*	%	*N*	%	*N*	%
I agree	2	25.0	12	**75.1**	27	**56.3**	20	**66.7**	24	**63.2**
I am not sure	3	37.5	2	12.5	19	39.6	10	33.3	12	31.6
I disagree	1	12.5	2	12.5	2	4.2			2	5.2

N—number of respondents, %—percentage of respondents.

In terms of responses to the statement "The ideal time for extraction of a tooth with a poor prognosis is 3 weeks before the start of oncology treatment.", there was a wide range of responses. The highest percentage of "I agree" answers was offered by students from Rijeka (87.6%) and Zagreb (81.6%), and the highest percentage of negative answers was offered by students from Ljubljana (37.5%).

Responses to the statement "Endodontic treatment on an avital tooth with symptoms must be performed at least 7 days before the start of oncology therapy." are shown in Table 6. Most students from Split and only half of the students from Sarajevo answered "I agree".

Table 6. Frequency and percentage of respondents regarding the answers to the statement "Endodontic treatment on an avital tooth with symptoms must be performed at least 7 days before the start of oncology therapy." for five selected faculties of dental medicine.

	Ljubljana		Rijeka		Split		Sarajevo		Zagreb	
	N	%	*N*	%	*N*	%	*N*	%	*N*	%
I agree	5	62.5	9	60	31	**64.6**	15	**50**	23	60.5
I am not sure	2	25.0	4	26.7	13	27.1	7	23.3	8	21.1
I disagree	1	12.5	2	13.3	4	8.4	8	26.7	7	18.5

N—number of respondents, %—percentage of respondents.

Even greater variance in results, both within each faculty and between faculties, was shown in the answers to the statement "If a single-visit endodontic procedure cannot be performed on a tooth, extraction of that tooth is required.". Students from Rijeka agreed for the most part (62.5% of them), while students from Zagreb offered the most "I disagree" answers (44.8%).

To the statement "Dentists also recommend alcohol-based mouthwashes.", most respondents from Rijeka (75.0%) and the least respondents from Sarajevo answered "I disagree" (33.3%).

To the question "Would you recommend removing fixed orthodontic appliances before starting oncological treatment?" (Table 7) the highest percentage of respondents from Sarajevo and the lowest percentage of respondents from Zagreb answered affirmatively. A relatively large percentage of "I do not know" answers was offered by students from all faculties, mostly students from Zagreb.

Table 7. Frequency and percentage of respondents regarding the answers to the question "Would you recommend removing fixed orthodontic appliances before starting oncological treatment?" for five selected faculties of dental medicine.

	Ljubljana		Rijeka		Split		Sarajevo		Zagreb	
	N	%	*N*	%	*N*	%	*N*	%	*N*	%
Yes	6	75.0	12	75.0	33	68.8	26	**86.7**	19	**50.0**
No					2	4.2	1	3.3	6	15.8
I do not know	2	25.0	4	25.0	13	27.1	3	10.0	13	**34.2**

N—number of respondents, %—percentage of respondents.

To the question "Do you think that it is best for the patient not to wear mobile prosthetic replacements during the oncology therapy?", most respondents from Rijeka answered affirmatively (75.0%), and the most negative answers were offered by respondents from Zagreb (42.1%).

To the question "Can implants osseointegrate into the irradiated maxilla/mandible?", the largest percentage of positive answers was offered by respondents from Rijeka (43.8%), while the largest percentage of negative answers was offered by respondents from Ljubljana (50.0%).

Most respondents from Rijeka (81.3%) answered affirmatively to the question "Do you think that supragingival and subgingival scaling should be delayed for some time after the end of oncology therapy?", and the most negative answers were offered by respondents from Ljubljana (87.5%).

With the general regression model of 10 selected dependent variables representing students' knowledge of dental care in oncology patients, four of them showed a weak, statistically significant correlation with predictor variables: "There is no proven higher incidence of caries in oncology patients." ($R = 0.25$; $p = 0.0373$), "The ideal time for extraction of a tooth with a poor prognosis is 3 weeks before the start of oncology treatment." ($R = 0.25$; $p = 0.0376$), "If a single-visit endodontic procedure cannot be performed on the tooth, extraction of that tooth is required." ($R = 0.20$; $p = 0.0462$), and "Dentists also recommend alcohol-based mouthwashes." ($R = 0.24$; $p = 0.0419$) (Figures 1–4).

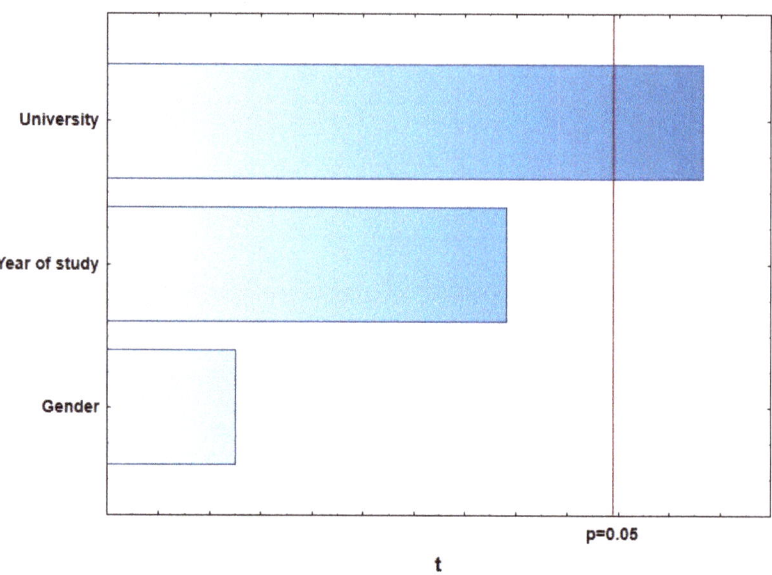

Figure 1. A higher incidence of caries in oncology patients has not been proven.

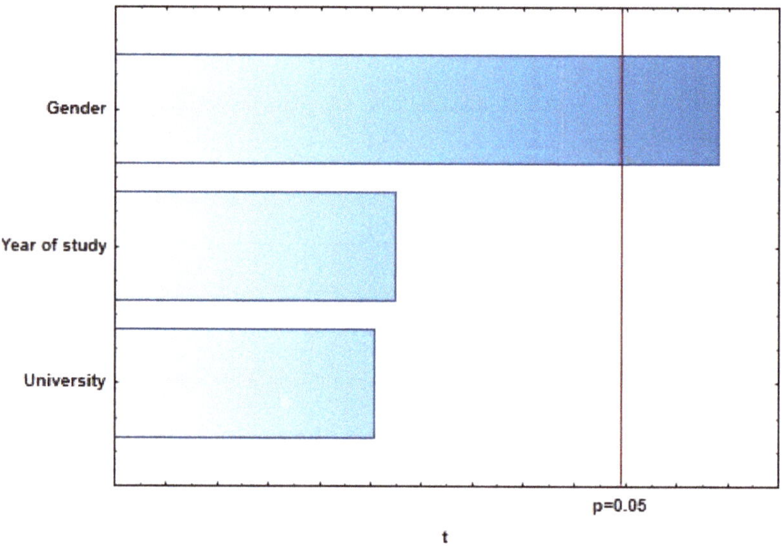

Figure 2. The ideal time to extract teeth with a poor prognosis is 3 weeks before starting oncology treatment.

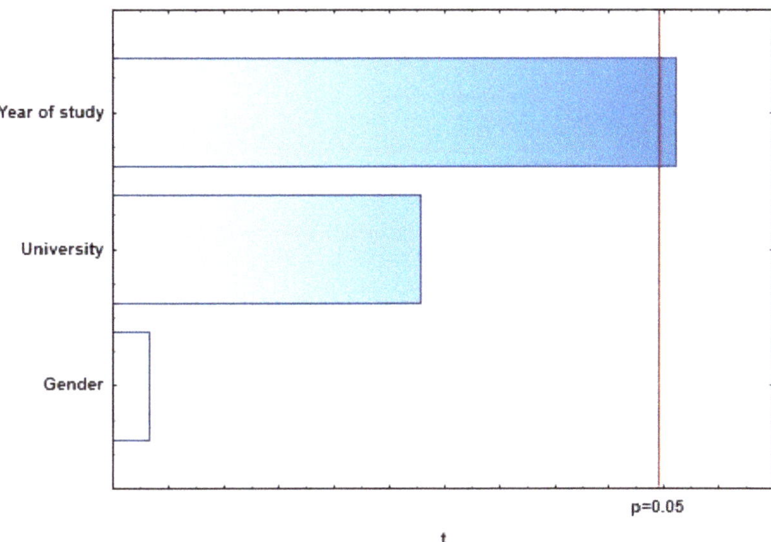

Figure 3. If a single-visit endodontic procedure cannot be performed on a tooth, extraction of that tooth is required.

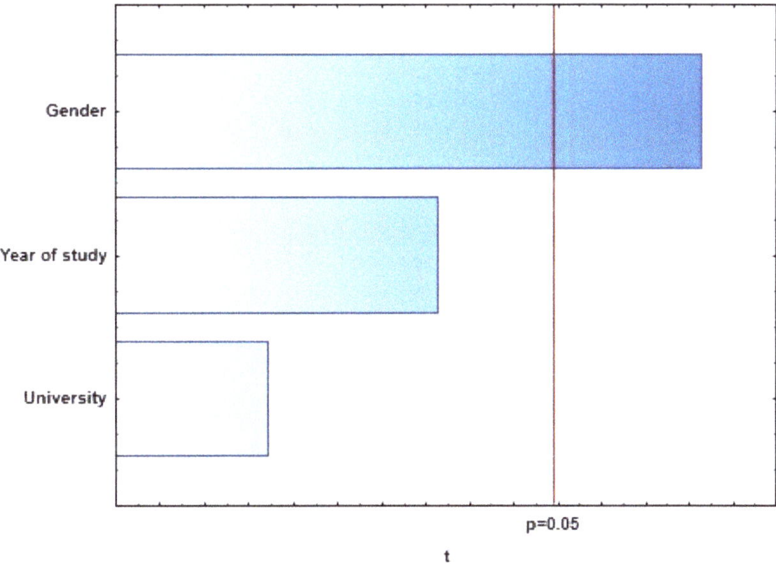

Figure 4. Dentists also recommend alcohol-based mouthwashes.

Although certain differences in the level of knowledge across faculties were observed, they were not statistically significant when applied in the Kruskal–Wallis ANOVA test.

4. Discussion

The main goal of this study was to determine whether the students of dental medicine from five different universities from three neighboring countries have enough knowledge about dental care of patients on oncology therapy. School programs are quite similar across all dental faculties. Respondents were mainly female students, and the majority of respondents were students in their fourth year of study. It seems that the younger students are more willing to respond to surveys or are more willing to test their knowledge. Older colleagues are either uninterested in completing surveys or overburdened with learning and have no desire to spend time completing surveys. We expected just the opposite, i.e., more responses from older years, as one form of testing their knowledge before graduation. According to the answers of 140 students from the last 3 years of studies, a conclusion is that they did not learn enough about this specific topic. Similar results were reported by Walton et al. in their study from 1992 when they examined the quality of dental students' education in the field of oncology. Students' knowledge about oncological patients was assessed on the basis of an exam results after a summer course at UCLA for 2 consecutive years of third-year dental students (1990 and 1991). In the same study, students were asked about risk factors for developing squamous cell carcinoma; 69% of students in 1990 and 77% in 1991 offered the correct answer [6]. This study showed similar results, whereby students showed good knowledge about the incidence of head and neck tumors cancer and the histological type of the cancer. They also knew that two-thirds of head and neck tumors occur in men. On questions about the prevention and treatment of complications of head and neck cancer treatment (ORN), 69% of students in 1990, and 77% in 1991 offered the correct answer [7].

The 2007 study conducted in Great Britain [8] investigated the differences in awareness of oral cancer between future doctors of medicine and dentistry. According to the answers on the 12-question questionnaire that included questions about an oral examination of patients, knowledge about risk factors and advising patients about them, the clinical appearance of oral precancerous lesions and oral cancer, and clinical care procedures of oncology patients, the authors concluded that respondents did not have enough knowledge [8]. In this research, to the question "Do you think you have enough knowledge to provide dental care for cancer patients?", 45.7% of students from Split, Zagreb, Rijeka, Sarajevo, and Ljubljana answered that they think they are not educated enough. Nevertheless, there was a willingness for additional education on dental care for oncology patients.

In this study, the statement "Potentially long-lasting and most serious side-effect of radiotherapy is osteoradionecrosis (ORN)", 81.4% of respondents answered correctly by choosing the answer "I agree with the statement". Poorer knowledge was shown regarding radiation doses effects on ORN development and the potential antibiotic prophylaxis of ORN. To the claim "A total radiation dose greater than 40 Gy poses a risk to ORN.", most of the answers offered were "I am not sure" (47.9%). To the question "Do you think that, before tooth extraction after oncology therapy, a patient is safe from ORN?", only 55% of all respondents agreed that this was not true. According to these results, it is evident that knowledge about ORN as the most serious consequence of treatment is not satisfactory, and there is a need for additional education of students on this topic.

As for blood cell counts values and their importance for dental care of oncological patients, the research of Walton et al. [7] reported that approximately 64% of students showed a good knowledge of blood cell counts. Comparing results with this study, 73.6% of respondents answered that they agree to the statement "Before oral surgical treatment of a patient on chemotherapy, analysis of CBC and WBC counts is mandatory.", and 64.3% of respondents answered affirmatively to the statement "In case an emergency invasive dental procedure must be performed, and the platelet count is less than 50000 cells/mm^3, platelet transfusion is required.", which is a similar finding to Walton's study. Furthermore, to the statement "During chemotherapy, if the granulocyte count is less than 2000 cells/mm^3, antibiotic prophylaxis is required.", 60.7% of respondents answered affirmatively. It is evident that students are aware of the need to analyze CBC and WBC counts of patients.

A study by Alpöz et al. conducted in 2013 on Turkish final-year dental students examined students' knowledge of oral complications that occur in oncology patients and their treatment, as well as the role of dentists in implementing necessary dental care protocols. Oral complications of chemotherapy and head and neck radiotherapy were accurately recognized by 87% of students [9]. This study obtained similar results; 84.3% of respondents answered correctly to the statement "Mucositis is an acute consequence of head and neck radiotherapy.". The study by Singh et al. [10] reported that, due to radiation, some of the cells of oral mucosa die during or at the end of second week of therapy. Due to this fact, the mucous membrane will become red and inflamed. This clinical condition is known as mucositis. After the completion of radiotherapy, the mucosa begins to heal rapidly, and most healing is complete by about 2 months [11,12].

Radiation caries, a rampant form of dental decay, occurs in individuals who receive a course of radiotherapy that includes exposure of the salivary gland [10]. In a Turkish study on the question "Do dental caries progress faster after head and neck radiotherapy?", 84.4% of students offered the correct answer. Our students also showed good knowledge by responding to the statement "There is no proven higher incidence of caries in oncology patients.", whereby 77.9% disagreed with the statement. Moreover, 92.9% of students agreed with the statement "Pre-therapy assessment of an oncology patient must include a detailed clinical examination of the oral cavity and radiological imaging.", thus showing a high level of knowledge about pre-therapy guidelines.

The guidelines presented by the Multinational Association of Supportive Care in Cancer (MASCC) and the International Society of Oral Oncology (ISOO) suggest the use of a soft toothbrush, dental floss with wax, and mouthwash several times after brushing your teeth [13]. Similarly, the guidelines of the British Society for Disability and Oral Health from 2018 recommend the use of a manual or electric brush with medium bristles, with the additional use of dental floss and interdental brushes. If brushing becomes too painful, the toothbrush can be replaced with a soft one, but they pointed out that soft toothbrushes are not as effective in controlling plaque [4]. Turkish students are not so familiar with pre-therapeutic oral patient evaluation, while students in this study were familiar with the instructions in oral hygiene and as many as 85% agreed with the statement "Patients undergoing head and neck radiotherapy should use soft brushes.".

To the question about the ideal period for oral surgery before the start of oncological treatment, only 27.3% of Turkish students offered the correct answers. To the statement "The ideal time for extraction of a tooth with a poor prognosis is 3 weeks before the start of oncology treatment.", 65.7% of students in this study answered affirmatively. The correct answer to the statement "Endodontic treatment on an avital tooth with symptoms must be done at least 7 days before the start of oncology therapy." was offered by 59.3% of respondents. To the statement "If a single-visit endodontic procedure cannot be performed on a tooth, extraction of that tooth is required.", 39.3% of students agreed.

In conclusion we can state that, although dental students learned about oncological therapy, their knowledge and readiness for providing dental care to oncological patients is still not enough. Most students are familiar with the incidence and most common type of head and neck tumors, while knowledge about tumor treatment and the side-effects of radiation therapy and/or chemotherapy is weak. Students did not show satisfactory knowledge about osteoradionecrosis, which is the most serious side-effect of radiotherapy; therefore, the emphasis on additional education should be the greatest in this area.

A good thing is that the surveyed students are aware of their lack of knowledge, and they want to learn more. Teaching staff should be aware of the situation and try to offer more information and practice in providing dental care for oncology patients. Perhaps the best way for that is to introduce courses to the curriculum that will prepare future dentists to work with oncology patients.

The limitations of this study were the small number of participants and the large difference in the number of responses per university. A similar study with a greater number of participants is needed to gain better insight into the dental students' knowledge.

Author Contributions: Conceptualization, I.P., L.C. and I.M.M.; methodology, I.P., D.K.G. and I.M.M.; validation, R.B. and R.G.; formal analysis, R.G.; investigation, I.P.; resources, K.V., R.B. and R.G.; data curation, I.P. and K.V.; writing—original draft preparation, I.P. and I.M.M.; writing—review and editing, L.C., D.K.G. and I.M.M.; visualization, L.C. and I.M.M.; supervision, I.M.M. All authors read and agreed to the published version of the manuscript.

Funding: This research received no external funding.

Institutional Review Board Statement: The study was conducted according to the guidelines of the Declaration of Helsinki and approved by the Ethics Committee the University of Split, School of Medicine (003-08/20-03/0005, 2181-198-03-04-20-0006, 30 January 2020).

Informed Consent Statement: Informed consent was obtained from all subjects involved in the study.

Acknowledgments: The authors would like to thank Ivana Brekalo Prso from the School of Dental Medicine, University of Rijeka, Croatia, Alma Konjhodzic from the Faculty of Stomatology, University of Sarajevo, BiH, Valentina Brzovic Rajic from the School of Dental Medicine, University of Zagreb, Croatia, and Asst. Jana Krpez from the School of Medicine, University of Ljubljana, Slovenia for their help with sharing of question forms.

Conflicts of Interest: The authors declare no conflict of interest.

References

1. Trybek, G.; Chruściel-Nogalska, M.; Machnio, M.; Smektała, T.; Malinowski, J.; Tutak, M.; Sporniak-Tutak, K. Surgical extraction of impacted teeth in elderly patients. A retrospective analysis of perioperative complications—The experience of a single institution. *Gerodontology* **2016**, *33*, 410–415. [CrossRef]
2. Little, J.W.; Miller, S.C.; Rhodus, N.L. *Little and Falace's Dental Management of the Medically Compromised Patient*, 9th ed.; Elsevier: St. Louis, MO, USA, 2017; pp. 480–514.
3. Topić, B. *Interdisciplinarity in the Diagnosis and Treatment of Premalignant and Malignant Lesions of the Oral Mucosa: Dentist, Member of the Oncology Team in Radio (Chemo) Therapy of the Head and Neck*, 1st ed.; Academy of Science, Dental Chammber FBiH: Sarajevo, Bosnia and Herzegovina, 2016; pp. 133–150.
4. Levi, L.E.; Lalla, R.V. Dental Treatment Planning for the Patient with Oral Cancer. *Dent. Clin. N. Am.* **2018**, *62*, 121–130. [CrossRef] [PubMed]
5. Kumar, N.; Burke, M.; Brooke, A.; Chan, F.; Ali, S.; Doughty, J.; Shaw, J.; Duggal, M.; Lewis, D.; Fiske, J.; et al. *The Oral Management of Oncology Patients Requiring Radiotherapy, Chemotherapy and/or Bone Marrow Transplantation: Clinical Guidelines [Internet]*; The Royal College of Surgeons of England: London, UK, 2018; Available online: https://www.rcseng.ac.uk/-/media/files/rcs/fds/publications/rcs-oncology-guideline-update--v36.pdf (accessed on 25 June 2021).
6. Trybek, G.; Rydlińska, J.; Aniko-Włodarczyk, M.; Jaroń, A. Effect of Platelet-Rich Fibrin Application on Non-Infectious Complications after Surgical Extraction of Impacted Mandibular Third Molars. *Int. J. Environ. Res. Public Health* **2021**, *18*, 8249. [CrossRef] [PubMed]
7. Walton, L.; Silverman, S.; Ramos, D., Jr.; Costa, C.R. Dental student education in oncology: Design and assessment of an undergraduate course. *J. Cancer Educ.* **1992**, *7*, 221–225. [CrossRef] [PubMed]
8. Carter, L.M.; Ogden, G.R. Oral cancer awareness of undergraduate medical and dental students. *BMC Med. Educ.* **2007**, *7*, 44. [CrossRef] [PubMed]
9. Alpöz, E.; Güneri, P.; Epstein, J.B.; Cankaya, H.; Osmic, D.; Boyacıoğlu, H. Dental students' knowledge of characteristics and management of oral complications of cancer therapy. *Support. Care Cancer* **2013**, *21*, 2793–2798. [CrossRef] [PubMed]
10. Singh, G.; Sood, A.; Kaur, A.; Gupta, D. Pathogenesis, Clinical Features, Diagnosis, and Management of Radiation Hazards in Dentistry. *Open Dent. J.* **2018**, *12*, 742–752. [CrossRef] [PubMed]
11. White, S.C.; Pharaoh, M.J. *Oral Radiology: Principles and Interpretation*, 2nd ed.; Mosby, Inc.: St. Louis, MO, USA, 2014.
12. Iannucci, J.; Howerton, L.J. *Laura Jansen Howerton. Dental Radiology Principles and Technique*, 3rd ed.; Saunders Elsevier: Philadelphia, PA, USA, 2006; p. 526.
13. Oral Care Education. Available online: https://www.mascc.org/oral-care-education (accessed on 25 June 2021).

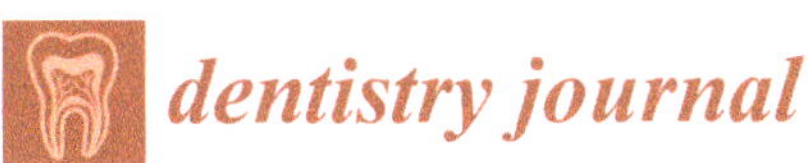 MDPI

Article

Use of a Knowledge-Based Governance Approach to Plan a Post-COVID-19 Predoctoral Dental Curriculum

Natasha M. Flake [1,*], Daniel C. N. Chan [2], Arthur C. DiMarco [2,3] and Bruce D. Silverstein [4,5]

1 Department of Endodontics, University of Washington School of Dentistry, Seattle, WA 98195, USA
2 Department of Restorative Dentistry, University of Washington School of Dentistry, Seattle, WA 98195, USA; dcnchan@uw.edu (D.C.N.C.); adimarco@ewu.edu (A.C.D.)
3 Department of Dental Hygiene, Eastern Washington University, Spokane, WA 99202, USA
4 Department of Medicine, University of Washington School of Medicine, Seattle, WA 98195, USA; brucesil@uw.edu
5 Department of Oral Medicine, University of Washington School of Dentistry, Seattle, WA 98195, USA
* Correspondence: nflake@uw.edu

Abstract: COVID-19 abruptly changed dental education, forcing educators out of their comfort zones and into using new technologies and teaching approaches. At the University of Washington School of Dentistry, a task force evaluated the curricular changes that resulted from COVID and made recommendations for the future predoctoral dental curriculum. This manuscript reports the process employed, the findings of the task force, and how these findings will impact the curriculum. A knowledge-based governance (KBG) approach was employed. KBG focuses on gathering all relevant information and identifying all choices. It separates dialogue from deliberation. Information was gathered via literature review, focus group interviews, electronic surveys, and other metrics. The task force evaluated: (1) delivering didactic content remotely; (2) administering assessments remotely; (3) duplicating preclinical simulation lab courses due to social distancing; and (4) the conversion from a numerical to a credit/no credit grading scale. Key recommendations resulted from focus groups and electronic surveys that allowed any student or faculty member an opportunity to provide input. Some topics were relatively non-controversial and strong recommendations were evident. The most controversial issue was which grading scale should be utilized. A KBG approach is an effective means to address mega issues in the dental school environment.

Keywords: undergraduate dental education; postgraduate dental education; specialty training; teaching methodology; online education; student survey; knowledge-based governance; curriculum

Citation: Flake, N.M.; Chan, D.C.N.; DiMarco, A.C.; Silverstein, B.D. Use of a Knowledge-Based Governance Approach to Plan a Post-COVID-19 Predoctoral Dental Curriculum. *Dent. J.* **2021**, *9*, 142. https://doi.org/10.3390/dj9120142

Academic Editors: Jelena Dumancic and Božana Lončar Brzak

Received: 29 August 2021
Accepted: 5 November 2021
Published: 1 December 2021

1. Introduction

The COVID-19 pandemic caused dental schools worldwide to change the way they teach students and assess their skills and knowledge. Academicians were forced to significantly rework teaching methodologies and assessment techniques on very short timelines due to dental school closures and social distancing requirements [1,2]. The Association for Dental Education in Europe assessed the initial response of European Academic Dental Institutions to the pandemic and found widespread modifications throughout 69 dental schools [3]. Likewise, dental schools in the United States faced similar challenges and made adjustments to administration, teaching, and learning [4]. Students in one dental school reported they appreciated online learning, but they missed educational experiences and had concerns about independent clinical practice after graduation due to the pandemic [5].

It is likely that some of the curricular changes instigated out of the necessity of the pandemic will find a place in dental school curricula of the future. At the University of Washington School of Dentistry (UWSOD), a task force was charged with evaluating the curricular changes that resulted from the COVID-19 pandemic. The task force evaluated what worked well, what worked poorly, and what aspects should be kept going forward.

The following pandemic-induced changes were assessed: (1) delivering didactic courses remotely; (2) administering exams and other assessments remotely; (3) duplicating courses in the preclinical simulation lab due to social distancing requirements; and (4) the conversion to a credit/no credit (Cr/NC) grading scale from a numerical grading scale. This manuscript reports the process employed, the findings of the task force, and how these findings will impact the predoctoral dental curriculum.

2. Process

A knowledge-based governance (KBG) approach was employed to assess the curricular changes triggered by COVID-19 [6–8]. KBG is a philosophy of governance and decision-making used by professional associations. It values the quality of the information on which decisions are made, rather than who makes the decisions. It focuses on gathering all relevant information and identifying all choices, rather than focusing on the conclusion. The advantages and disadvantages of each choice are considered. KBG separates dialogue from deliberation. Dialogue seeks to inform and ensure common understanding of the information that impacts a decision, including consideration of all available options. Deliberation focuses on evaluation, decisions, and conclusions.

A KBG process asks four key questions [6,8]. Adapted for the dental school setting, these are: (1) What do we know about our stakeholders' needs, wants, and preferences that is relevant to this decision? (2) What do we know about the current reality and evolving dynamics of our school and profession that is relevant to this decision? (3) What do we know about the capacity and strategic position of our school that is relevant to this decision? (4) What are the ethical implications of our choices?

The task force prioritized the success of the school as a whole over individual agendas and was motived by the long-term future, not just the next academic year. To achieve this, a four-pronged approach to information gathering was implemented: (1) literature review; (2) focus group interviews; (3) surveys; and (4) metrics.

Thirteen focus group and individual interviews were conducted (Table 1). Participation by all stakeholders was voluntary. Student recruitment for focus group participation was facilitated by student leaders. Focus groups were held online using the Zoom platform. Standardized questions addressing all topics of interest were used for the interviews of students, foundations faculty, preclinical faculty, Clerkship Directors, and Associate Deans. Questions specific to staff expertise were used for staff interviews. Staff were interviewed who had knowledge and experience in scheduling, information technology, educational technology, and managing preclinical laboratory courses. Questions for the Graduate Program Directors focused on grading scales and graduate program admissions.

Table 1. Focus group interviews. Standardized questions were asked for the student, foundations faculty, preclinical faculty, Clerkship Directors, and Associate Dean interviews. Questions specific to expertise were asked for staff and Graduate Program Directors interviews.

Students	Faculty
Class of 2021 Class of 2022 Class of 2023 Class of 2024	Foundations faculty Preclinical faculty Clerkship Directors Graduate Program Directors
Staff	Administration
Scheduler Director of Information Technology Educational Technology Specialist Preclinical Lab Support	Associate Dean of Academic Affairs and Associate Dean of Student Services and Admissions

Electronic surveys were sent to all students, faculty, and Graduate Program Directors. Survey questions were based on comments heard in the focus groups. Standardized questions addressing all topics were used for student and faculty surveys, with a few questions that differed or differed in wording depending on the target audience. The Graduate Program Directors survey specifically addressed the impact of grading scales on graduate program admissions. All surveys consisted of a series of statements grouped by topic, and participants were instructed to rate their level of agreement with the statement as: "strongly agree", "agree", "neutral", "disagree", "strongly disagree", or "not applicable/don't know". All electronic surveys also invited open-ended comments. Course directors were also asked for any metrics that could compare their pre-COVID-19 and COVID-era course to provide supporting data that might aid in formulating recommendations.

3. Findings

We report the results of the surveys and relate them to the focus group findings and metrics from course directors. Survey response demographics are reported in Table 2. For the narrative, we considered responses of "strongly agree" and "agree" as supporting a statement, and responses of "neutral", "disagree", "strongly disagree", and "not applicable/don't know" as not supporting a statement. The complete results of the survey are detailed in Appendix A. The recommendations of the task force are included in the Discussion section.

Table 2. Demographics of electronic survey responses. Age and gender identity were asked as optional, open-ended questions. Regular appointment faculty include both full-time and part-time faculty. Affiliate faculty volunteers are paid a nominal stipend, typically one or less day per week.

Faculty Demographics	Student Demographics
Total faculty responses, n = 42	Total student responses, n = 74
Regular faculty appointments, n = 33	Class of 2021, n = 8
Affiliate faculty appointments, n = 9	Class of 2022, n = 23
Time worked in dental education:	Class of 2023, n = 12
0–5 years, n = 8	Class of 2024, n = 31
6–10 years, n = 4	Students reporting age, n = 55
11–20 years, n = 10	Median age = 25 years
>20 years, n = 20	Mean age = 26 years
Teach in these predoc settings:	Age range = 21–44 years
Foundations, n = 9	Students reporting gender identity, n = 55
Preclinical dental courses, n = 21	Female/woman, n = 32
Clinical dental courses, n = 21	Male/man, n = 22
Clinic, n = 18	Genderqueer/non-binary, n = 1
Other, n = 1	
Do not teach predoc, n = 3	
Teach in >1 predoc setting, n = 18	
Course director for predoc course, n = 22	
Faculty reporting age, n = 30	
Median age = 57 years	
Mean age = 55 years	
Age range = 29–75 years	
Faculty reporting gender identity, n = 29	
Female/woman, n = 13	
Male/man, n = 16	

3.1. *Delivering Didactic Courses Remotely*

The UWSOD academic calendar is based on academic quarters. All in-person courses ceased in the last week of winter quarter 2020 due to the pandemic. Didactic courses have remained remote since that time, with an anticipated return to in-person courses in autumn quarter 2021.

Students and faculty share concerns about the social impacts of remote learning (Figure 1): 81% of faculty and 53% of students agree or strongly agree that remote learning has impacted class dynamics (Figure 1A). Sixty-one percent of students feel disconnected from their classmates, and 45% feel disconnected from faculty, while 67% of faculty feel disconnected from students (Figure 1C). The social effects also impact learning: 76% of faculty and 47% of students think that remote learning decreases student ability to learn from classmates (Figure 1B). Faculty (95%) and students (61%) agree that in-person interactions with faculty promote professional development (Figure 1D).

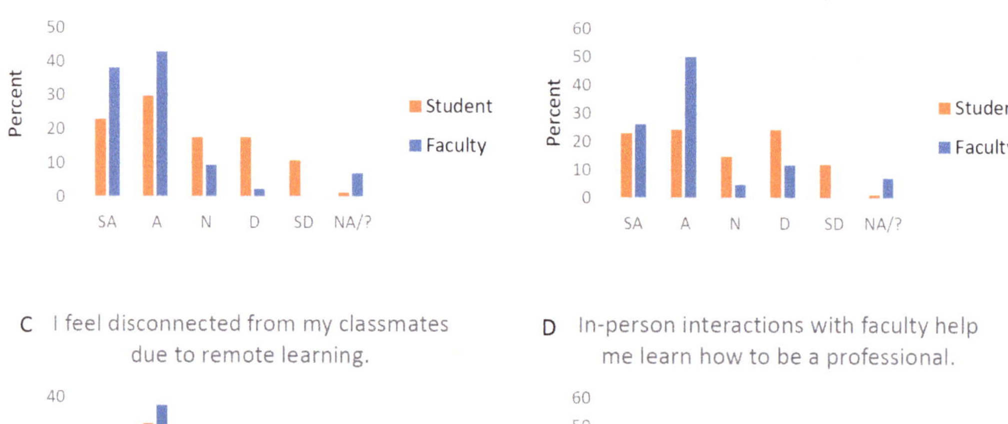

Figure 1. Social impacts of remote learning. All students and faculty were asked about the social impacts of remote learning. Graph titles reflect wording asked of students, but wording was customized for students and faculty. For example, the statement for students was "Remote learning has weakened my class dynamic", and the statement for faculty was "Remote learning has weakened dental student class dynamics". SA, strongly agree; A, agree; N, neutral; D, disagree; SD, strongly disagree; NA/?, not applicable/don't know.

The majority of faculty generally prefer in-person didactics. Faculty understand student level of comprehension and can "read the room" and adjust teaching in real-time better when didactics are in person. They find that students are more likely to ask a question or speak up in person, and that students do not actively engage in Zoom sessions. While only 7% of faculty generally prefer pre-recorded asynchronous lectures, 55% like the flexibility of this format. They do think it takes more time to prepare a quality pre-recorded lecture than to deliver an in-person lecture. Faculty also are concerned about students not viewing assigned lectures, which can be corroborated by statistics in the learning management software.

Students are more split than faculty, with 39% generally preferring in-person didactics, and 51% preferring pre-recorded asynchronous lectures. Approximately half (51%) of students find it difficult to focus during Zoom sessions, and 27% say they log on but do not typically actively engage. One-third (34%) of students are more likely to ask a question or speak up during an in-person didactic session. A large majority (88%) of students like the flexibility of asynchronous pre-recorded lectures, though over half (55%) also like to be able to ask questions in real-time.

The class of 2021 focus group, the most experienced student cohort, unanimously agreed that pre-recorded asynchronous lectures are convenient, but that in-person formats are best for learning. They stated that pre-recorded lectures are fine if the goal is to pass a test, but in-person interactions are best for learning to become a dentist. These students explained that in-person didactics are more organic and foster more questions, discussion, and learning.

3.2. Administering Assessments Remotely

Almost all faculty adapted their exam format for remote administration, but the adaptations varied. For example, some faculty increased the number of essays, while others increased the number of multiple-choice questions. Some faculty proctored exams remotely via Zoom or via automated software; others did not proctor and relied on the honor system or gave open-book exams.

Approximately one-half (52%) of faculty think students study less when an exam is open-book, and one-third (33%) think students learn less when an exam is open-book. From the student perspective, 38% say they study less, and 22% say they learn less when an exam is open-book.

Importantly, 62% of faculty and 32% of students are concerned about academic dishonesty when exams are not proctored. Students are more comfortable than faculty with remote proctoring, but still only 41% of students are comfortable with a Zoom proctor and 28% with proctoring by automated software. Twenty-seven percent of students say it is difficult to find a suitable (quiet, private) space to take a remote exam.

3.3. Split Shift in the Preclinical Simulation Lab

Social distancing requirements allow only one-half of a class in the preclinical simulation lab at once. Thus, all courses in the preclinical lab are held in two shifts. In addition, lectures, quizzes and exams are prohibited in the preclinical lab and must be completed remotely. This necessitates a complex scheduling puzzle, where one-half of the class attends lab and the other half of the class remains offsite during any class period.

Feedback from course directors strongly supports a return to the entire class in the lab at once. Course directors adapted to the split shift in varied ways, including covering some content only didactically, shifting content to other courses, focusing on hands-on experience at the expense of didactics, and increasing student practice time after hours. The most compelling reason to return to a single lab session is the reduction in time for hands-on experience during class for students with the split shift. Further, scheduling for the split shift is a logistical challenge that impacts other courses. From the student perspective, 65% feel disconnected from classmates who do not share the same lab time, and 31% are concerned about imbalanced experiences between the two groups of students.

3.4. Conversion to Credit/No Credit Grading from a Numerical (4.0) Grading Scale

The UWSOD historically utilizes a numerical (4.0) grading scale for most required predoctoral dental courses and calculates a class rank based on academic performance. Starting spring quarter 2020, predoctoral courses were temporarily converted to a Cr/NC (i.e., pass/fail) grading scale. Courses are scheduled to return to their pre-COVID-19 grading scales in autumn quarter 2021. The rationale for Cr/NC grading was primarily due to concerns with remote learning. Concerns for students included internet connectivity difficulties, family responsibilities, and discrepancies among students in their housing and economic resources. Apprehension over the ability to verify academic integrity with distance learning also contributed. Overall, Cr/NC grading was intended to alleviate stress and help students cope with the uncertainties of the time. Given the circumstances, the decision to temporarily implement Cr/NC grading had wide, though not universal, support from both students and faculty.

The issue of Cr/NC versus 4.0 grading scales was the most polarizing subject the task force addressed. Individual stakeholders have strong and diverse opinions on the subject. From the perspective of class culture, 50% of faculty think numerical grades foster healthy competition, and 26% think numerical grades foster toxic competition within a class (Figure 2A,B). In contrast, 16% of students think numerical grades foster healthy competition, and 74% think numerical grades foster toxic competition (Figure 2A,B). Further, 74% of students are more likely to collaborate with classmates when a course is graded Cr/NC.

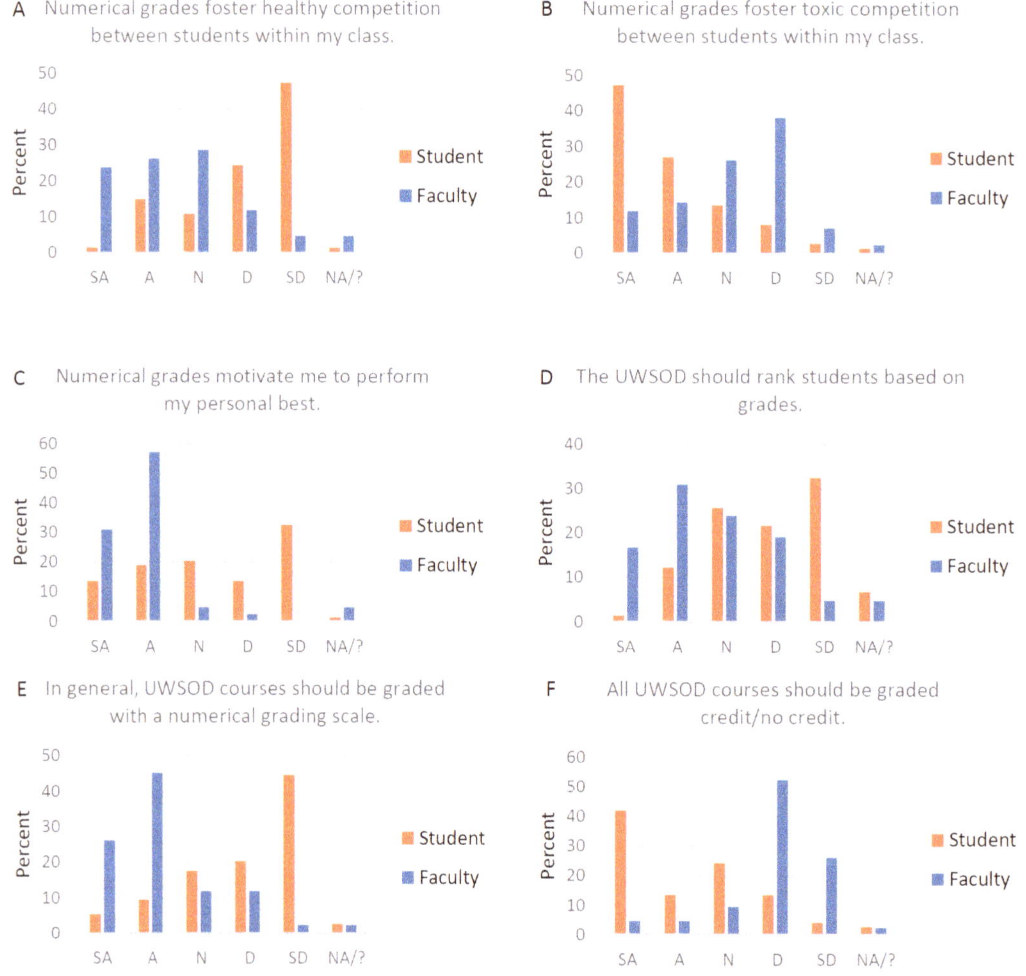

Figure 2. Faculty and student responses regarding grading scales. All students and faculty were asked about numerical and credit/no credit grading scales. Graph titles reflect wording asked of students, but wording was customized for students and faculty. For example, the statement for students was "Numerical grades motivate me to perform my personal best", and the statement for faculty was "Numerical grades motivate students to perform their personal best". SA, strongly agree; A, agree; N, neutral; D, disagree; SD, strongly disagree; NA/?, not applicable/don't know; UWSOD, University of Washington School of Dentistry.

From an academic perspective, faculty strongly prefer numerical grades. The differential effort that students put into courses with a numerical versus Cr/NC grading scale was raised by both faculty and students. Historically, when students had Cr/NC and 4.0 scale courses concurrently, they put less effort into Cr/NC courses, and even stopped attending once they had earned enough points to pass a Cr/NC course. Most faculty (88%) believe numerical grades motivate students to perform their personal best

(Figure 2C). Ninety percent say students study more, and 57% say students learn more in a numerically-graded course. Overall, 71% of faculty think that in general, courses should be graded with a numerical grading scale, while only 10% think all courses should be Cr/NC (Figure 2E,F). Finally, 76% of faculty agree or strongly agree that numerical grades foster academic excellence.

From an academic perspective, students favor Cr/NC grades, though not quite as strongly as faculty favor numerical grades. Approximately one-third (32%) of students say numerical grades motivate them to perform their personal best (Figure 2C). Approximately one-third (32%) of students study more, and 14% say they learn more, in a course with a numerical grade. Overall, 15% of students think that in general, courses should be graded with a numerical grading scale, while 55% feel all courses should be graded Cr/NC (Figure 2E,F).

A common concern about Cr/NC grading is its impact on graduate program admissions. Graduate Program Directors reported they consider both GPA and class rank in the admissions process. They relate it is difficult to assess applicants who went to a dental school that does not issue grades. All Graduate Program Directors who responded are concerned that a switch to Cr/NC grading might impact student matriculation to graduate programs.

Class rank can be considered separately from grades, as it is possible to calculate grade point average but not student rank. Forty-eight percent of faculty think students should receive a class rank based on grades (Figure 2D). One-fifth (20%) of students are motivated by class rank, and 14% feel that the school should rank students (Figure 2D). However, 5 of 8 Graduate Program Directors say if they could have only one piece of objective data for applicants, it would be class rank.

Each class of students has a different perspective, since they have experienced different time and grading formats. Even the class of 2021, who have the most experience and yet no personal stake in the decision, were conflicted. Students in this focus group were split on whether they preferred Cr/NC versus numerical grades; however, they agreed they studied less, and probably learned less, for a Cr/NC course.

4. Recommendations and Discussion

4.1. Delivering Didactic Courses Remotely

The task force recommends that the method of delivering didactic content ultimately be decided by course directors. In-person interactions and learning are highly valued. Faculty and students agree that personal interactions with faculty help students learn to be professionals, the "hidden" curriculum [9]. However, some content can be effectively delivered remotely, and some courses or content within a course are more amenable to remote delivery. The strengths and limitations of remote learning cited by students are similar to those reported by students in other countries [10–12].

Asynchronous remote didactics have the advantage of offering students multiple, flexible review opportunities. In cases where content is delivered by pre-recorded lectures or other asynchronous methods, the task force recommends they be followed-up with interactive sessions such as question and answer sessions, case reviews, etc. The task forces also recommends checkpoints throughout a course to ensure students are learning content in a timely manner (e.g., quizzes or other exercises).

A clearly successful example of the use of synchronous remote learning at UWSOD is the Regional Initiatives in Dental Education (RIDE) program. Synchronous remote methods have been used successfully with the RIDE program for many years, where dental students in Spokane, Washington actively participate in courses that are delivered in Seattle. Students are together in a classroom with an instructor in both Seattle and Spokane. This differs from the remote synchronous didactics started during the pandemic, which are often experienced as lecturing to "black boxes" on Zoom. With some exceptions, the task force has little enthusiasm for synchronous remote lectures, due to low student engagement. These methods also lack the flexible timing offered by asynchronous methods.

For all methods, the task force recommends that faculty be trained in effective teaching, and that they have protected time to dedicate to this training. Though nearly all the feedback received on remote asynchronous didactics related to pre-recorded lectures, other modalities are available. There is ample evidence that online teaching can be effective in higher education [13]. It is a matter of identifying which methods are useful for individual courses and providing faculty the training and time to implement these methods.

4.2. *Administering Assessments Remotely*

The task force strongly recommends that exams be administered in person under proctored conditions. The convenience of administering exams remotely does not outweigh the concerns over academic integrity, either real or perceived. Exceptions to this recommendation would be those exam formats that were administered as take-home exams prior to COVID.

4.3. *Split Shift in the Preclinical Simulation Lab*

The task force strongly recommends that the preclinical lab courses return to all students attending at the same time. The only recognized advantages of the split shift are potential lower student:faculty and/or student:equipment ratios. Improved ratios could also be achieved by deploying additional faculty or procuring additional equipment for preclinical courses, though this may be unfeasible.

4.4. *Conversion to Credit/No Credit Grading from a Numerical (4.0) Grading Scale*

The advantages and disadvantages of both Cr/NC and numerical grading scales are compelling. The task force recommends that the SOD resume its pre-COVID-19 grading scales for the foreseeable future. This means a numerical grading scale for most courses, with exceptions for courses that were graded Cr/NC prior to the pandemic. The task force recommends that, if a global change to Cr/NC grading is to be considered, more deliberate preparation is needed. Namely, a change to Cr/NC would require: (1) a culture that emphasizes excellence, rather than passing, and a mindset that the objective of the curriculum is to prepare students to be clinicians rather than test takers; and (2) faculty buy-in.

The attitudes of faculty and students regarding Cr/NC grading reflect those described in the literature [14]. In a point/counterpoint article, Jham, Cannella, and Abdibi support the position that a pass/fail system improves learning experiences for students [15]. They argue that pass/fail grades positively impact students' psychological well-being, that academic performance of health care students can be successfully evaluated using pass/fail grades, and that pass/fail grades promote self-directed and collaborative learning [15]. Austin, Allareddy, and Petrie support the position that a traditional grading system provides more objectivity and reliability in student evaluation [15]. They argue that traditional grades motivate student performance, provide objectivity and validity in performance assessment, and are important objective criteria for evaluation of graduate program applicants [15]. Ramaswamy et al. argue in favor of pass/fail grading, citing promotion of student well-being, intrinsic motivation, and competency-based education [16]. Further, comments provided by students in our focus groups and surveys are consistent with those of other dental students [17–19].

The question of how advanced dental education programs can best evaluate candidates has increased in importance in the past decade with the change to pass/fail scores on national board exams, particularly for applicants who attend a pass/fail dental school [20,21]. The Advanced Dental Admission Test (ADAT) was developed to provide a metric for use in graduate program admissions [22]. Each graduate program has its own process, but program directors consider many interacting factors when selecting candidates for graduate programs. The Graduate Program Directors reported they consider both GPA and class rank in the admissions process, consistent with published literature [23–25]. Clinical grades, dental school class rank, and dental school GPA were the three most important factors considered by pediatric dentistry program directors [24]. Among endodontic program directors, dental school class rank was the second most important factor, while dental school clinical grades, endodontic grades, and basic science grades were ranked sixth through eighth in importance [23]. For periodontics graduate programs, dental school clinical grades and dental school periodontics grades ranked second and third, while dental school class rank was the seventh most important factor considered in admissions [25].

4.5. Limitations

The KBG approach was effective overall, though there are limitations associated with the methods employed. First, a limitation of the electronic surveys is the risk of response bias, particularly because participants likely understood the purpose of the survey. Second, course directors were asked for any metrics that could be used to compare their course in pre-COVID-19 and COVID-19 times. We were aware that there would be caveats associated with any data collected. With the method of delivering content, the assessment method, and the grading scale changing simultaneously in most cases, it would be difficult to tease out the individual impact of these factors. Third, different cohorts of students have different lived experiences in dental school. For example, students in the class of 2024 provided input on a grading scale that they had not experienced in dental school, as pandemic-related changes occurred prior to their matriculation. In comparison, the class of 2021 had the greatest experience with different methods of teaching and learning in dental school and had the least personal stake in any decision about the curriculum. Although the focus group for this class was extremely insightful, the class also had the lowest participation rate in the electronic survey. A final caveat of note is the timeline of the process related to the course of the pandemic. During the time of information gathering and analysis, pandemic-related restrictions at the University were relaxed, followed by a return to more restrictive social distancing rules. This highlights the need for dental schools to have alternative educational methods in reserve and ready to implement as needed due to fluctuations in the pandemic or other impactful factors.

5. Conclusions

Use of the KBG approach to plan changes to a predoctoral dental curriculum was successful. Focus groups followed-up by electronic surveys allowed any student or faculty member the opportunity to provide input. Focus group and individual interviews also facilitated input from staff with valued expertise relevant to the decisions at hand. Some topics were relatively non-controversial and strong recommendations were evident, while other topics generated more divisive opinions. The KBG approach allowed for transparency and assurance of thorough vetting of difficult decisions. A KBG approach is an effective means to address mega issues in the dental school environment.

Author Contributions: Conceptualization, N.M.F., D.C.N.C., A.C.D. and B.D.S.; investigation, N.M.F., D.C.N.C., A.C.D. and B.D.S.; writing—original draft preparation, N.M.F.; writing—review and editing, D.C.N.C., A.C.D. and B.D.S.; supervision, N.M.F.; project administration, N.M.F. All authors have read and agreed to the published version of the manuscript.

Funding: This research received no external funding.

Institutional Review Board Statement: Not applicable.

Informed Consent Statement: Not applicable.

Data Availability Statement: Not applicable.

Acknowledgments: The authors thank Jeina Montgomery for help with electronic surveys.

Conflicts of Interest: The authors declare no conflict of interest.

Appendix A

Electronic survey results. Standardized questions were asked for the all-student and all-faculty surveys. Questions specific to graduate program admissions were asked on the Graduate Program Directors surveys. Data represent the number of respondents who answered with each response.

Table A1. Electronic survey results.

ALL-FACULTY AND ALL-STUDENT SURVEY RESULTS						
Statements Related to Social Impacts of Remote Learning.						
	SA	A	N	D	SD	NA/?
FACULTY						
Remote learning has weakened dental student class dynamics.	16	18	4	1	0	3
Remote learning has decreased student's ability to learn from their classmates.	11	21	2	5	0	3
I feel disconnected from students due to remote learning.	12	16	10	2	1	1
In-person interactions with faculty help students learn how to be a professional.	21	19	2	0	0	0
STUDENT						
Remote learning has weakened by class dynamic.	17	22	13	13	8	1
Remote learning has decreased my ability to learn from my classmates.	17	18	11	18	9	1
I feel disconnected from my classmates due to remote learning.	20	25	11	7	11	0
I feel disconnected from faculty due to remote learning.	20	13	16	17	8	0
I have formed study groups during remote learning.	13	19	10	18	12	2
In-person interactions with faculty help me learn how to be a professional.	24	21	13	9	4	3
Statements related to didactics. Didactics can be lectures or small group seminars/discussions. Didactics can be in-person, remote synchronous (i.e., Zoom), or remote asynchronous (i.e., pre-recorded).						
	SA	A	N	D	SD	NA/?
FACULTY						
Students log on to my Zoom sessions, but typically do not actively engage in them.	5	11	8	5	2	11
I prefer students to have their cameras ON during Zoom sessions.	18	11	4	0	1	8
Technical difficulties often hinder my Zoom sessions.	1	4	5	18	5	9
I understand students' level of comprehension better when didactics are in-person.	13	17	3	2	3	4
I am able to read the room and adjust my teaching in real time better during in-person didactics.	16	19	1	1	0	5
Students are more likely to ask questions or speak up during an in-person didactic session (versus a Zoom session).	14	15	3	2	1	6
I like students to be able to ask questions in real time.	19	18	3	0	0	2
I appreciate the flexibility of pre-recorded asynchronous lectures.	6	17	5	5	2	7
It takes me longer to prepare a quality pre-recorded lecture than it does to deliver an in-person lecture.	15	7	7	6	0	7
In general, I prefer in-person didactics.	17	13	6	3	1	2
In general, I prefer pre-recorded asynchronous lectures (versus in-person lectures or Zoom lectures).	0	3	11	15	10	3
STUDENT						
I log on to Zoom sessions, but typically do not actively engage in them.	22	16	12	15	9	0
It is difficult to focus during Zoom sessions.	4	16	12	30	12	0
I prefer to have my camera OFF during Zoom sessions.	19	29	20	6	0	0
I often have technical difficulties that hinder Zoom sessions.	1	5	10	27	31	0
Faculty understand my level of comprehension better when didactics are in-person.	16	20	11	10	9	8
I am more likely to ask a question or speak up during an in-person didactic session (versus a Zoom session).	16	9	7	18	21	3
I like the ability to ask questions in real time.	19	22	22	9	2	0
I appreciate the flexibility of pre-recorded asynchronous lectures.	47	18	6	2	1	0
In general, I prefer in-person didactics.	19	10	14	12	17	2
In general, I prefer pre-recorded asynchronous lectures (versus in-person lectures or Zoom lectures).	26	12	19	10	7	0

Table A1. *Cont.*

ALL-FACULTY AND ALL-STUDENT SURVEY RESULTS						
Statements related to remote exams. This could also mean quizzes.						
	SA	A	N	D	SD	NA/?
FACULTY						
Students study less when an exam is open-book.	10	12	8	6	1	5
Students learn less when an exam is open-book.	4	10	14	7	2	5
I have concerns about academic dishonesty when exams are not proctored.	8	18	5	6	0	5
I am comfortable with the use of remote proctoring via a Zoom proctor.	1	6	9	6	6	14
I am comfortable with the use of remote proctoring via automated software (e.g., Proctorio).	1	5	9	7	5	15
STUDENT						
I study less when an exam is open-book.	6	22	10	28	8	0
I learn less when an exam is open-book.	6	10	10	29	19	0
I have concerns about academic dishonesty when exams are not proctored.	8	16	17	20	12	1
I am comfortable with remote proctoring via a Zoom proctor.	7	23	15	18	11	0
I am comfortable with remote proctoring via automated software (e.g., Proctorio).	4	17	15	14	22	2
It is difficult for me to find a suitable (quiet, private) space to take a remote exam.	11	9	11	25	18	0
Statements related to course grading schemes: numerical grades (4.0 scale) versus credit/no credit grades.						
	SA	A	N	D	SD	NA/?
FACULTY						
Numerical grades foster healthy competition between students within a class.	10	11	12	5	2	2
Numerical grades foster toxic competition between students within a class.	5	6	11	16	3	1
Numerical grades motivate students to perform their personal best.	13	24	2	1	0	2
Credit/no credit grades motivate students to perform "good enough".	8	18	11	2	2	1
Students study more in a course with a numerical grading scale.	16	22	2	0	0	2
Students learn more in a course with a numerical grading scale.	6	18	10	1	3	4
I am concerned credit/no credit grades may impact students' post graduation plans	11	16	7	3	2	3
Students are more likely to contest individual points on an assessment in a course with a numerical grading scale.	12	22	3	1	0	4
I am concerned about calibration of graders in a course with a numerical grading scale.	5	21	9	4	0	3
Numerical grades foster academic excellence at the UWSOD.	11	21	5	3	0	2
The UWSOD should rank students based on grades.	7	13	10	8	2	2
In general, UWSOD courses should be graded with a numerical grading scale.	11	19	5	5	1	1
All UWSOD courses should be graded credit/no credit.	2	2	4	22	11	1
STUDENT						
Numerical grades foster healthy competition between students within my class.	1	11	8	18	35	1
Numerical grades foster toxic competition between students within my class.	35	20	10	6	2	1
Numerical grades motivate me to perform my personal best.	10	14	15	10	24	1
Credit/no credit grades motivate me to perform "good enough".	6	18	7	17	24	2
I study more in a course with a numerical grading scale.	7	17	12	13	21	4
I learn more in a course with a numerical grading scale.	6	4	10	22	29	3
I am concerned credit/no credit grades may impact my post-graduation plans.	4	9	13	16	30	2
I am more likely to contest individual points on an assessment in a course with a numerical grading scale.	36	18	10	6	4	0
I am concerned about calibration of graders in a course with a numerical grading scale.	36	22	9	2	1	4
The UWSOD should rank students based on grades.	1	9	19	16	24	5
I am motivated by class rank.	4	11	10	12	37	0

Table A1. *Cont.*

ALL-FACULTY AND ALL-STUDENT SURVEY RESULTS Statements related to course grading schemes: numerical grades (4.0 scale) versus credit/no credit grades.						
	SA	**A**	**N**	**D**	**SD**	**NA/?**
STUDENT						
I am more likely to collaborate with my classmates when a course is graded credit/no credit.	30	15	12	12	3	2
I typically study for the grade in a course with a numerical grading scale, rather than studying to become a good dentist.	26	24	5	11	7	1
In general, UWSOD courses should be graded with a numerical grading scale.	4	7	13	15	33	2
All UWSOD courses should be graded credit/no credit.	31	10	18	10	3	2
Statements related to courses in the preclinical simulation lab.						
	SA	**A**	**N**	**D**	**SD**	**NA/?**
FACULTY						
There is a disconnect between students in the two lab groups.	3	4	2	2	1	30
I am concerned about imbalanced experiences between two groups of students in the lab.	1	3	4	4	1	29
Students get greater personal attention from faculty with the split shift in the lab.	3	7	3	0	2	27
It is easier for students to use shared equipment with the split shift in the lab.	2	7	3	0	1	29
I spend more time preparing and teaching with the split shift in the lab.	3	3	3	2	0	31
Teaching the same course twice detracts from my other responsibilities as a faculty member.	5	9	3	3	0	22
STUDENT						
I feel disconnected from classmates who do not share the same lab time as me.	32	16	5	6	3	12
I am concerned about imbalanced experiences between two groups of students in the lab.	9	14	11	17	9	14
I get greater personal attention from faculty with the split shift in the lab.	20	16	6	3	4	25
It is easier to use shared equipment with the split shift in the lab.	26	17	5	2	2	22
GRADUATE PROGRAM DIRECTOR SURVEY RESULTS						
	SA	**A**	**N**	**D**	**SD**	**NA/?**
I consider GPA when assessing applicants to my graduate program.	4	4	0	0	0	0
I consider class rank when assessing applicants to my graduate program.	5	2	1	0	0	0
It is difficult to assess an applicant who went to a dental school that does not issue grades.	4	4	0	0	0	0
I prefer that applicants to my graduate program report GPA.	6	2	0	0	0	0
I prefer that applicants to my graduate program report class rank.	6	2	0	0	0	0
Class rank is a poor metric for applicants, because students within a class are separated by extremely small differences in GPA.	0	1	3	3	1	0
Class rank is a valuable metric for applicants, because GPAs are elevated by grade inflation.	2	3	1	1	0	1
I am concerned that a switch to credit/no credit grades at UWSOD may impact our students' matriculation to graduate programs.	3	5	0	0	0	0
I am concerned that eliminating class rank at UWSOD may impact our students' matriculation to graduate programs.	4	3	0	1	0	0
	Class rank		**GPA**		**Standardized test score**	
If you could have only one piece of objective data when assessing applicants to your graduate program, which would it be?	5		3		0	

References

1. Advancing Through Innovation in a Challenging Time. *J. Dent. Educ.* **2021**, *85*, 877. [CrossRef]
2. Escontrias, O.A.; Istrate, E.C.; Stewart, D.C.L. *Resilient Dental Schools, Better Oral Health Care for the Underserved: The Impact of the COVID-19 Pandemic on U.S. Dental Schools*; ADEA Policy Research Series; American Dental Education Association: Washington, DC, USA, 2021.
3. Quinn, B.; Field, J.; Gorter, R.; Akota, I.; Manzanares, M.C.; Paganelli, C.; Davies, J.; Dixon, J.; Gabor, G.; Mendes, R.A.; et al. COVID-19: The immediate response of european academic dental institutions and future implications for dental education. *Eur. J. Dent. Educ.* **2020**, *24*, 811–814. [CrossRef] [PubMed]

4. Iyer, P.; Aziz, K.; Ojcius, D.M. Impact of COVID-19 on dental education in the United States. *J. Dent. Educ.* **2020**, *84*, 718–722. [CrossRef] [PubMed]
5. Hattar, S.; AlHadidi, A.; Sawair, F.A.; Alraheam, I.A.; El-Ma'Aita, A.; Wahab, F.K. Impact of COVID-19 pandemic on dental education: Online experience and practice expectations among dental students at the University of Jordan. *BMC Med. Educ.* **2021**, *21*, 151. [CrossRef] [PubMed]
6. Association Forum. *Professional Practice Statement on Association Strategic Governance, Part II: Characteristics*; Association Forum: Chilago, IL, USA, 2015.
7. Schwella, E. Knowledge Based Governance, Governance as Learning: The Leadership Implications. *Int. J. Leadersh. Public Serv.* **2014**, *10*. [CrossRef]
8. Tecker International. Knowledge-Based Decision Making. 2012. Available online: http://www.tecker.com/wp-content/uploads/2012/10/TIKBDMJan12.pdf (accessed on 4 April 2021).
9. Masella, R.S. The hidden curriculum: Value added in dental education. *J. Dent. Educ.* **2006**, *70*, 279–283. [CrossRef] [PubMed]
10. Schlenz, M.A.; Schmidt, A.; Wöstmann, B.; Krämer, N.; Schulz-Weidner, N. Students' and lecturers' perspective on the implementation of online learning in dental education due to SARS-CoV-2 (COVID-19): A cross-sectional study. *BMC Med. Educ.* **2020**, *20*, 354. [CrossRef] [PubMed]
11. Shrivastava, K.J.; Nahar, R.; Parlani, S.; Murthy, V.J. A cross-sectional virtual survey to evaluate the outcome of online dental education system among undergraduate dental students across India amid COVID-19 pandemic. *Eur. J. Dent. Educ.* **2021**. [CrossRef] [PubMed]
12. Varvara, G.; Bernardi, S.; Bianchi, S.; Sinjari, B.; Piattelli, M. Dental Education Challenges during the COVID-19 Pandemic Period in Italy: Undergraduate Student Feedback, Future Perspectives, and the Needs of Teaching Strategies for Professional Development. *Healthcare* **2021**, *9*, 454. [CrossRef] [PubMed]
13. Bartlett, T. Online Learning: What Does the Reserach Say? In *Online 2.0: How to Lead a Large-Scale Transformation of Virtual Learning*; The Chronicle of Higher Education: Congers, NY, USA, 2020.
14. Zmiyiwsky, M.; Allen, N.; Yoon, T.; Zeller, K.; Lamichhane, P. Individual Preferences on Grading Systems in Dental Schools. *Online J. Dent. Oral Health* **2018**, *1*. [CrossRef]
15. Jham, B.C.; Cannella, D.; Adibi, S.; Austin, K.; Allareddy, V.; Petrie, C.S. Should Pass/Fail Grading Be Used Instead of Traditional Letter Grades in Dental Education? Two Viewpoints: Viewpoint 1: Pass/Fail Grading Improves Learning Experiences for Students and Viewpoint 2: Traditional Letter Grading Provides Objective Evaluation for Dental Education. *J. Dent. Educ.* **2018**, *82*, 1258–1264. [PubMed]
16. Ramaswamy, V.; Veremis, B.; Nalliah, R.P. Making the case for pass-fail grading in dental education. *Eur. J. Dent. Educ.* **2020**, *24*, 601–604. [CrossRef] [PubMed]
17. Cuculino, L. How Pass/Fail Grading Can Impact the Dental School Experience. ASDA Blog. December 2019. Available online: https://www.asdablog.com/how-pass-fail-grading-can-impact-the-dental-school-experience/ (accessed on 4 April 2021).
18. McCarty, B. P's Get Degrees: Pass/Fail Grading in Dental School. ASDA Blog. March 2015. Available online: https://www.asdablog.com/ps-get-degrees-pass-fail-grading-in-dental-school/ (accessed on 4 April 2021).
19. Oak, S. A Review of Dental School Pass/Fail Curriculum. ASDA Blog. July 2020. Available online: https://www.asdablog.com/a-review-of-the-dental-school-pass-fail-curriculum/ (accessed on 4 April 2021).
20. Valachovic, R. Making the Grade in a Pass/Fail Environment: What It Means for Students. ADEA Charting Progress. December 2014. Available online: https://adeachartingprogress.wordpress.com/2014/12/15/making-the-grade-in-a-passfail-environment-what-it-means-for-students/ (accessed on 4 April 2021).
21. Valachovic, R. Making the Grade in a Pass/Fail Environment: Challenges for Advanced Dental Education Programs. ADEA Charting Progress. January 2015. Available online: https://adeachartingprogress.wordpress.com/2015/01/ (accessed on 4 April 2021).
22. Eidelman, A.S.; Whitmer, T. Is the Advanced Dental Admission Test (ADAT) the Metric Needed to Assist with Postgraduate Admissions? Two Viewpoints: Viewpoint 1: The ADAT Provides a Viable Solution to Help Postgraduate Programs Differentiate Applicants and Viewpoint 2: The ADAT Has Questionable Utility and Value for Postgraduate Admissions. *J. Dent. Educ.* **2017**, *81*, 685–690. [PubMed]
23. Bell, L.T.; Sukotjo, C.; Yuan, J.C.-C.; Johnson, B.R. Applicant selection procedures in endodontic specialty programs in the United States: Program director's perspective. *J. Endod.* **2014**, *40*, 797–804. [CrossRef] [PubMed]
24. Justema, R.B.; Majewski, R.F.; Salzmann, L.; Murdoch-Kinch, C.A.; Boynton, J.R. Contemporary appraisal of factors influencing pediatric dental program directors' selection of residents. *J. Dent. Educ.* **2020**, *84*, 742–748. [CrossRef] [PubMed]
25. Khan, S.; Carmosino, A.J.; Yuan, J.C.-C.; Lucchiari, N.; Kawar, N.; Sukotjo, C. Postdoctoral Periodontal Program Directors' Perspectives of Resident Selection. *J. Periodontol.* **2015**, *86*, 177–184. [CrossRef] [PubMed]

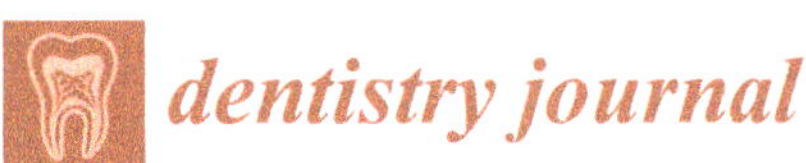

MDPI

Article

A Qualitative Exploration of Existing Reflective Practices Used by Undergraduate Dental Students in Paediatric Dentistry

Faith Campbell [1], Kirsten Jack [2] and Helen Rogers [3,*]

[1] Academic Unit of Oral Health, Dentistry and Society, School of Clinical Dentistry, University of Sheffield, Sheffield S10 2TA, UK; faith.campbell@sheffield.ac.uk

[2] Faculty of Health and Education, Manchester Metropolitan University, Manchester M15 6GX, UK; k.jack@mmu.ac.uk

[3] School of Dental Sciences, Newcastle University, Newcastle upon Tyne NE2 4AZ, UK

* Correspondence: Helen.Rogers@newcastle.ac.uk

Abstract: Background: Reflection is increasingly significant for dental students and professionals and is a continuing requirement of dental regulatory bodies. There is a paucity of evidence regarding how best to facilitate deep reflection for dental students. This study explored whether the use of clinical logbooks in undergraduate clinical attachments in Paediatric Dentistry was facilitating deep reflection. **Methods:** This qualitative study used individual interviews for data collection. This was conducted at the University of Sheffield with third year undergraduate dental students and clinical teaching staff. Interviews were immediately transcribed verbatim. A reflexive approach to thematic analysis was used to co-constitute the data, enabling the development of the thematic framework. **Results:** The sample compromised 10 students and 4 educators. Thematic analysis generated 4 key themes: understanding of reflection, preparation for reflection, importance of learning through experience, and suggestions for development. The findings indicated that students perceived that they were not being supported in engaging in deep reflection by the use of a clinical logbook and that greater preparation for reflection would be beneficial. **Conclusions:** The current study revealed that using clinical logbooks during clinical attachments in Paediatric Dentistry was not facilitating deep reflection. Further research is required to explore how deep reflection can be facilitated for undergraduate dental students undertaking clinical learning.

Keywords: education; dental; graduate; education; dental continuing; teacher training

Citation: Campbell, F.; Jack, K.; Rogers, H. A Qualitative Exploration of Existing Reflective Practices Used by Undergraduate Dental Students in Paediatric Dentistry. *Dent. J.* **2022**, *10*, 1. https://doi.org/10.3390/dj10010001

Academic Editors: Jelena Dumancic and Božana Lončar Brzak

Received: 2 November 2021
Accepted: 17 December 2021
Published: 23 December 2021

1. Introduction

Reflective thought may be defined as 'the active, persistent and careful consideration of any belief, or supposed form of knowledge in the light of grounds that support it and the further conclusion to which it tends' [1]. It enables one to direct their actions with foresight and to know what we are about when we act [1]. Reflection enables healthcare professionals to think critically about practice, supporting the development of their professional identity and enabling identification of learning needs. It can support self-awareness development, which enables self-monitoring and regulation within the healthcare culture [2]. Reflection can be undertaken in action, which occurs during experience where one can respond by modifying behaviour immediately and reflection on action after the experience, with consideration of the event with thought and feeling on this [3].

Reflective practice can help learners to bridge the gap between theory and practice, allowing them to find answers that they are unable to access through formal learning whilst exploring their emotions associated with their learning experience [3]. This is pertinent in workplace-based learning where learners may feel anxious or insecure regarding their contribution to patient care and their role within the healthcare team [4]. This may in turn present as a barrier to learning. Deeper and more meaningful reflection has been associated with improved self-awareness, supporting holistic and lifelong learning [5].

This is in contrast to superficial reflection, which is descriptive and less critical. Critical reflection demonstrates an awareness that actions and events are not only located within and explicable by multiple perspectives but are located in and influenced by multiple historical and socio-political contexts [6].

Deep reflection involves purposeful critical analysis of knowledge and experience in order to achieve deeper meaning and understanding [2]. These deeper levels of reflection are more difficult to reach and less frequently demonstrated [2]. It is helpful to engage in this deeper state of reflection because it has been proposed as the key to moving between surface and deep approaches to learning, and a deep approach to learning and reflection appears to be both fundamentally related and mutually beneficial [2].

Deep reflective thought can also engage the emotions [7]. This is important because positive emotions enhance the learning process and can help a learner to persist in challenging situations and provide a basis for new learning, whilst negative emotions can lead to irrationality, denial of future learning opportunities, and a failure to extract the learning that a given situation provides [7]. Negative emotions may also lead to increased dropout rates and negatively affect the students' physical and psychological wellbeing [8]. Specifically in healthcare courses, the anxiety induced by a negative experience in a clinical placement can lead to increased attrition from the course [9]. These negative emotions may continue to be experienced when a learner is placed in the same situation. Through reflection, learners can acknowledge negative emotions, reducing the likelihood that they will disrupt future learning experiences [7]. This is important in Paediatric Dentistry, a speciality which can invoke additional anxiety in comparison to other dental attachment experiences [10].

Many international regulators of dental professionals require practitioners to demonstrate maintenance of their practice and knowledge according to current best practice as part of their standards for practitioners [11–13]. It is globally acknowledged that the development and maintenance of professional standards and skills involves rigorous self-assessment and reflection on one's current practice [14,15].

Within the United Kingdom (UK), this idea has been developed further with greater incorporation of reflective practice within regulatory standards. Upon registration with the General Dental Council (GDC), registrants are required to undertake meaningful experiential learning on an ongoing basis, and should be able to explain the importance of critical reflection [16]. Furthermore, the GDC encourages dentists to be reflective practitioners, whereby they should consider their experiences to gain insight into their practice to support the continual improvement of the quality of their care. In 2018, the GDC introduced the Enhanced Continuing Professional Development Scheme (eCPD), a new cycle that changed the way that dental practitioners must undertake their continuing professional development (CPD) [17]. A key component of this cycle is reflection, with all practitioners required to keep an eCPD record including mandatory demonstration of reflection [17]. Outside of the UK, providers of dental education must support students to improve their performance by providing regular feedback and encouragement of reflecting on their practice [18,19].

Reflective practice is essential for undergraduate students throughout their dental education, with this being included in regulatory policy documents [18,20]. At the School of Clinical Dentistry (SCD), the University of Sheffield, UK, students must complete a formal written self-reflection in their personal logbook for every patient contact during clinical attachments in Paediatric Dentistry.

Anecdotally, reflections in the logbooks are rarely used by students, and hence it has been questioned whether this is the most effective method in facilitating. There is limited evidence regarding how to appropriately support students in their reflective practice; an area that the present study intended to address.

This study aims to explore staff and student perspectives on reflective practice by answering the research question; are current methods for reflection effective in facilitating the learning and personal and professional growth of undergraduate students undertaking clinical attachments in Paediatric Dentistry. The study focused on paediatric dental clinics, as students have described Paediatric Dentistry as invoking additional anxiety, and is therefore an area where the development of reflective practices may be particularly beneficial [10].

2. Materials and Methods

2.1. Context and Participant Recruitment

Ethical approval for this study was granted by the Ethics Committee at the University of Sheffield (reference: 034416).

A qualitative approach was used, through semi-structured interviews with students and staff, which was followed by thematic analysis.

Staff and students were purposively sampled to ensure that they had experience of using the logbook for reflective practice as a learner or educator, during the third year Bachelor of Dental Surgery (3BDS) clinical attachments in Paediatric Dentistry during the academic year 2019–2020 at the University of Sheffield. At this stage in their course students had passed clinical assessments on phantom heads to perform basic procedures on children, they had also provided dental care for patients for a year, including assessments, restorative procedures, dentures, and extractions on adults, but notably had no contact with child patients. During this previous year of clinical contact with patients, students had used a logbook for their reflective practice after each patient contact, so they were familiar with the current process of reflection. Reflection is a key requirement of the undergraduate course throughout the five years; thus students had been engaging in reflective writing through reports and verbal reflection.

Both staff and student participants were recruited as they would have different but important experiences of the current method of reflective practice. This ensured that important data would not be missed and that future research resulting from this study could use data from both groups to inform any changes to reflective practice.

The logbook contains a blank space for an unstructured written reflection, which is completed on an open clinic at the end of a clinical session, during time which is not protected for this purpose and may overrun into personal time. This logbook is then handed in to SCD at the end of the rotation (Figure 1).

Students receive one lecture on the use of the clinical logbook and reflection prior to commencing clinical attachments. Clinical tutors who facilitate reflection receive no formal training on reflection or how to engage students in this using a logbook. These tutors are of varying backgrounds and include general dental practitioners, specialty trainees and consultants in paediatric dentistry.

A General Data Protection Regulation (GDPR)-compliant, open-ended invitation to participate was sent by an administrative assistant to all eligible staff and students with no time limit, whilst further advertising was undertaken through social media. The participant information sheet was shared with the invitational email, and students were assured that their progress on the course would not be affected by their decision regarding participation.

An online interview was arranged for those who responded to the invitation, following completion of a written consent form. Staff and students were advised that they would receive a £5 shopping voucher on completion of the interview, to thank them for their time.

2.2. Data Collection

All interviews were conducted through Google Meet (©Google, LLC, Mountain View, CA, USA) in a private room at the lead researchers' home, in June and July 2020, due to the ongoing COVID-19 pandemic prohibiting physical interviews. The stages of student and staff recruitment are summarized in Figure 2. Interviews were chosen over focus groups to provide the opportunity to gain a deeper insight into individual participant perspectives on reflective practice, with group discussion not being necessary to illuminate the research topic.

Patient ID [ ] **Recorded on Portfolio** ☐

Child Patient ☐ **CSLE** ☐ **Date** [ ] **Clinic** [ ]

Description

Procedure	Tooth	Notes/comments on individual procedure	Competency			
			Student		Tutor	
			O A		O A	
			B L		B L	
			C P		C P	
			O A		O A	
			B L		B L	
			C P		C P	
			O A		O A	
			B L		B L	
			C P		C P	
			O A		O A	
			B L		B L	
			C P		C P	
			O A		O A	
			B L		B L	
			C P		C P	
			O A		O A	
			B L		B L	
			C P		C P	
			O A		O A	
			B L		B L	
			C P		C P	

Overall Student Reflection

Professionalism	1 2 3 4 5 6	Patient Management	1 2 3 4 5 6

Overall Tutor Summary Feedback and Action Points

Professionalism	1 2 3 4 5 6	Patient Management	1 2 3 4 5 6
Tutor Name		**Tutor Signature**	

Figure 1. Sample page from the student logbook showing the unstructured space for reflection. CSLE—Clinical Skills Learning Environment, O—Observed, A—Assisted, B—Beginner, L—Learner, C—Competent, P—Proficient.

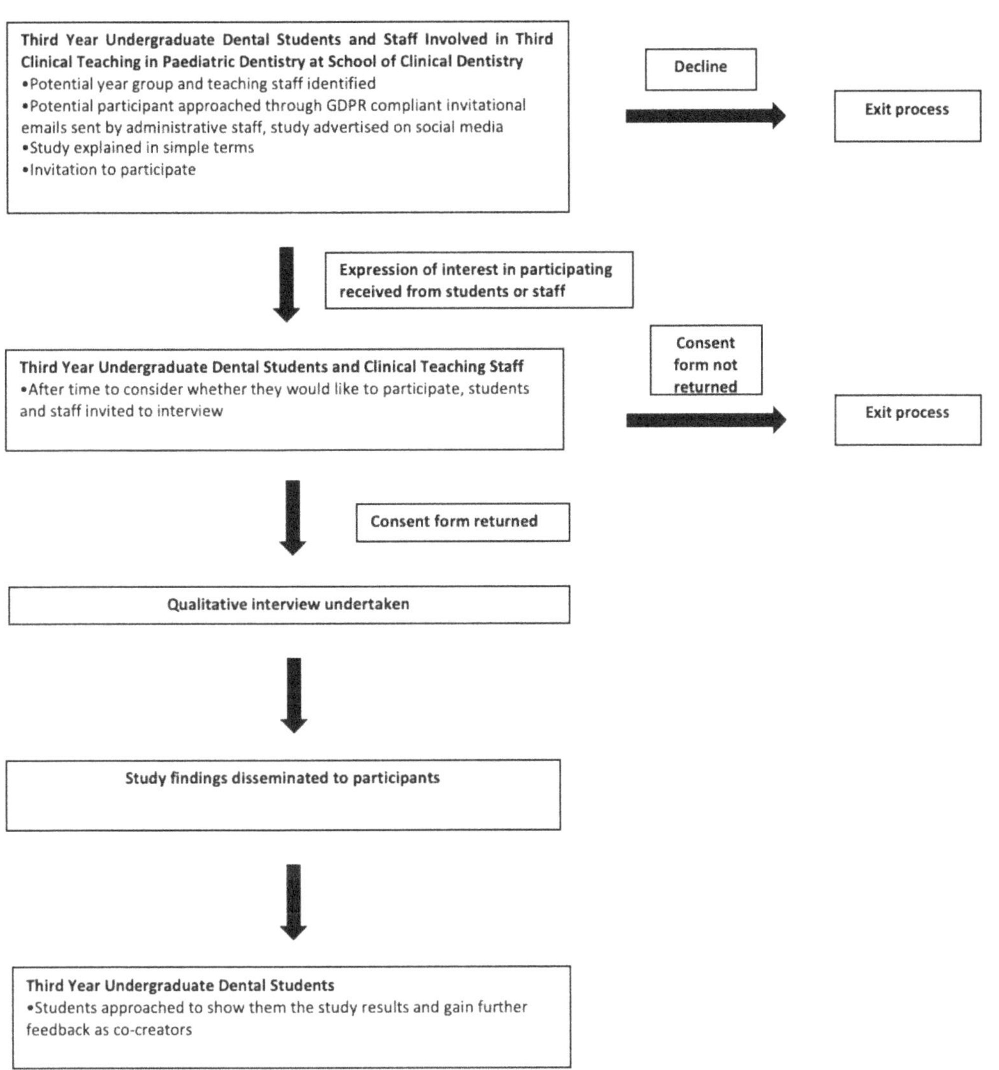

Figure 2. Participant recruitment flowchart.

The study was explained to participants verbally prior to the interview, and consent was confirmed and recorded. Participants were advised that they could discontinue the interview or withdraw from the study at any time. Hermeneutic (interpretive) phenomenology was chosen as the approach for this research, as it enables understanding of the participants' values, beliefs, feelings, and actions lived against the backdrop of their environment [21]. This 'lifeworld' approach contrasts with those which split participants from the world in which they live and is based on the philosophy of Heidegger [22]. Heidegger suggested that it is essential to understand the person's lifeworld if we are to understand them as individuals [22]. This approach is in contrast to the descriptive phenomenological approach, which uncovers a 'truth' which is free from the researcher's pre-suppositions [23]. Using the researcher's interpretative lens enables understanding that might not be reached by bracketing off our pre-suppositions. This process is grounded in Heidegger's description of the hermeneutic circle [22]. We start with our initial 'whole' of understanding, which is then exposed to the 'parts' of the student data. A different 'whole' is then reached and based on what we know already about the topic, combined with the student data. This circular process enables not only a description of student thoughts but also attempts to uncover the meaning behind them [24]. This is important in this study, for example, when considering the multiple contextual influences on students' lives and how they reflect on their experiences. This approach has been used with success when researching reflective practices in other disciplines, for example, Nursing and Dental Technology [25,26].

Topic guides were developed to explore staff and student perceptions of the current method of reflecting within the paediatric dental clinic. The topic guides were piloted during the first interviews where both members of the interviewing team were present, and adjusted as necessary to produce a more logical structure, and minimise repetition. The topic guide was subsequently developed iteratively after each interview to prompt exploration of new themes.

Any students who had been taught by the interviewer involved with 3BDS teaching (FC) were interviewed by the alternative interviewer (HJR). Interviewers were both female, and at the time of study one was a post CCST specialist and honorary clinical lecturer in Paediatric Dentistry and the other was a clinical teacher in Paediatric Dentistry, with participants being aware that they were both staff members, the interviewers had a working relationship with staff members but no relationship with any student participants. The former has experience and formal training in qualitative interviewing, whilst the latter did not. The participants were aware that the intention of the interviews was to gain insight into their views on reflection. Interviewers wore non-clinical attire for the interviews. Both interviewers had interest but no bias relating to the research topic.

Consideration was given to potential power issues between the researchers conducting the interviews and participants, to minimise conflict of interest the researcher involved in teaching at 3BDS level did not conduct any interviews with any students whom they had taught. The researchers were and are not involved in student progress committees or any senior level of student management. Staff participants were known to the researchers.

A digital voice recorder and the recording function in Google Meet were both used to record the interviews, which were subsequently, transcribed verbatim. Field notes were made during every interview. Participants were recruited and interviews undertaken until no new ideas emerged and it was agreed that data saturation had been reached.

2.3. *Data Analysis*

Thematic analysis was conducted on the transcripts of the interviews, which were organised using NVivo version 12 (©QSR International PSY Ltd., Melbourne, Australia) software by one of the researchers (FC) following data familiarisation. This was undertaken immediately after each interview, alongside use of a saturation grid. Data were initially analysed independently by two researchers (FC and KJ). One researcher is a Professor of Nursing Education and is a National Teaching Fellow and an experienced qualitative researcher of the topic area. The lead researcher has practical experience of teaching and facilitating reflection with undergraduate dental students. Both researchers discussed their analysis to reach agreement on themes using a constant comparative approach until consensus on the meaning of the data was reached [27]. The final results of the analysis were then shared with experienced academics at The School of Clinical Dentistry at the University of Sheffield. We applied the standards for rigour as described by van Manen, which included the presentation of a clear audit trail and the use of verbatim quotes, which enabled the meaning and context of the participants' experiences to be clearly described [28].

A reflexive approach to analysis enabled the combination of experiences of the research team with those of the participants, to co-constitute the data [22]. This enabled the development of the thematic framework. This approach required the team to move from the whole of the data to individual parts and then back again, to develop a different understanding of the phenomenon. Throughout the process, all explanations of the data were considered through discussion and the main elements of each theme were explored and described using original data excerpts. Using a 'whole-parts-new whole' approach enabled the team to discover new meanings about the phenomenon of dental student reflective practices, and how they are experienced by both students and educators. Key themes were identified and relayed back to the participants to ensure their statements have been interpreted as intended.

3. Results

There were ten student respondents, and all were interviewed. Any that had been taught by members of the research team (FC) were interviewed by HJR, who had no involvement in teaching 3BDS. Four staff members, excluding members of the research team who had taught 3BDS during clinical attachments in Paediatric Dentistry, responded, and all were interviewed. No repeat interviews were conducted. There were no non-participants and nobody from either group dropped out of the study. Data saturation was reached when all four suitable staff participants and ten student participants had been interviewed. The transcripts and associated themes were returned to the participants, and all felt that their experiences were accurately represented in each. Participant characteristics can be seen in Table 1.

Table 1. Participant and Interview Characteristics.

	Student Participants	Staff Participants
Experience	All 3 BDS	Clinical Tutor in Paediatric Dentistry Specialty Trainee and Clinical Tutor in Paediatric Dentistry Clinical Tutor and Specialist in Paediatric Dentistry Professor and Consultant Paediatric Dentistry
Number of Participants	10	4
Gender (F/M)	8/2	4/0
Mean and Range Interview Length (Mins)	25:87 (17:59–33:23)	12:10 (8:57–16:20)

Several of the participants from both staff and student groups had a basic understanding of reflective practice, in terms of exploration of what went 'right or wrong'. Many students described the logbook as being unhelpful to support deep learning from experience. However, several participants were able to articulate the importance of reflective learning and offered suggestions about how this could be supported in the programme.

Analysis of these qualitative data resulted in four overarching themes (Table 2):

1. Understanding of Reflection
2. Preparation for Reflection
3. Importance of Learning Through Experience
4. Suggestions for Development

Table 2. Summary of themes.

Understanding of Reflection	Preparation for Reflection	Importance of Learning through Experience	Suggestions for Development
• Descriptive learning task • Identifies improvements • Therapeutic process	• Informal process • Uncertainty about logbook • Inadequate time • Safety aspects	• Improvement to patient care • Educator/Student relationship • Peer feedback	• Formal preparation • Optional activity • Online options

3.1. Understanding of Reflection

The data revealed a varied understanding of reflective practice. Several participants described the concept in basic terms, for example, to think about what had gone well or badly in their clinical sessions. All participants described reflection as something that occurred after an experience. The following participants described reflection as a descriptive task and one which could serve as an aide memoire for future:

> *I write something first about what I think has happened, and, bits that I think had gone well, bits that have gone badly or things, usually I like to pick out something which was ... where it's something new to me, and which I just learnt, so, because it'll help me remember better, and then the tutor then looks at it, and then gives me feedback based on my reflections*
>
> (Participant 2, student)

> *I think that reflection is pretty much just us writing in our clinic books ... I find it quite useful to look back sometimes ... we don't have 'paeds' very often so I look before my next rotation if I have the book ... generally, I just try and write something I learned in the session to trigger my memory next time*
>
> (Participant 3, student)

> *Reflect on what we've done on clinic and reflect on how you feel like it's gone with the patient ... the treatment, what you actually did and if that was any good*
>
> (Participant 5, student)

For the following participants, reflection was an opportunity to identify improvements which could be made to their practice and ensuring that positive aspects of practice could continue to be developed. For the educator, reflection enabled not only identification of positive practice, but also a consideration of the reason why something went well:

> *So I suppose it's looking at what you've done on the clinic, your actions and clinical work and sort of seeing how you could have, what you did well, what you didn't do so well and sort of trying to act on what you didn't do so well to make it better for next time, so it's more about trying to improve future clinical practice*
>
> (Participant 6, student)

> *So, you can look back and look at everything that went well and that didn't so go well, and how you go on from that ... also, so not just improve on the stuff that went wrong but keep on doing things right*
>
> (Participant 7, student)

> *Just about how you ... when you've done a job ... and then it's, why did it go well, what have I done different ... so reflection to me is just checking yourself, looking back at what you've done, trying to put into place things that you can follow to make it better next time*
>
> (Participant 3, staff)

For the following participants, reflection was viewed as a therapeutic process although this was determined by the actions of the educator during the joint discussion. Reflection enabled students to track growth in their confidence and this process was either supported by positive and constructive comments or reduced by the educators focussing only on negative aspects:

> *Sometimes ... you might beat yourself (up) or just putting yourself down and sometimes, reflection can be positive as well, almost like a mini counselling session*
>
> (Participant 1, student)

> *I think that to somehow track how your confidence grows ... be able to get a better overall picture ... because I know ... everyone knows that we're probably nervous. (Laughter) Yeah, I think it might be helpful as well to the tutors that may look at it afterwards and see that, read, 'Oh, I was really worried about that' and then they could either silence*

those worries and say, 'Well, you know, you did okay,' or, 'Actually, well, if you do it like that next time,' and you might not feel so worried or whatever

(Participant 5, student)

... it depends which tutor you have. Sometimes, they just focus on what you've done badly, and I think a lot of people, myself included, find that quite off-putting ... you shouldn't take it as a personal attack but it almost is because it's nice to begin with a positive and have the bit that you need to improve on and then end with a positive as well because I think people engage with a bit more than if you're just told, "Right, so you didn't do this well," and that's it

(Participant 6, staff)

3.2. Preparation for Reflection

None of the student participants could remember having any formal support to develop their reflective thinking, describing it as something they picked up from their peers. This left some participants unsure about the standard and depth of their required reflective thinking. Within the course students do not presently have formal preparation for reflection in the logbook, a lecture on logbooks is given but there is no specific teaching on the importance of reflection and how to do this:

It's just something you develop whilst you're on clinic work, whether it be actually treating the patient or seeing my peers work on patients and then seeing how they discuss the performance with the tutor ... it's just sort of something you pick up. In terms of formal teaching, I don't recall having marks on it

(Participant 4, student)

... we're not taught how deep to go with it. So I think with myself I go quite, I try and be quite detailed with it because it's only the more detail we put in, the more I can identify what I've done wrong but I think a lot of people don't really take it very seriously or they don't go that much in detail so some people I'd seen on clinics say I'll be better at this next time but they haven't said how they need to be better at it. And I think that a lot of people just go very superficially into it

(Participant 6, student)

I feel like I make it up as I go along. I thought like (laughter) you know, when you're at school and it's like two stars and a wish. I feel like (laughter) it's a little bit ambiguous, and we just ... I kind of just write anything down.

(Participant 2, student)

The following participants described the logbook as a way to document observations rather than reflection on their practice and were unclear about how this method of reflection should be used. Further to their lecture on clinical logbooks, students are advised on how to use their logbook during their clinical induction to clinics on Paediatric Dentistry by their clinical tutor, therefore this is dependent on the educator understanding and explaining how to use the book for effective reflective practice. There was also uncertainty about the role of the educator and the type of feedback they were meant to provide to develop the students' reflections, and educators are currently not formally prepared on the use of the logbook to reflect and develop these skills:

A lot of the time ... I've written, "observed child communication and assisted full assessment and learned about hypomineralised molars and the appearance of them". I suppose that is an observation rather than a reflection. And I know that that's something I'm guilty of doing in all of my logbooks ...

(Participant 6, student)

I think there is confusion among tutors and the students about what exactly you're meant to put in there, and what the tutors- what feedback the tutor's meant to give you as well

(Participant 2, student)

The reflective process occurred at the end of a clinic and led to a rushed, unmeaningful experience for the students. The timing meant that students were left with no time to prepare their reflective thinking to enable them to share it with the educator. This led to students finding the reflective experience stressful and needing more time to prepare for the conversation:

> *... you feel like you have to get something down in order to leave the clinic, and so, when you haven't had, you know, that maybe a session wasn't as interesting or it's something that you've already done before, the fact that you have to, you know, it's compulsory to reflect in order to leave, you just think, 'Oh, okay. I don't really have anything to say ... ' reflection for me, it's more of a ... I don't know, maybe I'm being too philosophical, but it's more of a personal thing. And so, yeah, sometimes, I don't feel like reflecting*
>
> (Participant 1, student)

> *It depends on how rushed they all feel because they will leave it to the last, oh, I put it on the book, can you sign all these papers, and then it's all stressful, ... you don't have time to talk to them, you don't have time, you just- they write their reflection, you write yours, you're there for like a 2-min chat, it's not ... that's not ideal I don't think, ... so you just haven't got time. It'd be nice to have plenty of time to do it*
>
> (Participant 3, staff)

In contrast, the next participant felt that the logbook facilitated conversations with students, was useful for prompting learning points, and enabled immediate feedback on practice. The preceding clinical sessions were adequate preparation for the reflective conversation, although in this excerpt this is described as feedback rather than a joint reflective process:

> *Sometimes things happen during the sessions that you maybe need to really brought up that ... think about this, so I think there's lines that they need—it's important that if something important happens in that session that really needed to be given feedback on*
>
> (Participant 2, staff)

For the following participants, there were concerns about the safety of reflecting at the end of the clinic session when their peers and other educators might be present. The timing and environment led some to conceal reflection on their feelings with concerns about confidentiality:

> *... you got a queue of people waiting to get their books signed and waiting to speak to the tutor ... and, you know, how you felt if you're feeling a bit emotional or upset, you may not feel like it's a safe environment to disclose those things ... your peers who, you know, are behind, you don't want them to know how you're feeling or see that you're upset or bothered by things*
>
> (Participant 1, student)

> *They probably do socially modify what they write if I'm standing over them. But they tend to just write it themselves, and they write very grey stuff. I don't think they write enough for anybody to judge them on*
>
> (Participant 1, staff)

Only one student participant disagreed about the need for a safer space to reflect:

> *... because I know tutors, at the end of the day, they just want you to improve; they're not going to criticise you for being negative or picking up things that you can improve on. So, I don't really think it would make a difference (having a safer space)*
>
> (Participant 4, student)

3.3. Importance of Learning through Experience

The following participants understood the importance of reflective practice, although tended to view it to make improvements to patient care, rather than an exploration of their personal thoughts and feelings:

I think it helps you with being able to provide better care for your patients. So, as I said before, areas that you need to improve on can be highlighted through your reflection if you do it properly. And that's only going to advantage all the patients and the people that you interact with. And, you know, it could highlight that you need to do more CPD or go on courses . . .

(Participant 1, student)

We have a standard professionally that we need to fulfil when treating all of our patients. So, once you have a standard in mind, that is really valuable to see where you measure up against it. Whether you're just passing it or you need to work on something or everything's going well, it's always important to make sure that the patient gets that standard of care and you're trying your best to provide it

(Participant 4, student)

Because we need to improve. I think you need to reflect, look at what actually you could have done better and what did go well? And so, you can sort of build up on that

(Participant 5, student)

I think a lot of people think that the review and assessment bits and reflection is all about just making yourself better but people I don't think realise that it's actual requirement of the GDC through professional development

(Participant 6, student)

The learning depended to a great extent on the partnership between the students and the educators. Opportunities for deep reflection were lost if educators provided superficial feedback. Engaging in peer feedback was viewed as a helpful way to identify improvements which could be made to practice, in contrast to feedback from educators:

. . . You could think that you've done an amazing job. But really, the tutor hasn't really looked at it, you know, doesn't have anything else to say other than, 'Oh yeah, good.' And so, the opportunity to reflect on a deeper level isn't always there I'd say, because, you know, your knowledge on what's good and what's bad as a student isn't always, you know, as good as it could be obviously

(Participant 1, student)

I'll talk about how I think it is then, but then often the tutor will be able to point things out to me, and then I guess it's a nice feedback they give me as well, it gives me a better understanding of what I've done, yeah

(Participant 2, student)

I think a lot of the time, people find it difficult to identify what they have done wrong in the session so they need to have some element of peer review. So maybe that partner would sit with them and talk to them honestly about what they think they didn't do so well as well what I did well . . .

(Participant 6, student)

3.4. Suggestions for Development

Several participants had suggestions about how preparation and support for reflective learning could be enhanced. For the following participants, a more formal structure would be beneficial to support deep reflection:

For me, maybe just having maybe just a little bit of guidance or like a point on, okay, something, what went well, what didn't go well. Just something like that, just something to hint you to think a little bit more deeply, and just to make it a bit more something that is sit down, and ... yeah, just think about it a bit more instead of just a gap. To keep the gap as well just for any other random comments, but more of a guided reflection perhaps

(Participant 1, student)

I think a breakdown of the reflection box ... what went well, what didn't go well, what did you learn today that forces you to write something. But I like the idea of, well, potential idea of not having to do it every session, doing it so many times a session. Because then, it's not like a forced, 'Well, I've got to write something because,' you know. So, I think that would take that away. And actually, then, you'd maybe have, I don't know, like for a four-week rotation, have two really good things you've actually found really interesting ...

(Participant 5, student)

I suppose I write in the reflections what I need to, what things I've learnt about and what things I need to go away and learn about myself and I suppose that greater awareness of what knowledge you're lacking so that you can work on it. It does improve your work a bit more. But I think, the reflections, if we're told how to properly reflect could be more valuable than they are at the moment

(Participant 6, student)

Making reflective activity optional or having the opportunity to reflect with peers were suggestions from the following participants:

Is it compulsory to reflect on every clinic? Maybe just making it, you know, an optional thing that I have a reflection. You know, the tutor can always give comments ... Do you want to reflect on this procedure or ... ? Yeah, maybe making it an optional thing

(Participant 1, student)

One thing that would be more useful with the peers, is that peers see you all the time. Whereas the staff members, is looking after two to four units at a time. So, I think the peer review would be more valuable because they've seen you from when you've brought the patient in to when you've sent them out

(Participant 6, student)

For the following participants, having the flexibility of an app or having an online option were suggestions to engage students further in reflective practices:

So, I don't know if you've heard of these apps. So, the applications where you just basically track what you eat during the day ... on the e-portfolio, I can see the number of treatments, professionalism, patient management, in a similar way like in a kind of a chart representation. So, something like this in terms of the layout on the e-portfolio like, yeah, the professionalism, average management; if that could be translated into something that we could access really quickly like an app, that might be another option

(Participant 1, student)

As more and more things go online if these things can be done online and they can submit them there. And the tutors could have access to look at things and to help them because it means they can go away and do it in their own time. I don't necessarily reflect straightaway because if something happens on clinic that I haven't, if I haven't had a great experience I'm a bit wound up at the time so, my thinking's not particularly clear so I wouldn't think about it until later when I'm a lot more calm and reasonable and I think that would be better for the students because they've got time and they can access something where they can look at the questions and start to think about it

(Participant 4, staff)

4. Discussion

This study has explored student and staff perceptions on current methods used to facilitate reflective practice for undergraduate dental students undertaking clinical attachments in Paediatric Dentistry. This was done using qualitative semi-structured interviews and thematic analysis. The participants had a limited understanding of reflection, and their experiences suggest that the logbooks do not support deep reflection.

There are a number of strengths to this study; notably, the rigour of the study design, and the experience and varied skills of the research team. Furthermore, this novel study highlights the importance of reflective practice in supporting students to deal with stress and anxiety, which is likely to be further exacerbated by the COVID-19 pandemic. Whilst this study focused on the use of reflection in paediatric dental rotations, the findings may be relevant for other undergraduate rotations that use a similar reflective process.

The existing relationship between the interviewers and staff participants was an unavoidable limitation in this study, in that it may have precluded open discussion. Furthermore, as all members of the research team had prior and ongoing experience of undertaking reflection in a clinical setting as learners and educators, respectively, the questions asked and interpretation of responses may have been subject to bias. Purposive sampling of one year group within one discipline in one dental school restricted the diversity of potential participants. There was an imbalance in the gender of the participants, as 8 of the 10 students and all four staff participants were female, which is 12 out of a total of 14 participants. This imbalance should be acknowledged when considering the findings.

It was evident that understanding of reflection was extremely varied, for some was elementary, focusing on improvement in clinical skills and knowledge, and performed by all on action as opposed to in action. Limited understanding appeared to be linked to a perceived lack of support for students in developing reflective skills. There is evidence that individuals with a more linear, superficial understanding of the reflective process failed to improve the quality of their reflection compared with those with a deep understanding, supporting the need for greater understanding of reflection within staff and student groups [2]. Moreover, it is acknowledged that reflection is a fundamental aspect of the learning cycle. Schon described the positive impact of teaching reflective practice to learners, to successfully equip them for their real-world practice [29]. As such, there is a need for reflective practice to be taught effectively to facilitate learners' professional development. Superficial approaches to the teaching of reflection have been linked to superficial levels of reflective thinking in students [1]. Approaches to the teaching of reflection are often inconsistent and generally misunderstood. Furthermore, there is little guidance to support educators in understanding reflective ability in learners, with students being found to suffer from an overload of reflection particularly in the early years of their learning programmes [30,31].

Participants appreciated the clinical logbook for prompting immediate feedback, discussions, and learning, though not for the intended purpose of deep and purposeful reflection. The focus of the reflective exercise was, in general, perceived as being for 'improvement' rather than the articulation of the development of relational skills, which are very important in dental practice. This is important, as these skills are enriched through discussion and reflection, and by not being aware of the purpose and benefit of this deep reflection, students were unable to access the occasion to develop. The opportunity to communicate with the clinical tutor was seen as valuable by both staff and student participants. It is acknowledged that logbooks facilitate immediate and ongoing communication between learner and educator in the clinical environment, alongside providing a feedback loop for evaluating the learning activity and a method of continuous assessment [32]. However, logbooks can often be inadequate for reasons such as a learner perception of logbooks being boring, bureaucratic, and an exercise in collecting signatures with no consequence for improper completion and a misalignment of clinical experience and logbook requirements [33]. This is found in the present study, where reflecting in the logbook was perceived as almost bureaucratic due to its compulsory nature, with the logbook feeling like a tick box exercise. Considering this alongside the feeling that there is not always something to be reflected upon, thus a desire for optional reflection, any interventions to change reflective practice should be flexible in how and when students reflect to respond to this feeling of reflection being laborious.

Lack of privacy, tutor engagement, and time were described as further barriers to engaging in deeper reflection. These findings concur with current literature that suggests that the setting and time available for reflection affect the depth of reflection undertaken [3]. Reflection was always discussed as occurring at the end of a clinical session rather than during. This therefore suggests that there may be value in dedicating specific time within and during clinical teaching sessions for reflection to be undertaken so that it is given greater importance and not perceived as an afterthought, as it was described by many participants, allowing both reflection in and on action to occur. Reflection in action is also described as 'thinking on our feet' and this is important, as it allows one to connect their feelings with experience and build an understanding of the situation in which they find themselves [3]. Continuing this practice can help to improve the quality of patient care. It is recommended by the NHS staff and learners' mental wellbeing commission that healthcare learners and professionals have protected time and access to safe spaces in which reflect on clinical experiences [9]. Some students felt that reflecting optionally and with peers if they wish would be beneficial, supported by literature stating that deeper reflective thinking can be fostered by mutual support of group members, the opportunity to consider experiences more deeply, and learn from the experience of others [2].

The study was undertaken in the paediatric dental clinic, where dental students are known to experience significant anxiety about performing their first paediatric procedures [10]. More broadly, dental students experience significant stress and anxiety throughout their studies, with a significant impact on their mental and physical wellbeing [34–36]. Moreover, students undertaking undergraduate healthcare courses often have increased stress due to the academic and clinical demands of their course and are less likely to report or seek health for mental health conditions, fearing the consequences of doing so [9]. Student anxiety can also be an indicator for poorer academic performance and may exacerbate patient anxiety during treatment [34,35]. During the current COVID-19 pandemic, dental students are experiencing heightened levels of anxiety and worry about their studies suffering [37]. Reflection was valued by staff and students and was described as providing a 'mini-counselling session' which helped with stress and worries about clinical encounters and performance.

Emotions can have significant effects on students' productivity and interpersonal perceptions, with negative emotions negatively affecting both the current and future learning experience and students' wellbeing [8]. Greater subjective wellbeing, defined as the cognitive and affective evaluations of ones' life, also correlates with higher academic performance in further education [38]. The regulation of emotions is also highlighted as a key skill for successful healthcare professionals in effectively delivering high quality care [9]. Thus, it is reasonable to assume that the exploration of emotions through deep reflection is a vital tool in fostering a healthy and effective learning environment.

With so many student participants already undertaking reflection in their personal lives, it became evident that participants recognise the importance of deep reflection. Suggestions for improvement included making a safer space for reflection and providing more formal guidance on reflection relating to the need for more formal support in developing knowledge and understanding of reflective skills. In this post-Bawa-Gaba era, following a key case whereby a doctor in training had their reflective records evidenced against them in court, healthcare professionals are finding written reflection to no longer be a safe space to reflect, and have called for the opportunity to use different methods [39].

Although the findings of this study may not be generalisable to entire student populations in all institutions, the most important aspect of the research was capturing the hermeneutic stories of the participants and thus the data speak for themselves. The findings of this study are valuable as they can now be used to justify and guide an intervention to effectively facilitate deep reflection for undergraduate dental students. Rolfe refers to 'wicked' problems, which are those complex challenges faced daily by healthcare practitioners which cannot simply be solved by simply applying best evidence to the situation, and cannot be fully understood until they attempt to solve it [40]. These situations are not amenable to simple application of past experience or current evidence, and reflective practice, specifically experimenting in action, is the best hope of successfully managing them [40]. Schön argued that when the practitioner reflects in action, they become their own researcher [3]. In an ever-demanding healthcare sector, where no amount of theory or knowledge of evidence will enable one to manage these problems, it is vital to create a generation of practitioners who are their own theorists and researchers by generating and testing hypotheses on the spot in the form of practice interventions [40].

5. Conclusions

The results of this study show that in its current form, the logbook is not facilitating students in engaging in deep reflection, with staff and students feeling that greater understanding of and support in reflection would be beneficial in improving clinical experience and learning.

Author Contributions: Conceptualization, F.C., K.J. and H.R.; methodology, F.C., K.J. and H.R.; formal analysis, F.C., K.J. and H.R.; writing—original draft preparation, F.C.; writing—review and editing, F.C., K.J. and H.R.; supervision H.R.; project administration, F.C. All authors have read and agreed to the published version of the manuscript.

Funding: This research received no external funding.

Institutional Review Board Statement: The study was conducted according to the guidelines of the Declaration of Helsinki, and approved by the University of Sheffield Ethics Committee (reference: 034416).

Informed Consent Statement: Informed consent was obtained from all subjects involved in the study.

Data Availability Statement: Anonymized data obtained through this study are available upon reasonable request to the corresponding author. Data are not publicly available for privacy reasons.

Acknowledgments: The authors would like to thank administrative staff and all student and staff participants.

Conflicts of Interest: The authors declare no conflict of interest.

References

1. Dewey, J. *How We Think: A Restatement of the Relation of Reflective Thinking to the Educative Process*; D.C. Heath and Company: Boston, NY, USA, 1933.
2. Mann, K.; Gordon, J.; MacLeod, A. Reflection and Reflective Practice in Health Professions Education: A Systematic Review. *Adv. Health Sci. Educ. Theory Pract.* **2007**, *14*, 595–621. [CrossRef] [PubMed]
3. Schön, D. *The Reflective Practitioner: How Professionals Think in Action*; Basic Books: New York, NY, USA, 1983; pp. 68–69.
4. Reeson, M.G.; Walker-Gleaves, C.; Jepson, N. Interactions in the Dental Team: Understanding the Theoretical Complexities and Practical Challenges. *Br. Dent. J.* **2013**, *215*, 1–6. [CrossRef] [PubMed]
5. Boud, D. Avoiding the traps: Seeking good practice in the use of self-assessment and reflection in professional courses. *Soc. Work. Educ.* **1999**, *18*, 121–132. [CrossRef]
6. Hatton, N.; Smith, D. Reflection in teacher education: Towards definition and implementation. *Teach. Teach. Educ.* **1995**, *11*, 33–49. [CrossRef]
7. Boud, D.; Keogh, R.; Walker, D. *Reflection: Turning Experience into Learning*; Kogan: London, UK, 1985.
8. Pekrun, R. Inquiry on emotions in higher education: Progress and open problems. *Stud. High. Educ.* **2019**, *44*, 1806–1811. [CrossRef]
9. NHS Health Education England. NHS Staff and Learners' Mental Wellbeing Commission. 2018. Available online: https://www.hee.nhs.uk (accessed on 1 May 2021).
10. Piazza-Waggoner, C.A.; Cohen, L.L.; Kohli, K.; Taylor, B.K. Stress Management for Dental Students Performing Their First Pediatric Restorative Procedure. *J. Dent. Educ.* **2003**, *67*, 542–548. [CrossRef] [PubMed]
11. General Dental Council. *Standards for the Dental Team [Internet]*, 1st ed.; General Dental Council: London, UK, 2013. Available online: https://standards.gdc-uk.org/Assets/pdf/Standards%20for%20the%20Dental%20Team.pdf (accessed on 1 May 2021).
12. Dental Council New Zealand. *Standards Framework for Oral Health Practitioners [Internet]*, 1st ed.; Dental Council New Zealand: Wellington, New Zealand, 2015; Available online: https://www.dcnz.org.nz/assets/Uploads/Practice-standards/Standards-Framework-for-oral-health-practitioners.pdf (accessed on 1 May 2021).

13. Dental Board of Australia. *Code of Conduct for Registered Health Practitioners [Internet]*, 1st ed.; Dental Board of Australia: Melbourne, Australia, 2014. Available online: https://www.dentalboard.gov.au/Codes-Guidelines/Policies-Codes-Guidelines/Code-of-conduct.aspx (accessed on 1 May 2021).
14. Asadoorian, J.; Schönwetter, D.J.; Lavigne, S.E. Developing reflective health care practitioners: Learning from experience in dental hygiene education. *J. Dent. Educ.* **2011**, *75*, 472–484. [CrossRef] [PubMed]
15. Dempsey, M.; Halton, C.; Murphy, M. Reflective learning in social work education: Scaffolding the process. *Soc. Work. Educ. Int. J.* **2001**, *20*, 631–641. [CrossRef]
16. General Dental Council. *Preparing for Practice. Dental Team Learning Outcomes for Registration*, 2nd ed.; General Dental Council: London, UK, 2015; p. 25. Available online: https://www.gdc-uk.org/docs/default-source/quality-assurance/preparing-for-practice-(revised-2015).pdf?sfvrsn=81d58c49_2 (accessed on 30 March 2020).
17. General Dental Council. *Enhanced CPD Scheme 2018 Guidance [Internet]*, 2nd ed.; General Dental Council: London, UK, 2018. Available online: https://www.gdc-uk.org/docs/default-source/enhanced-cpd-scheme-2018/enhanced-cpd-guidance-for-professionals.pdf?sfvrsn=edbe677f_4 (accessed on 1 May 2021).
18. General Dental Council. *Standards for Education Standards and Requirements for Providers [Internet]*, 2nd ed.; GDC: London, UK, 2015. Available online: https://www.gdc-uk.org/docs/default-source/quality-assurance/standards-for-education-(revised-2015).pdf?sfvrsn=1f1a3f8a_2 (accessed on 1 May 2021).
19. American Dental Association. *Accreditation Standards For Dental Education Programs [Internet]*, 1st ed.; American Dental Association: Chicago, IL, USA, 2019. Available online: https://www.ada.org/~{}/media/CODA/Files/predoc_standards.pdf?la=en (accessed on 1 May 2021).
20. Chief Executives of Statutory Regulators of Health and Care Professionals. *Benefits of Becoming a Reflective Practitioner A Joint Statement of Support from Chief Executives of Statutory Regulators of Health and Care Professionals [Internet]*, 1st ed.; Health and Care Professionals Council: London, UK, 2019. Available online: https://www.gdc-uk.org/docs/default-source/reflective-practice/benefits-of-becoming-a-reflective-practitioner-joint-statement-2019.pdf?sfvrsn=3c546751_2 (accessed on 1 May 2021).
21. Polit, D.F.; Beck, C.T. *Nursing Research: Principles and Methods*, 7th ed.; Lippincott, Williams & Wilkins: Philadelphia, PA, USA, 2009.
22. Heidegger, M. *Being and Time*; Stambaugh, J., Translator; SUNY Press: New York, NY, USA, 1927.
23. Husserl, E. *Logical Investigations*; Findlay, J., Translator; Humanities Press: New York, NY, USA, 1970.
24. Lopez, K.; Willis, D. Descriptive versus interpretive phenomenology: Their contributions to nursing knowledge. *Qual. Health Res.* **2014**, *14*, 726–735. [CrossRef]
25. Jack, K. The meaning of compassion fatigue to student nurses: An interpretive phenomenological study. *J. Compassionate Healthc.* **2017**, *4*, 1–8. [CrossRef]
26. Lewis, J.; Jack, K. The use of the arts to encourage reflection in the dental professions—A commentary. *Eur. J. Dent. Educ.* **2018**, *22*, e648–e650. [CrossRef] [PubMed]
27. Ritchie, J.; Lewis, J.; McNaughton Nicholls, C.; Ormston, R. *Qualitative Research Practice*; Sage: London, UK, 2013.
28. Van Manen, M. *Researching Lived Experience: Human Science for an Action Sensitive Pedagogy*; State University of New York Press: Albany, NY, USA, 1990.
29. Schön. *Educating the Reflective Practitioner: Toward a New Design for Teaching and Learning in the Professions*; Jossey-Bass: San Francisco, CA, USA, 1987.
30. Coward, M. Does the use of reflective models restrict critical thinking and therefore learning in nurse education? What have we done? *Nurse Educ. Today* **2011**, *31*, 883–886. [CrossRef] [PubMed]
31. Moon, J. *A Handbook of Reflective and Experiential Learning: Theory and Practice*; Routledge Falmer: London, UK, 2004.
32. Patil, N.G.; Lee, P. Interactive logbooks for medical students: Are they useful? *Med. Educ.* **2002**, *36*, 672–677. [CrossRef] [PubMed]
33. Schüttpelz-Brauns, K.; Narciss, E.; Schneyinck, C.; Böhme, K.; Brüstle, P.; Mau-Holzmann, U.; Lammerding-Koeppel, M.; Obertacke, U. Twelve Tips for Successfully Implementing Logbooks in Clinical Training. *Med. Teach.* **2016**, *38*, 564–569. [CrossRef] [PubMed]
34. Cecchini, J.J.; Fridman, N. First-year dental students: Relationship between stress and performance. *Int. J. Psychosom.* **1987**, *34*, 17–19. [PubMed]
35. Freeman, R.E. Dental students as operators: Emotional reactions. *Med. Educ.* **1985**, *19*, 27–33. [CrossRef] [PubMed]
36. Lloyd, C.; Musser, L.A. Psychiatric symptoms in dental students. *J. Nerv. Ment. Dis.* **1989**, *177*, 61–69. [CrossRef] [PubMed]
37. Hung, M.; Licari, F.W.; Hon, E.S.; Lauren, E.; Su, S.; Birmingham, W.C.; Wadsworth, L.L.; Lassetter, J.H.; Graff, T.C.; Harman, W.; et al. In an Era of Uncertainty: Impact of COVID-19 on Dental Education. *J. Dent. Educ.* **2021**, *85*, 148–156. [CrossRef]
38. Chattu, V.K.; Sahu, P.K.; Seedial, N.; Seecharan, G.; Seepersad, A.; Seunarine, M.; Sieunarine, S.; Seymour, K.; Simboo, S.; Singh, A. Subjective well-being and its relation to academic performance among students in medicine, dentistry, and other health professions. *Educ. Sci.* **2020**, *10*, 224. [CrossRef]
39. Bradshaw, P. E-portfolios, reflections and the case of Dr Bawa-Garba. In *MA Healthcare*; Mark Allen Group: London, UK, 2018.
40. Rolfe, G. Rethinking reflective education: What would Dewey have done? *Nurse Educ. Today* **2014**, *34*, 1179–1183. [CrossRef]

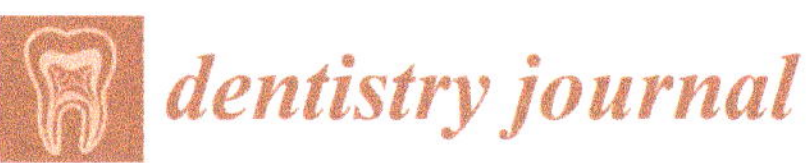

dentistry journal

MDPI

Review

Understanding Motor Skill Learning as Related to Dentistry

Mohamed El-Kishawi [1,*], Khaled Khalaf [1] and Tracey Winning [2]

[1] Preventive and Restorative Dentistry Department, College of Dental Medicine, University of Sharjah, Sharjah P.O. BOX 27272, United Arab Emirates; kkhalaf@sharjah.ac.ae

[2] School of Dentistry, the University of Adelaide, Adelaide, SA 5000, Australia; tracey.winning@adelaide.edu.au

* Correspondence: melkishawi@sharjah.ac.ae; Tel.: +971-65057382

Abstract: Learning dental procedures is a complex task involving the development of fine motor skills. The reported use of theories and/or evidence for designing learning activities to develop the fine motor skills needed for dental practice is limited. The aim of this review is to explore the available body of knowledge related to learning motor skills relevant to dentistry. Evidence from studies investigating motor skill learning highlights the negative impact of self-focus and self-regulation on learning outcomes, particularly during the early stages of learning. The development of activities and schedules that enable novices to demonstrate characteristics similar to experts, without the reported long period of 'deliberate practice', is clearly of value. Outcomes of learning implicitly are important in dentistry because working under stressful conditions is common, either during undergraduate study or in practice. It is suggested that learning implicitly in the simulation stage can reduce disrupted performance when transitioning to clinical settings. Therefore, further investigation of effective methods for learning dental fine motor skills is indicated, using approaches that result in robust performance, even under stressful conditions.

Keywords: motor skills; learning theories; dentistry; self-consciousness; working memory

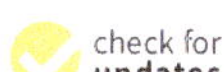

Citation: El-Kishawi, M.; Khalaf, K.; Winning, T. Understanding Motor Skill Learning as Related to Dentistry. *Dent. J.* **2021**, *9*, 68. https://doi.org/10.3390/dj9060068

Academic Editors: Jelena Dumancic and Božana Lončar Brzak

Received: 9 April 2021
Accepted: 8 June 2021
Published: 11 June 2021

1. Introduction

Procedural and cognitive skills are essential abilities for clinical dental practice. Students learn these skills during simulated clinical activities designed to ensure that they achieve a satisfactory level prior to proceeding to direct patient care. These simulated activities have associated high costs in terms of staffing and facilities [1–3]. To optimize learning in these settings, the design of relevant learning activities needs to be informed by theory and based on evidence.

However, there has only been limited research conducted in relation to the design of the most effective and efficient methods for learning the complex cognitive and fine motor skills required for patient care in dentistry [1,4–6]. Similarly, there are few publications discussing the rationale and design of simulation and clinical endodontic learning activities [7–9].

Other than investigation of the design and diameter of hand file handles and the effect of the fit of gloves on performance [10–12], there has been limited use of learning theories to explicitly inform the design of simulation and clinical dental learning activities [6,13–15]. The purpose of this review is to explore the available body of knowledge related to learning motor skills in dentistry. The review also aims to familiarize the reader with definitions and theoretical explanations concerning motor skill learning based on extensive research. Please see Table 1 below describing terms used in this article.

Table 1. Description of terms used in this article.

Term	Description
Augmented (extrinsic) feedback	Supplementary or reinforcing feedback received from the surrounding environment related to the movement outcome and the quality of the executed movement.
Block practice	Performing a motor task in a repetitive manner without variation in the practice (e.g., AAA, BBB, CCC).
Chunking	Dividing large pieces of information into smaller elements that are easier to store in the short-term memory.
Cognitive knowledge	Acquiring factual existing information and discovering new knowledge through human thinking.
Declarative knowledge	Descriptive information stored in memory that is static in nature which describes things, events, or processes.
Errorful learning	Learning by loading the learning environment (e.g., instructions, skill difficulty) aiming to increase errors.
Errorless learning	Learning by constraining the learning environment (e.g., instructions, skill difficulty) aiming to reduce errors.
Explicit learning	Learning which generates verbal knowledge of movement performance (i.e., facts and rules) that is dependent on working memory.
External focus	Occurs when the learner's focus of attention is directed toward the effect of the motor task (e.g., final shape of the cavity preparation).
Extraneous cognitive load	Dependent on how movement information is presented to learner and controlled by the design of instructions.
Generalized motor program	Stored muscle general rules that may be applied to different environmental or situational contexts.
Germane cognitive load	The work put into processing, construction, and automation of movement knowledge to create a permanent store in memory.
Hypothesis testing	Learning by repetitive attempt to perform a task by detecting and correcting errors.
Implicit learning	Learning with minimal increase in verbal knowledge (i.e., facts and rules) of movement resulting in skills that are unconsciously retrieved from memory.
Inherent (intrinsic) feedback	Feedback related to information about motor task gained through sensory channels during or after the execution of the movement.
Internal focus	Occurs when the learner's focus of attention is directed toward the action of the motor task (e.g., hand movement or bur angulation).
Intrinsic cognitive load	Directly related to learning task and defined by the number and interaction of the processed elements.
Random practice	Performing a motor task in a random manner with variation in the practice (e.g., ABC, BCA, CAB).
Sensory memory	Type of short-term memory that is able to process and recall information related to sensory input.
Working memory	Short-term memory that can store small amount of information for the execution of cognitive processes.

2. Materials and Methods

The following electronic databases were searched to identify relevant articles to our topic: Google scholar, Scopus, PubMed, and Medline until October 2020. The search was carried out by two investigators to eliminate any potential bias in selecting the relevant articles. The following keywords were used to conduct a comprehensive search so that no key studies were missed during the search: motor skills, learning theories, dentistry, working memory, and self-consciousness, as well as, MeSH terms i.e., "dentistry", "motor skills", "learning" were used to conduct our comprehensive search. Inclusion criteria: all types of studies investigating motor skill learning as related to dentistry and discussing definitions and theoretical concepts concerning motor skill learning.

3. Motor Skill Learning Theories

Fine motor skill learning requires the control and integration of a range of stimuli and responses to be able to perform the desired motor task. How can we explain, support, or predict how people learn these skills? Several learning theories have been developed to explain how learning motor skills occurs and what stimulates individuals to learn and change. In dentistry, understanding relevant learning theories is essential for dental educators to be able to design effective learning activities, with a clear rationale that supports their dental students' learning. Below, we will discuss five key theories that have relevance to learning procedural skills and declarative knowledge in dentistry. Specifically, these are Schema theory, Cognitive Load theory, OPTIMAL theory of motor learning, the Novice-Expert continuum and deliberate practice principles, and Reinvestment theory (Table 2).

3.1. Schema Theory

Theories of motor skill acquisition were initially conceptualized by behavioral psychologists based on the associations between stimuli and responses [21]. The role of cognition in motor skill acquisition was first emphasized by Adams [22]. Adams postulated that motor skill learning included a combination of motor behavior with a variety of cognitive processes in addition to the development of strategies that can be used to execute a motor task.

The way in which feedback and error detection affect learning was a fundamental element of Adams' [22] theory of motor control. According to this theory, learners usually hold a reference of accuracy that determines a desired outcome of the movement and a feedback process that perceives error between the learner's desired movement and the actual movement produced [22]. Research findings suggested that Adams' views were true for movements that are relatively slow [16]. Slow movements provided learners with a chance to evaluate their performance and to detect any error between the desired movement and the actual movement by way of a feedback mechanism. Adams' theory has several limitations [16]. It does not explain how rapid movements are learned and controlled. To achieve rapid movements, a motor plan needs to be structured in advance, which does not allow for feedback during the movement. Another reported limitation is the effect of random practice on the accuracy of the perceptual recall of movement stored in the central nervous system [23]. Despite these limitations, Adams' theory represented a step forward in understanding motor skill learning and paved the way for newer theories.

Schema theory, first proposed by Schmidt [16], suggested that a motor program (i.e., stored muscle commands) contains general rules that may be applied to different environmental or situational contexts through the contribution of an open-loop control process and generalized motor programs (GMP). Schema contain the common rules that generate the spatial, temporal muscle behavior designed to achieve a specified movement [24]. Therefore, when learning new movements, a person may produce a new GMP based on the choice of parameters (e.g., to reduce issues with the novel movement), or improve an existing GMP (which helps minimize the storage problem of multiple GMP), depending on previous experience with the movement and task context.

Table 2. Summary of motor learning theories relevant to dentistry.

Theory	Description	Points in Favor	Points Against
1. Schema Theory [16]	Motor learning involves ongoing processes that update the recall and recognition of proprioceptive information from limbs and fingers. The response parameters (e.g., speed and force) are specified according to stored knowledge of the results.	- Commonly used theory. - Used to explain procedural skill development.	- No longer valid for understanding motor skill learning. - Unable to describe learning through observation. - Unable to explain the role of augmented feedback.
2. The OPTIMAL theory of motor learning [17]	Focuses on discovering the correct instructional approach to support motivation and direction of motor learning to the desired outcome of the motor task.	- Supports simplifying movement instructions. - Positive impact on instructional design. - Reduces the load on the working memory.	- Limited evidence addressing complex fine motor skill learning.
3. Cognitive Load Theory [18]	Based on the assumption that cognitive system is limited as working memory can only store and process a small amount of information for a few seconds.	- Knowledge build up by combining simple elements can result in development of more complex results. - Reduces the load on working memory. - Positive impact on instructional design.	- Lacks conceptual clarity and validity of instrument used. - Lack generalizability in different contexts. - Uses self-reported survey to measure cognitive loads.
4. Novice-Expert continuum and deliberate practice principles [19]	Development of expert motor performance depends on continuous deliberate practice improved by trial-and-error learning and supported by appropriate supervision.	- Supports gradual buildup and improvement of motor skills. - Supports safe and low risk buildup of competency.	- Does not address individual's cognitive, attentional and perceptual abilities. - Requires a long deliberate practice to achieve expert level.
5. Reinvestment Theory [20]	Based on the distinction between individual's movement self-consciousness features related to movement processing and decision making.	- Commonly used theory. - Implicit learning reduces the load on the working memory. - Supports simplifying movement instructions. - Implicit learning maintains robust performance under multi-tasking and stressful conditions.	- Limited evidence addressing complex fine motor skill learning. - Lack of consensus related to the role of observational learning as an implicit learning approach. - Uses self-reported survey to measure the level of reinvestment.

Schema theory proposed that after generation of a movement, four components are usually stored in memory: (a) the initial conditions (i.e., the proprioceptive information of the limbs and body); (b) the response specifications for the motor program, which are the parameters used in the generalized motor program (e.g., speed and force); (c) the sensory consequences of the response produced, which consist of information about how the movement felt, looked and sounded; and (d) the outcome of that movement with knowledge of the results [16]. Schema theory proposes that motor learning involves ongoing processes that update the recall and recognition schemas with every movement that is performed [24]. For example, initial motor movements related to a dental procedure (e.g., cavity preparation) are usually stored from proprioceptive information gathered from clinical examination. This would activate a memory recall of previous clinical experience related to hand/fingers speed and forces required to achieve the motor task (i.e., caries excavation). The result of this movement would depend on the stored knowledge about the desired procedure outcome (i.e., cavity outline form) of this dental procedure (Figure 1). Despite its deficiencies, schema theory has triggered the development of alternative ideas and provided a model from which new theoretical positions have been proposed. Schema theory is the most commonly used theory, either explicitly or implied that has been used to explain procedural skill development in dentistry [25].

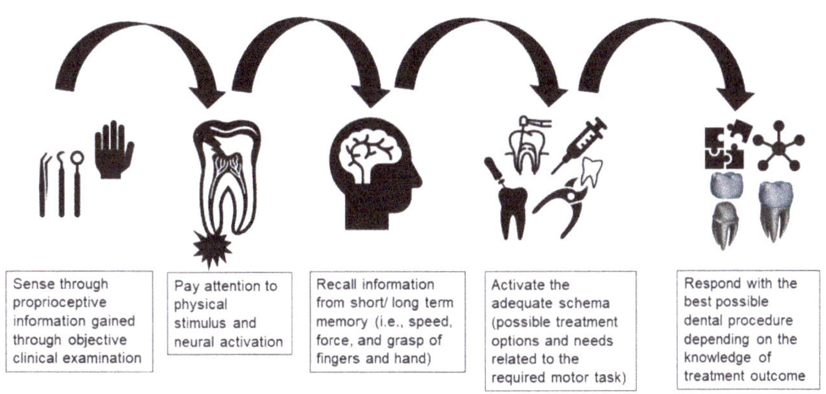

Figure 1. Schema theory as relevant to dentistry.

However, for many scholars, including Schmidt himself, Schema theory no longer provides a satisfactory theoretical basis for understanding motor skill learning. In particular, more recent findings cast doubt on the cognitive-based assumptions of Schema theory, and it can only provide incomplete explanations of how motor skills are acquired [23,26]. For example, this theory is unable to describe how people are capable of learning through observation in the absence of cutaneous sensory feedback or movement [27].

Another issue related to Schema theory is the theoretical role of augmented feedback, when retention and transfer tests are conducted [28]. Feedback about motor movement can be divided into inherent (intrinsic) feedback, and augmented (extrinsic) feedback [28]. Specifically, inherent feedback is related to information about a motor task gained by the performer through various sensory channels during or after the execution of a motor movement, depending on the nature of the task. Augmented feedback, on the other hand, is related to information provided about a movement task that is supplementary to, or that reinforces, the inherent feedback [28]. Studies conducted by Lai and Shea [29,30]. showed that manipulation of feedback about performance results under different practice conditions did not result in consistent improvement in skill. Specifically, reducing the frequency of results feedback, achieved better performance stability and enhanced the learning of the motor tasks during random practice using a mixture of variable motor tasks during a practice session (i.e., ABC, BCA, CBA). In contrast, repetition of a single task during a practice session (block practice; i.e., AAA, BBB, CCC) resulted in an improvement of the motor task learning [15]. Therefore, Schema theory is not able to explain the effect related to manipulations of frequency of feedback on performance outcomes on motor task variables. In addition, this theory is limited in regards to the kind of characteristics in a motor program that are affected by manipulations of feedback about results of performance (e.g., timing, pattern and movement sequence), and the influence of variability and order of practice on the acquisition of the motor skills [26].

3.2. The OPTIMAL Theory of Motor Learning

The OPTIMAL (Optimizing Performance Through Intrinsic Motivation and Attention for Learning) theory considers the social and cognitive nature of motor behavior [17]. The application of the OPTIMAL theory for enhancing motor performance and learning in clinical settings involves discovering the correct approaches to support motivation and directing attention to the desired outcome of the fine motor task. In a typical dental training setting, the clinical instructor decides on the task to be practiced, describes how to perform the movements of the task, provides corrective instructions and feedback that relate to the orientation of the hand/finger's movements. These instructions often include descriptions of the movements of a particular part(s) of the hand or fingers in relation to other body parts [31]. Instructions focusing on specific body movements, is described as having an 'internal focus'. On the other hand, instructions that direct a learner's attention to the effect of the movement are described as having an 'external focus' [32]. Literature on attentional focus effects have shown that slight modifications in the provided instructions can have a major effect on learning and performance [31]. When applying this concept in endodontics, it appears that providing instructions characterized by an external focus of attention (e.g., cleaning and shaping root canal space, and advancing the instrument) has more learning advantages, contrary to an internal focus of attention (e.g., angulation of the hand instrument inside the canal, movement or grasp on a hand instrument).

3.3. Cognitive Load Theory

Many contemporary theories of motor skill learning identified the importance of cognitive processes during motor skill acquisition, particularly in the initial stages of learning [33,34]. The initial stage of motor skill learning (i.e., cognitive stage/declarative stage) involves cognitive processing of verbal/visual instructions related to the task and rehearsal of the task in working memory. This cognitive processing facilitates the interpretation of the instructions required to perform the task [35]. Cognitive load theory (CLT) is related to working memory characteristics and instructional design [36]. It was developed to provide guidelines to assist in presenting instructional material in a way that facilitates learning motor activities and optimizes performance [37]. The history of this theory goes back to the 1950s when Miller [21] first described the limited nature of working memory and noted that humans are only able to hold seven, plus or minus two, pieces of information in their short-term memory. Subsequently, Sweller [18] further developed cognitive load theory to inform instructional design principles and strategies supported by a model of human cognitive architecture.

CLT is based on the assumption that the human cognitive system is limited by the fact that working memory (i.e., short-term memory) can only store and process a small amount of information for a few seconds [38]. This limitation in working memory capacity and duration is restricted to new information retrieved through sensory memory [39]. However, if information is obtained from long-term memory, these limitations do not exist. As reviewed by Sweller et al. [39], long-term memory is believed to store information as cognitive schemas, which may vary in complexity and automation. Expertise in humans is achieved by knowledge built up by these schemas. Careful and gradual combining of simple ideas to become more complex can result in the development of expertise in novice learners. The organization of knowledge by schemas can extensively reduce working memory load as highly complex schemas can be processed as a single element in working memory [40].

Limitation in the capacity of memory arises when handling completely new and unorganized information [41]. This limitation might be related to the increased number of elements to be organized, which increases the number of possible combinations of elements required to be tested during any problem solving process [40]. This memory overload problem can be compensated for by limiting the number of information units that are processed at the same time. This can be achieved by organizing information in long-term memory using schema construction processes, therefore reducing the extraneous cognitive load [40]. During problem solving processes, schemas can be built up by putting elements together (i.e., chunking), and/or combining new elements with already existing schemas in long-term memory [42]. Schemas can then be handled as a single element in working memory, which can significantly reduce cognitive load related to the performance of future tasks. Properly designed instructions should support schema construction, as well as encourage schema automation, which can help free working memory capacity for other activities.

The load on working memory may be influenced by the intrinsic environment of the learning tasks (*intrinsic load*), by the way tasks are presented (*extraneous load*), and by the actual learning that occurs (*germane load*) when handling intrinsic load [40].

Based on cognitive load theory, both intrinsic and extraneous cognitive loads are added and related when learners are presented with a task [40]. If intrinsic load is low, a high extraneous load resulting from poor instructional design might not be detrimental to learning as the total cognitive load is within the limits of working memory. When teaching complicated tasks (e.g., root canal preparation) involving greater interaction between elements involved in a task (i.e., motion, sequence, force, and tactile sensation in root canal preparation), the combined intrinsic and extraneous loads are likely to exceed working memory capacity and result in overload. The more that extraneous cognitive load is reduced, the more working memory resources can be dedicated to intrinsic cognitive load, which enables easier induction of a germane cognitive load for learning [40].

Cognitive Load theory has had a major impact on educational research and instructional design [43]. However, some critical questions have been raised concerning its conceptual clarity, validity of instruments used to measure cognitive load, and generalizability of its outcomes in different contexts and populations [36]. For example, there remains a lack of clear distinction between intrinsic, extraneous, and germane cognitive load. Moreover, measurement of cognitive load using self-reported questionnaires is often presented with no standard format and with differences in the number of items used for the survey. However, these measures cannot be used to measure cognitive overload (i.e., when working memory capacity is exceeded) [36].

3.4. Novice Expert Continuum and Deliberate Practice Principles

To develop expert understanding and skillful performance, Dreyfus et al., [19] suggested a five-stage development continuum beginning with novice level, moving through advanced beginner, to competent, proficient, and expert (Figure 2). A learner in training for a professional role develops from a true novice (a beginner) through a sequence of stages where capacities are gradually improved by trial-and-error learning and continual approximation supported by appropriate supervision. Dreyfus and colleagues [19] identified that the safe practitioner stage (competent) is a stage where the learner can perform the basic tasks related to a professional role and resolve common problems without assistance. This stage is the starting point for obtaining smooth, consistent, and accurate performance that is characteristic of true expertise [33].

The development of a graduate from a professional education program to become competent, proficient or even hold some aspects of expertise, depends on many factors [33]. These factors include the difficulty of the skills to be acquired, practice frequency, prospects for gradually increasing levels of challenge and responsibility for the task, and mentor availability to act as an instructor and role model [44]. Dental school graduates will generally not have the ability to perform as experts immediately after graduation, but hopefully can perform at a competent level for the essential skills associated with general dentistry [33]. With further practice and progress, it is anticipated that they will become experts.

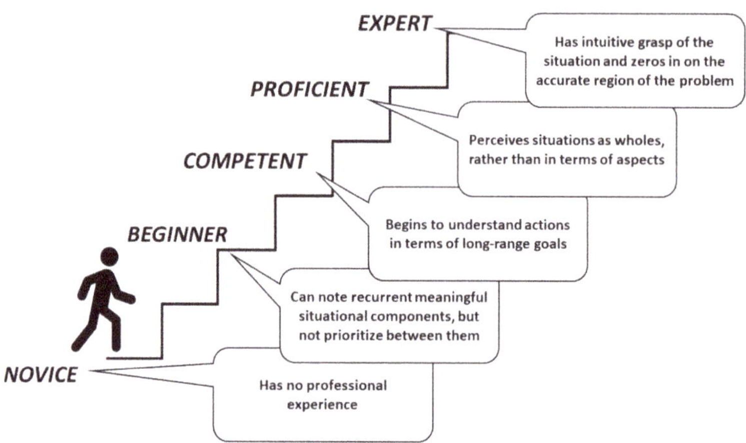

Figure 2. Pedagogical Needs and Limitations.

Differences between experts and novices are often related to how they structure, analyze, and use information [45]. Expert practitioners have integrated neural networks that enable instant recovery of information related to task performance or assessment of a problem [38]. Novice learners, on the other hand, find it difficult to bring together isolated pieces of information. Novices use an ineffective trial-and-error method because of the deficiency in their pre-existing networks [33]. Students may possess some information (i.e., from textbooks or manuals), but the information is isolated and often not related to other topics. To develop problem solving ability, students need to convert their disorganized acquired information (i.e., pieces of data) from textbooks and lectures into connected chains of networked knowledge, which have meaning, significance, and recognized value that can be described in an individual's own words [46].

Research studies have highlighted that novices can benefit from learning motor skills with minimal conscious involvement as performance is maintained when high levels of cognitive effort are required [47]. Furthermore, it is evident that novices who learn without attending to and monitoring their movements demonstrate characteristics that are similar to the performance of professionals with comprehensive knowledge and skills (i.e., experts). The development of activities and schedules that enable novices to demonstrate characteristics similar to experts, without the reported long period of 'deliberate practice', is clearly of value [45].

3.5. Reinvestment Theory

The general distinction between conscious and non-conscious features of motor learning processes is considered a starting point to explain a variety of motor learning models [48]. Research into motor skill acquisition has demonstrated that motor skill learning is often disrupted by distraction and self-focus, especially under stressful conditions [49,50]. When distracted, the attention of the performer becomes focused on stimuli that are not related to the motor task. Self-focus, on the other hand, can direct attention in a way that involves self-regulation and self-evaluation in an attempt to match the required standard of performance [51]. Masters (1992) grouped the range of views of self-focus control behaviors under the term 'reinvestment' [51,52].

The theory of reinvestment relates to the conscious attempts by performers to ensure the quality of their performance, by observing (i.e., movement self-consciousness) and controlling (i.e., conscious motor processing) their own movements using explicit processes involving working memory [51]. As a result, of this observation and control, disruption of automated execution of some motor skill components can occur, which results in poor movement quality, and subsequent breakdown of performance [20].

The difficulty of the task also influences the level of disruption from reinvestment. Propensity to reinvest has been suggested to be associated with more complex tasks rather than simple tasks [53]. This is relevant to learning how to prepare root canals or access cavity, as these are complex tasks involving different procedures that require cognitive access to both procedural knowledge (related to stages of treatment, sequence of instruments and materials, and different mechanical techniques used) and declarative knowledge (related to the anatomy of the root canal system, diagnosis of the case, and choice of the most suitable material and instrument in relation to the tooth/patient condition). Therefore, the impact of reinvestment during complex dental procedures might be more disruptive for performance.

Implicit and Explicit Learning

The negative effect of reinvestment can potentially be prevented by emotion control training, training performers to avoid conscious control of their behaviour, distraction techniques, or directing performers to an external focus of attention [51]. Another possible way to prevent reinvestment is by using implicit methods for learning motor skills. Implicit learning of motor skills includes learning skills without the accumulation of conscious verbal knowledge (e.g., rules) about motor task performance, such that these "implicitly learned skills are (unconsciously) retrieved from implicit memory" [48]. Therefore, by learning implicitly, the aim is to limit the accumulation of movement-specific knowledge, decrease dependence on declarative knowledge structures during motor task performance, and minimize testing of hypotheses related to movements that are aimed at improving performance [54]. Studies have found that the value of implicit motor learning in novices exceeds the expected objective of acquiring motor skills by also showing robust performance under conditions of stress conditions, fatigue and when high levels of cognitive effort are required (e.g., when performing an additional or secondary task) [55].

An implicit approach contrasts with the conventional approach to learning motor skills in dentistry and surgery, namely learning explicitly by consciously following detailed textual, visual, and/or verbal instructions related to carrying out a motor skill task [56]. An explicit learning process consists of cognitive (declarative) stages and depends on involvement of working memory [48]. Research on motor skill learning during laparoscopy procedures has indicated that using explicit learning approaches disrupts neural efficiency of the brain compared with implicit approaches [57]. While this explicit framework of instruction is routine, it was proposed recently that a shift to more implicit (less explicit) training strategies might be beneficial, particularly in the initial stages of learning [58].

In a study using the Delphi technique to explore opinions by experts regarding descriptions for implicit and explicit learning methods, there was a lack of agreement among experts regarding the application of explicit and implicit motor skill learning [59]. However, there was agreement that certain methods can promote more implicit or more explicit motor learning depending on instructions, limitations in the environment, type of motor task, and personal abilities. Various implicit and explicit motor skill learning strategies have been reported in the literature [48,59]. Methods for learning more implicitly include learning motor skills under secondary task conditions [13] learning without errors [13,60], learning with physical 'guidance' [61] [e.g. suture and knot tying; 61], learning by analogy [55] [e.g. table tennis; 55]), or learning from observation [62] [e.g. suture and knot tying. 62]). The efficacy of these various approaches for learning motor skills has been demonstrated in dentistry. For example, in restorative dentistry, using a procedure to reduce the production of errors (i.e., errorless learning: learning from simple to complex task), has been shown to result in significantly higher levels of performance during both learning and testing phases compared with learning explicitly via increasing errors (errorful: from complex to simple task) [6,13]. Errorless (implicit) learning is thought to result in motor skill performance that does not require working memory resources. In contrast, deterioration of performance in the errorful (explicit) learning might be related to an extra load on working memory resources that was needed for completing the dental procedure (Figure 3). Faculty involved in teaching and learning of dental students should be aware of this finding to improve students' learning as this would impact on their readiness to practice independently in their future career.

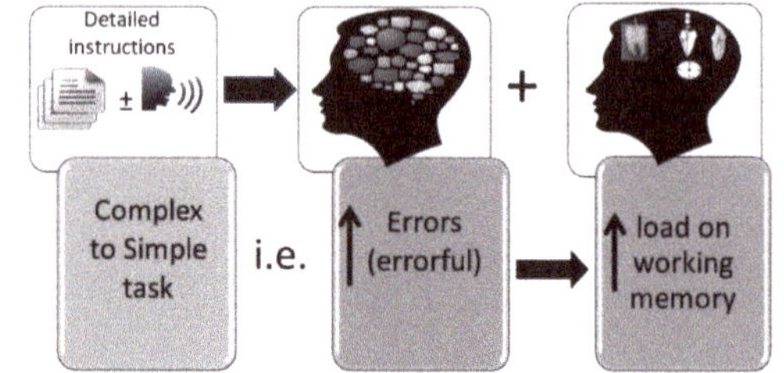

Figure 3. Application of implicit and explicit approaches. (**a**). Implicit learning, (**b**). Explicit learning.

Implicit learning tends to minimize hypothesis testing by participants [63]. Indeed, a core principle of implicit learning approaches is to develop learning protocols that minimize hypothesis testing and prevent participants learning from their errors [64]. Despite the increasing body of evidence supporting implicit approaches of motor task learning, most of these studies were related to simple gross motor learning (e.g., sports) [7,57,64] compared to a limited number of studies addressing complex fine motor tasks used in medicine and dentistry [6,13].

In general, motor skill learning strategies that result in high conscious awareness about how the motor task is articulated are used to promote motor learning that is more explicit; for example, by learning motor skills by increasing errors (errorful), trial-and-error learning, and learning by observation combined with instruction [59].

4. Conclusions

There is limited evidence regarding fine motor skill learning in dentistry, particularly in endodontics. It has been shown that learning implicitly when carrying out a motor skill may limit the effect of self-focus and self-regulation on subsequent performance.

Stressors related to dental students' transferring from simulation to clinical settings can result in deterioration of performance. It is suggested that learning implicitly in the simulation stage can reduce disruptions in performance when moving to clinical settings. Therefore, further investigation of effective methods for learning fine dental motor skills is indicated, using conditions that result in robust performance, even under multi-tasking or stressful conditions.

Author Contributions: M.E.-K.: Conceptualization, Methodology, Data Curation, Investigation, Funding acquisition, Writing—review & editing; K.K.: Validation, Methodology, Data curation, Investigation, Writing—original draft; T.W.: Validation, Investigation, Writing—review & editing. All authors have read and agreed to the published version of the manuscript.

Funding: This research received no external funding.

Conflicts of Interest: The authors declare no conflict of interest.

References

1. Tedesco, L. Issues in dental curriculum development and change. *J. Dent. Educ.* **1995**, *59*, 97–147. [CrossRef]
2. Glickman, G.; Gluskin, A.; Johnson, W.; Lin, J. The crisis in endodontic education: Current perspectives and strategies for change. *J. Endod.* **2005**, *31*, 255–261. [CrossRef]
3. McNally, M.; Dunning, D.; Lange, B.; Gound, T. A survey of endodontic residents' attitudes about a career in dental education. *J. Endod.* **2002**, *28*, 592–594. [CrossRef]
4. Knight, G.; Guenzel, P.; Feil, P. Using questions to facilitate motor skill acquisition. *J. Dent. Educ.* **1997**, *61*, 56–65. [CrossRef]
5. Wierinck, E.; Puttemans, V.; Swinnen, S.; van Steenberghe, D. Expert performance on a virtual reality simulation system. *J. Dent. Educ.* **2007**, *71*, 759–766. [CrossRef]
6. Winning, T.; Malhotra, N.; Masters, R. Investigating an errorless learning approach for developing dental operative technique skills: A pilot study. *Eur. J. Dent. Educ.* **2018**, *22*, e706–e714. [CrossRef] [PubMed]
7. Koedijker, J.; Poolton, J.; Maxwell, J.; Oudejans, R.; Beek, P.; Masters, R. Attention and time constraints in perceptual-motor learning and performance: Instruction, analogy, and skill level. *Conscious. Cogn.* **2011**, *20*, 245–256. [CrossRef] [PubMed]
8. Friedlander, L.; Anderson, V. A new predoctoral endodontic module: Evaluating learning and effectiveness. *J. Dent. Educ.* **2011**, *75*, 351–359. [CrossRef] [PubMed]
9. Sonntag, D.; Barwald, R.; Hulsmann, M.; Stachniss, V. Pre-clinical endodontics: A survey amongst German dental schools. *Int. Endod. J.* **2008**, *41*, 863–868. [CrossRef] [PubMed]
10. Chandler, N.; Shaw, J.; Treble, S. Effect of endodontic instrument handle diameter on operator performance. *J. Endod.* **1996**, *22*, 110–111. [CrossRef]
11. Chandler, N.; Ford, T.; Monteith, B. Pulp size in molars: Underestimation on radiographs. *J. Oral. Rehabil.* **2004**, *31*, 764–769. [CrossRef] [PubMed]
12. Min, L.; Yun-hui, L.; Qiang, H. An optimized haptic interaction model based on support vector regression for evaluation of endodontic shaping skill. In Proceedings of the IEEE International Conference on Robotics and Biomimetics (ROBIO), Sanya, China, 15–18 December 2007; pp. 617–622.
13. El-Kishawi, M.; Khalaf, K.; Masters, R.; Winning, T. Effect of errorless learning on the acquisition of fine motor skills in pre-clinical endodontics. *Aust. Endod. J.* **2021**, *47*, 43–53. [CrossRef]
14. El-Kishawi, M.Y.; Khalaf, K.; Odeh, R.M. Determining the impact of stressors on students' clinical performance in endodontics. *J. Taibah. Univ. Med. Sci.* **2021**. [CrossRef]
15. El-Kishawi, M.; Khalaf, K.; Winning, T. How to Improve Fine Motor Skill Learning in Dentistry. *Int. J. Dent.* **2021**, *2021*, 1–8. [CrossRef]
16. Schmidt, R. A schema theory of discrete motor skill learning. *Psychol. Rev.* **1975**, *82*, 225–260. [CrossRef]
17. Wulf, G.; Lewthwaite, R. Optimizing performance through intrinsic motivation and attention for learning: The OPTIMAL theory of motor learning. *Psychon. Bull. Rev.* **2016**, *23*, 1382–1414. [CrossRef]
18. Sweller, J. Cognitive load during problem solving: Effects on learning. *Cogn. Sci.* **1988**, *12*, 257–285. [CrossRef]
19. Dreyfus, H.; Dreyfus, S.; Zadeh, L. Mind over machine: The power of human intuition and expertise in the era of the computer. *IEEE Expert* **1987**, *2*, 110–111. [CrossRef]
20. Masters, R.; Polman, R.; Hammond, N. 'Reinvestment': A dimension of personality implicated in skill breakdown under pressure. *Pers. Individ. Dif.* **1993**, *14*, 655–666. [CrossRef]
21. Miller, G. The magical number seven, plus or minus two: Some limits on our capacity for processing information. *Psychol. Rev.* **1956**, *63*, 81–97. [CrossRef]
22. Adams, J. A closed-loop theory of motor learning. *J. Mot. Behav.* **1971**, *3*, 111–149. [CrossRef]
23. Schmidt, R. Motor schema theory after 27 years: Reflections and implications for a new theory. *Res. Q. Exerc. Sport* **2003**, *74*, 366–375. [CrossRef] [PubMed]
24. Schmidt, R.; Lee, T. The learning process. In *Motor Control and Learning: A Behavioral Emphasis*, 4th ed.; Human Kinetics: Champaign, IL, USA, 2005; pp. 401–431.
25. Hendricson, W.D. Changes in educational methodologies in predoctoral dental education: Finding the perfect intersection. *J Dent. Educ.* **2012**, *76*, 118–141. [CrossRef]
26. Sherwood, D.; Lee, T. Schema theory: Critical review and implications for the role of cognition in a new theory of motor learning. *Res. Q. Exerc. Sport* **2003**, *74*, 376–382. [CrossRef]
27. Rose, D.; Christina, R. *A Multilevel Approach to the Study of Motor Control and Learning*, 2nd ed.; Pearson/Benjamin Cummings: San Francisco, CA, USA, 2006.
28. Schmidt, R.; Lee, T. Augmented feedback. In *Motor Control and Learning: A Behavioral Emphasis*, 4th ed.; Human Kinetics: Champaign, IL, USA, 2005; pp. 364–400.
29. Lai, Q.; Shea, C. Generalized motor program (GMP) learning: Effects of reduced frequency of knowledge of results and practice variability. *J. Mot. Behav.* **1998**, *30*, 51–59. [CrossRef]
30. Lai, Q.; Shea, C. Bandwidth knowledge of results enhances generalized motor program learning. *Res. Q. Exerc. Sport* **1999**, *70*, 79–83. [CrossRef]
31. Wulf, G.; Shea, C.; Lewthwaite, R. Motor skill learning and performance: A review of influential factors. *Med. Educ.* **2010**, *44*, 75–84. [CrossRef] [PubMed]

32. Wulf, G.; Prinz, W. Directing attention to movement effects enhances learning: A review. *Psychon. Bull. Rev.* **2001**, *8*, 648–660. [CrossRef]
33. Hendricson, W.; Andrieu, S.; Chadwick, D.; Chmar, J.; Cole, J.; George, M.; Glickman, G.; Glover, J.; Goldberg, J.; Haden, N.; et al. Educational strategies associated with development of problem-solving, critical thinking, and self-directed learning. *J. Dent. Educ.* **2006**, *70*, 925–936.
34. Lam, W.; Masters, R.; Maxwell, J. Cognitive demands of error processing associated with preparation and execution of a motor skill. *Conscious. Cogn.* **2010**, *19*, 1058–1061. [CrossRef] [PubMed]
35. Anderson, J. Acquisition of cognitive skill. *Psychol. Rev.* **1982**, *89*, 369–406. [CrossRef]
36. de Jong, T. Cognitive load theory, educational research, and instructional design: Some food for thought. *Instr. Sci.* **2010**, *38*, 105–134. [CrossRef]
37. Sweller, J.; van Merrienboer, J.; Paas, F. Cognitive architecture and instructional design. *Educ. Psychol. Rev.* **1998**, *10*, 251–296. [CrossRef]
38. Robertson, L. Memory and the brain. *J. Dent. Educ.* **2002**, *66*, 30–42. [CrossRef]
39. Sweller, J.; Ayres, P.; Kalyuga, S. Interacting with the external environment: The narrow limits of change principle and the environmental organising and linking principle. In *Cognitive Load Theory*; Springer: Berlin/Heidelberg, Germany, 2011; pp. 39–53.
40. van Merrienboer, J.; Sweller, J. Cognitive load theory in health professional education: Design principles and strategies. *Med. Educ.* **2010**, *44*, 85–93. [CrossRef]
41. Cowan, N. Working Memory Underpins Cognitive Development, Learning, and Education. *Educ. Psychol. Rev.* **2014**, *26*, 197–223. [CrossRef]
42. Chase, W.; Simon, H. Perception in chess. *Cogn. Psychol.* **1973**, *4*, 55–81. [CrossRef]
43. Paas, F.; Ayres, P. Cognitive Load Theory: A broader view on the role of memory in learning and education. *Educ. Psychol. Rev.* **2014**, *26*, 191–195. [CrossRef]
44. Hendricson, W.; Kleffner, J. Curricular and instructional implications of competency-based dental education. *J. Dent. Educ.* **1998**, *62*, 183–196. [CrossRef]
45. Abernethy, B.; Poolton, J.; Masters, R.; Patil, N. Implications of an expertise model for surgical skills training. *ANZ J. Surg.* **2008**, *78*, 1092–1095. [CrossRef]
46. Hendricson, W.; Kleffner, J. Assessing and helping challenging students: Part one, why do some students have difficulty learning? *J. Dent. Educ.* **2002**, *66*, 43–61. [CrossRef]
47. Masters, R.; Poolton, J. Advances in implicit motor learning. In *Skill Acquisition in Sport: Research, Theory and Practice*, 2nd ed.; Hodges, N., Williams, M., Eds.; Routledge: London, UK, 2012; pp. 59–75.
48. Kleynen, M.; Braun, S.; Bleijlevens, M.; Lexis, M.; Rasquin, S.; Halfens, J.; Wilson, M.; Beurskens, A.; Masters, R. Using a Delphi technique to seek consensus regarding definitions, descriptions and classification of terms related to implicit and explicit forms of motor learning. *PLoS ONE* **2014**, *9*, e100227. [CrossRef]
49. Malhotra, N.; Poolton, J.; Wilson, M.; Ngo, K.; Masters, R. Conscious monitoring and control (reinvestment) in surgical performance under pressure. *Surg. Endosc.* **2012**, *26*, 2423–2429. [CrossRef]
50. Poolton, J.; Zhu, F.; Malhotra, N.; Leung, G.; Fan, J.; Masters, R. Multitask training promotes automaticity of a fundamental laparoscopic skill without compromising the rate of skill learning. *Surg. Endosc.* **2016**, *30*, 4011–4018. [CrossRef] [PubMed]
51. Masters, R.; Maxwell, J. The theory of reinvestment. *Int. Rev. Sport Exerc. Psychol.* **2008**, *1*, 160–183. [CrossRef]
52. Masters, R. Knowledge, knerves and know-how: The role of explicit versus implicit knowledge in the breakdown of a complex motor skill under pressure. *Br. J. Psychol.* **1992**, *83*, 343–358. [CrossRef]
53. Jackson, R.C.; Kinrade, N.P.; Hicks, T.; Wills, R. Individual propensity for reinvestment: Field-based evidence for the predictive validity of three scales. *Inter. J. Sport Psychol.* **2013**, *44*, 331–350.
54. Masters, R.; Maxwell, J. Implicit motor learning, reinvestment and movement disruption: What you. In *Skill Acquisition in Sport: Research, Theory and Practice*, 1st ed.; Williams, A., Hodges, N., Eds.; Routledge: London, UK, 2004; pp. 207–228.
55. Liao, C.; Masters, R. Analogy learning: A means to implicit motor learning. *J. Sports Sci.* **2001**, *19*, 307–319. [CrossRef]
56. Dubrowski, A.; Brydges, R.; Satterthwaite, L.; Xeroulis, G.; Classen, R. Do not teach me while I am working! *Am. J. Surg.* **2012**, *203*, 253–257. [CrossRef] [PubMed]
57. Zhu, F.; Poolton, J.; Wilson, M.; Hu, Y.; Maxwell, J.; Masters, R. Implicit motor learning promotes neural efficiency during laparoscopy. *Surg. Endosc.* **2011**, *25*, 2950–2955. [CrossRef]
58. Poolton, J.; Masters, R.; Maxwell, J. The relationship between initial errorless learning conditions and subsequent performance. *Hum. Mov. Sci.* **2005**, *24*, 362–378. [CrossRef] [PubMed]
59. Kleynen, M.; Braun, S.; Rasquin, S.; Bleijlevens, M.; Lexis, M.; Halfens, J.; Wilson, M.; Masters, R.; Beurskens, A. Multidisciplinary views on applying explicit and implicit motor learning in practice: An international survey. *PLoS ONE* **2015**, *10*, 1–15. [CrossRef] [PubMed]
60. Lam, W.; Maxwell, J.; Masters, R. Probing the allocation of attention in implicit (motor) learning. *J. Sports Sci.* **2010**, *28*, 1543–1554. [CrossRef]
61. Masters, R.; Poolton, J.; Abernethy, B.; Patil, N. Implicit learning of movement skills for surgery. *ANZ J. Surg.* **2008**, *78*, 1062–1064. [CrossRef]

62. Masters, R.; Lo, C.; Maxwell, J.; Patil, N. Implicit motor learning in surgery: Implications for multi-tasking. *Surgery* **2008**, *143*, 140–145. [CrossRef] [PubMed]
63. Seger, C. Implicit learning. *Psychol Bull* **1994**, *115*, 163–196. [CrossRef]
64. Maxwell, J.; Masters, R.; Kerr, E.; Weedon, E. The implicit benefit of learning without errors. *Q. J. Exp. Psychol. A* **2001**, *54*, 1049–1068. [CrossRef]

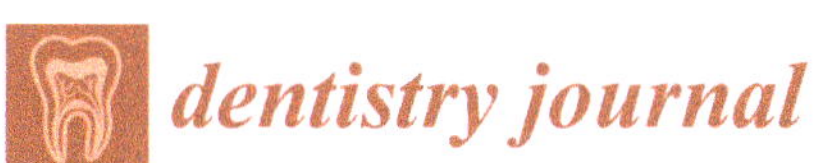 dentistry journal

MDPI

Brief Report

Psychometric Characteristics of Oral Pathology Test Items in the Dental Hygiene Curriculum—A Longitudinal Analysis

Mythily Srinivasan

Department of Oral Pathology, Medicine and Radiology, Indiana University School of Dentistry, Indiana University Purdue University at Indianapolis, Indianapolis, IN 46202, USA; mysriniv@iu.edu

Abstract: As the landscape of oral healthcare and the delivery of services continue to undergo change, the dental hygienist plays an increasing role in assisting dentists with oral diagnosis and preventive strategies. Hence, the dental hygiene curriculum standards require biomedical science instructions, including general and oral pathology. Student learning and cognitive competencies are often measured using multiple-choice questions (MCQs). The objectives of this study were to perform a longitudinal analysis of test items and to evaluate their relation to the absolute grades of the oral pathology course in the dental hygiene curriculum. A total of 1033 MCQs covering different concepts of oral pathology administered from 2015 through 2019 were analyzed for difficulty and discriminatory indices, and the differences between the years were determined by one-way ANOVA. Test reliability as determined by the average KR-20 value was 0.7 or higher for each exam. The mean difficulty index for all exams was 0.73 +/− 0.05, and that of the discriminatory index was 0.33 +/− 0.05. Wide variations were observed in the discriminatory indices of test items with approximately the same difficulty index, as well as in the grade distribution in each cohort. Furthermore, longitudinal data analyses identified low achieving cohorts amongst the groups evaluated for the same knowledge domain, taught with the same instruction, and using similar test tools. This suggest that comparative analyses of tests could offer feedback not only on student learning attributes, but also potentially on the admission processes to the dental hygiene program.

Keywords: dental hygiene; oral pathology; exam soft; item analysis

Citation: Srinivasan, M. Psychometric Characteristics of Oral Pathology Test Items in the Dental Hygiene Curriculum—A Longitudinal Analysis. *Dent. J.* **2021**, 9, 56. https://doi.org/10.3390/dj9050056

Academic Editors: Jelena Dumancic and Božana Lončar Brzak

Received: 25 March 2021
Accepted: 22 April 2021
Published: 13 May 2021

1. Introduction

Dental hygienists play an integral role in assisting individuals and groups in achieving and maintaining optimal oral health. Thus, the dental hygiene educational guidelines recommended by the Commission on Dental Accreditation (CODA) require instructions on biomedical sciences to ensure an understanding of the basic biological principles for comprehensive oral hygiene care [1]. The CODA standards specify that pathology class time hours should be classified in terms of general pathology and oral pathology. By description, the general pathology content areas focus on the nature of disease processes and the associated alterations in structure and function.

The oral pathology content emphasizes the etiopathogenesis of oral diseases, and the systemic pathology teaches the etiologies and host responses of organ systems [2]. Traditionally, dental hygiene education has relied on a teacher-delivered, lecture-based curriculum and a performance-based approach to clinical activities. In recent years, the lecture as an instructional format is supplemented with a variety of useful adjunct educational tools, such as videos, student-led discussions, and online activities that are incorporated into the curriculum. This ensures the proper transfer and acquisition of knowledge, preparing the students to understand and participate comprehensively in the delivery of oral healthcare [3].

Student learning is often evaluated using multiple choice questions (MCQs) that test cognitive competencies [4]. The assessment of learning is an important element of an instructional design process, which provides feedback on learning and teaching processes and enables the review and improvement of the whole process [5,6]. There have been few reports on the assessment of general and oral pathology instruction in terms of instructional content and student performance [7]. Various methods are used to assess multiple-choice tests to provide feedback on learning and teaching processes. Item analysis is one such method that examines student responses to individual test item. The Difficulty Index (DI) is the percentage of students who chose the correct answer, and is expressed as a fraction of 1 or as a percentage. The Discrimination Index (Disc-I), or point biserial correlation, measures how students who did well or poorly overall performed on an item. In other words, the discriminating measures evaluate how performance on a single item correlated with overall performance [8–10].

This study aims to determine the DI, Disc-I, or point biserial correlation of the MCQs administered as part of the oral pathology course in the dental hygiene bachelor's degree program offered through Purdue University at Indianapolis, Indiana. The MCQs were designed to test the student's comprehension of the content and its application to the practice of dental hygiene. The specific research objectives were to perform item analysis of MCQ test items in an oral pathology course to evaluate the relationship between the DI and Disc-I of multiple-choice questions and the distribution of grades in the oral pathology course in the dental hygiene curriculum; and (2) to compare the reliability of the MCQ exams assessing the same knowledge domain across multiple years.

2. Methods

Question cohort and participants: The study cohort consisted of 1033 MCQs (with four choices) that were included across twenty exams in the fall semesters of 2015–2019 at four exams per year, covering different concepts of oral pathology. The number of exam takers were 30 in each exam in 2015, 27 in each exam in 2016, 19 in each exam in 2017, and 20 in each exam in 2018 and in 2019.

Data collection: ExamSoft testing software (ExamSoft Worldwide, Dallas, TX, USA) was used to administer the MCQ exams [11]. Questions were presented as one question per screen. The exam takers were allowed one hour to complete the exam, and could advance to the next question, review previous questions, and change answers as desired. After completion, the exam takers uploaded the examination file to the ExamSoft database. All questions in each exam were used for data collection, and the raw score of each exam taker in terms of the total number of correct responses, the percentage of correct responses, and the letter grade based on a pre-determined range were obtained in the summary report. In ExamSoft, the internal consistency and reliability of each exam was measured by KR-20 (Kuder–Richardson Formula). It considers all dichotomous questions and how many exam takers answered each question correctly [12]. The ExamSoft statistical report for each item also included DI, Disc-I, and point biserial.

Data analysis: The mean DI, Disc-I, and point biserial were calculated for each of the four exams of each year. The difference in the mean scores of DI, Disc-I, and point biserial scores was assessed by one-way ANOVA and Tukey's post hoc analysis. A p-value of less than 0.05 was considered significant. An absolute grading system was used to provide a letter grade for the exam based on the average scores of all four exams at the end of the semester in each year on a scale of 90–100 points for A, 80–89 points for B, 70–79 points for C, and an F for points 69 and below [13,14].

3. Results

Course duration: In the current study, the format of didactic instruction in the pathology courses included thirty-two hours of lectures and online activities and sixty-four hours of individual student–instructor hours as needed. Each year, students were assessed by four MCQ tests over the course of 16 weeks. Table 1 gives examples of MCQs covering two distinct concepts of the oral pathology curriculum.

Table 1. Examples of MCQs and respective DI and Disc-I.

A 50-year-old ex-smoker is referred to the dentist by a cardiologist. Past history includes severe recurrent oral ulcerations affecting lateral borders of the tongue, labial mucosa, and soft palate. Ulcers are one or two at a time and persist for about eight weeks. Medical history showed use of a potassium channel activator (nicorandil) for unstable angina and aspirin (75 mg/day) since his myocardial infarction nine months ago. He has no eye, skin, or genital ulcerations. The most probable cause of the major RAS ulcers is		a. Aspirin burn b. Bechet's disease c. Nicorandil use (potassium channel blocker) d. Smoking cessation
Academic Year	**DI**	**Disc-I**
2015	0.65	0.4
2016	0.65	0.6
2017	0.63	0.6
2018	0.1	0.2
2019	0.35	0.0
A middle-aged man presented with a slowly growing swelling on the left side of the mandible. The X-ray showed driven snow appearance of mixed radio-opacity and radiolucency. The most likely diagnosis is		a. Odontogenic keratocyst b. Ameloblastoma c. Pindborg's tumor d. Compound odontoma
Academic Year	**DI**	**Disc-I**
2015	0.72	0.38
2016	0.76	0.4
2017	0.79	0.2
2018	0.75	0.4

The reliability of exams: The reliability of the examination was measured using KR-20; a high KR-20 indicates that if the same exam takers took the same assessment, there is a higher chance that the results would be the same. A low KR-20 means that the results would be more likely to be different [12]. A KR-20 value of <0.3 is considered poor, and a value of ≥0.7 is considered acceptable [15,16]. The mean and standard deviation of the KR-20 value for each of the four exams administered over five consecutive years is given in Table 2.

Table 2. The reliability score of each exam as determined by the Kuder–Richardson formula 20 coefficient (KR-20).

	KR-20 Values						
	2015	**2016**	**2017**	**2018**	**2019**	**Average**	**SD**
Exam 1	0.73	0.68	0.7	0.71	0.76	0.716	0.03
Exam 2	0.72	0.52	0.81	0.68	0.76	0.698	0.10
Exam 3	0.77	0.77	0.57	0.77	0.68	0.712	0.08
Exam 4	0.7	0.68	0.56	0.83	0.67	0.688	0.09
Average	0.73	0.6625	0.66	0.7475	0.7175		
SD	0.03	0.09	0.10	0.06	0.04		

The item analysis of exams: The mean DI of the examinations ranged from 63% in 2018 to 81% in 2015, that of the mean Disc-I ranged between 0.25 in 2019 to 0.43 in 2016, and that of the mean point biserial ranged between 0.25 in 2015 to 0.45 in 2016 (Table 3). The mean DI for all of the exams for the course in each year was 72 +/− 4.72%, a value that is widely considered acceptable. The overall mean Discriminatory Index was 0.33 +/−

0.05, and the overall mean point biserial was 0.34 +/− 0.05 (Table 2). The average DI was significantly higher in the year 2015 (77.8 +/− 2.9%) than that for the years 2017 (70.3 +/− 3.3%), 2018 (71.3 +/− 5.4%), and 2019 (70 +/− 3.54%). The Discriminatory Index and point biserial were significantly lower in 2017 compared to the values in 2015.

Table 3. Item analysis including the Difficulty Index, Discriminatory Index, and point biserial score of each exam.

A	**Difficulty Index**							
		2015	**2016**	**2017**	**2018**	**2019**	**Average**	**SD**
	Exam 1	0.78	0.71	0.67	0.7	0.73	0.72	0.04
	Exam 2	0.73	0.7	0.67	0.63	0.67	0.68	0.03
	Exam 3	0.79	0.77	0.74	0.77	0.66	0.75	0.05
	Exam 4	0.81	0.76	0.73	0.75	0.74	0.76	0.03
	Average	0.78	0.74	0.70	0.71	0.7	0.73	0.03
	SD	0.03	0.03	0.03	0.05	0.04		
B	**Discriminatory Index**							
		2015	**2016**	**2017**	**2018**	**2019**	**Average**	**SD**
	Exam 1	0.35	0.43	0.29	0.29	0.25	0.32	0.06
	Exam 2	0.3	0.33	0.37	0.41	0.37	0.36	0.04
	Exam 3	0.35	0.34	0.26	0.35	0.26	0.31	0.04
	Exam 4	0.28	0.4	0.3	0.34	0.31	0.33	0.04
	Average	0.32	0.375	0.305	0.35	0.3		
	SD	0.03	0.04	0.04	0.04	0.05		
C	**Point Biserial**						**Average**	**SD**
	Exam 1	0.34	0.4	0.25	0.31	0.28	0.32	0.05
	Exam 2	0.35	0.32	0.35	0.34	0.33	0.34	0.01
	Exam 3	0.32	0.45	0.27	0.37	0.32	0.34	0.06
	Exam 4	0.33	0.43	0.32	0.36	0.33	0.35	0.04
	Average	0.34	0.4	0.3	0.35	0.32		
	SD	0.01	0.04	0.04	0.02	0.02		

Course grade across five years: The exam takers were provided an absolute grade based on predetermined cutoff levels. Data showed that the letter grade A was achieved from 20% to 35% of exam takers in each of the four exams in 2015 and 2019. The letter grade B was the most common, obtained by >50% of the exam takers in all years except 2017, in which the common grade of exam takers was C (Figure 1A). The final grade for the course based on the average of four exams per year suggested that the most common grade for the course was B for all years except for 2017, with most exam takers obtaining a C. The percentage of exam takers with a grade F was higher in the years 2016–2018.

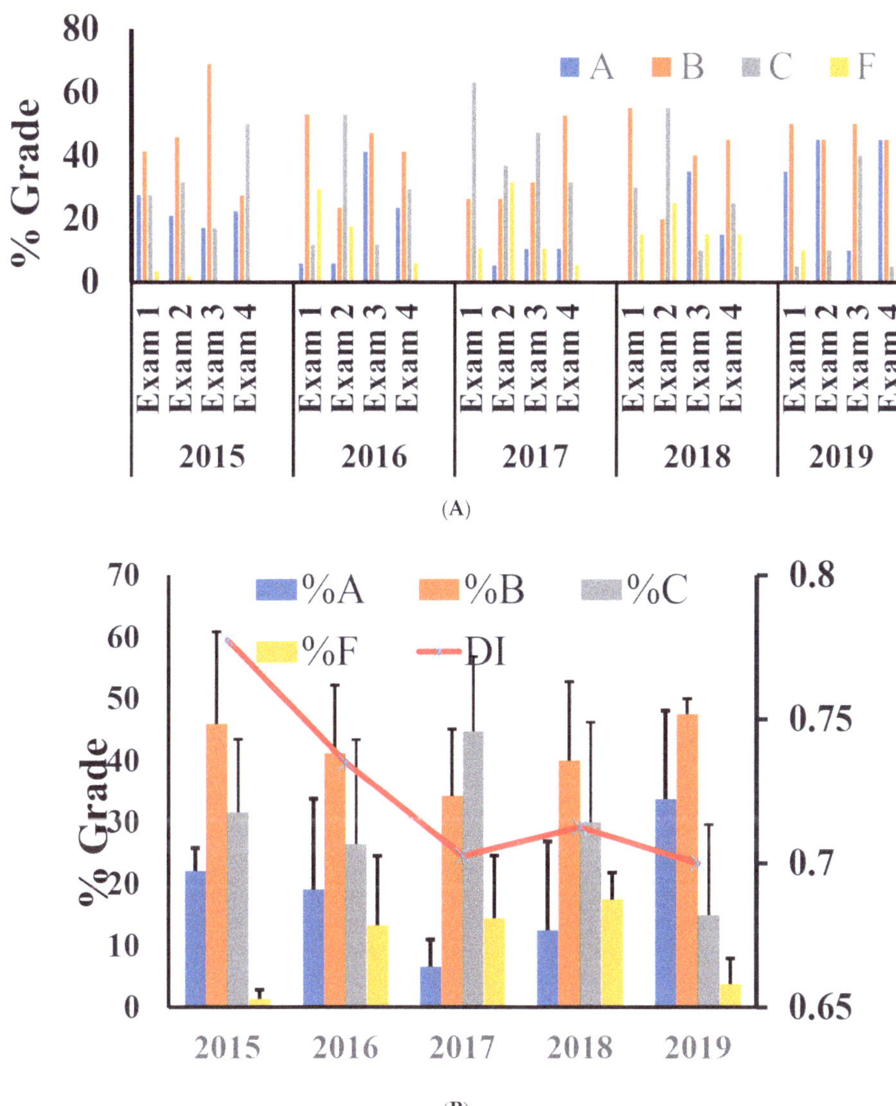

Figure 1. (**A**) Letter grade in each exam for each year. The students were provided a letter grade based on the percentage of their raw score against a fixed scale of absolute grading: 90–100% for A, 80–89% for B, 70–79% for C, and an F for points 69% and below. (**B**) The average of the four exams for each year was used as the final grade for the oral pathology course. The line graph is the average Discriminatory Index for all four exams of the indicated year.

Relationship between grade distribution and DI and Disc-I: As noted above, although the material taught, the instructor, and the multiple-choice question developer were the same across the years, the distribution of grading was different. The DI of 78% suggested that the 2015 cohort of exam takers found that the test items were relatively easy, and was reflected in the higher percentage of individuals achieving the letter grade A in 2015 (Figure 1B). The lower Disc-I and point biserial in the 2017 cohort suggested that the items were identified as relatively hard, and thereby was reflected the lower percentage of exam takers who achieved scores consistent with the letter grade A (Figure 2) [17].

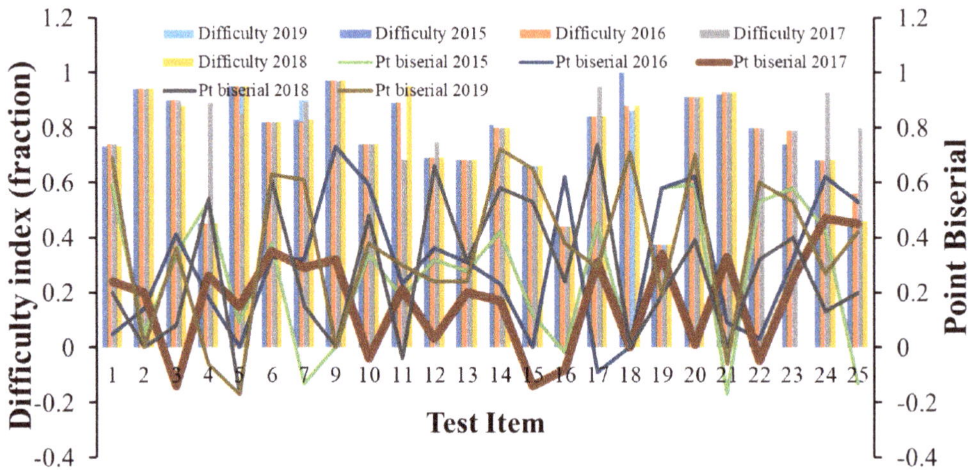

Figure 2. The relationship between the DI and point biserial of test items. Twenty-five test items included in the exams in each year with a similar DI were selected. Line graphs are the point biserial value of the indicated test item. The point biserial value (the broad brown line) indicates the values of the test time in 2017.

Next, the contribution of individual item characteristics, DI, Disc I, or point biserial, to the differences in the grade distribution was evaluated. Analysis of performance of twenty-five test items with approximately the same DI (+/− 0.05) showed that the test items exhibited varied Disc-I and point biserial indices, potentially reflecting the differences in the ability of the exam taker cohorts (Figure 2).

4. Discussion

One of the most challenging areas in dental and dental hygiene practice is the diagnostic process. The dental hygienist plays a key role in the preliminary evaluation and data collection of oral pathologic conditions for final diagnosis and management by the dentist [18]. Instruction in pathology content areas helps prepare the students of dental hygiene for this role. It has been stated that the knowledge gained from pathology instruction enables students to understand and participate comprehensively in the delivery of healthcare [3].

In addition to the content, the assessment of learning is an important element of an instructional design process. It provides feedback on learning and teaching processes and enables the review and improvement of the whole process [5,19]. Although some basic test statistics, including the mean, median, and mode, have been carried out routinely, there is a paucity of item analysis in specific subjects of the pathology course domain in dental hygiene education. This study examined the assessment of the oral pathology instructions in the dental hygiene program from two different perspectives: evaluating student learning using item analysis of MCQs and evaluating the test content in assessing student comprehension across multiple years. Furthermore, we discuss whether the data could be of value in a retrospective analysis of admission criteria to the dental hygiene program.

This study included only single best response MCQs designed specifically to assess broad domains of knowledge effectively and reliably [15,20,21]. In the present study, the mean DI value was 72.6 +/− 4.7%, which is widely considered an acceptable level of difficulty. Similarly, the mean Disc-I and point biserial values, 0.33 +/− 0.05 and 0.34 +/− 0.05, respectively, were also within an acceptable range. The Disc-I and point biserial coefficient values correlate with a dichotomous variable (a right or wrong response for a single item) and a continuous variable (the test score) [15,22,23]. The data showed that these values exhibited significant variations for items with similar levels of DI in different cohorts of exam takers. Although variations in discriminatory indices are often considered indicators of ambiguous wording, the wide scatter could also reflect some extent of guessing practices [8,24,25]. Pertinently, Dascalu et al. observed that, in a cohort of students in dental medicine, while the grades of MCQ tests followed a normal distribution, the average was significantly lower than that in traditional oral examinations [6]. A limitation of this study is that the analysis was restricted to one subject domain in the senior year of the dental hygiene curriculum, and may not be representative of the overall ability of the exam takers to succeed in other didactic or clinical courses.

Alternatively, variations in the Discriminatory Index and point biserial across the years could reflect the learning attributes of the exam taker cohort. It is observed that the analysis across five years showed that the Discriminatory Index for the same test item was consistently lower in the year 2017, and the average test grade for this cohort was one grade lower (C) than that of the other years. In this context, it is interesting to note that the KR-20 value for exams three and four in the year 2017 were 0.57 and 0.56, respectively. Since the calculation of KR-20 is based on the standard deviation and the proportion of students responding correctly and incorrectly, it appears that the lower Discriminatory Index for the year 2017 could at least be partially cohort specific. Typically, admissions to the dental hygiene program require at least one year of college and the completion of prerequisite courses, including anatomy, biology, chemistry, microbiology, and math. Interestingly, in a recent analysis of predictive factors for student success in dental school, Sabato et al. showed that the elements of undergraduate education could help identify students who are at risk for poor performance and require timely intervention [26].

5. Conclusions

As with other health professional training, the effective measurement of knowledge is an important component of both allied dental education and practice [20,27,28]. Well-designed, single-choice MCQs are excellent tools to align the evidence resulting from the tests with student achievement or cognition as reflected in the grades [4,15]. Our observations of a low-achieving cohort amongst the cohorts of five consecutive years evaluated for the same knowledge domain using similar test tools suggest that the comparative analyses of tests could offer some feedback not only on learning abilities, but also on the selection processes for admission to the dental hygiene program. It will be interesting to analyze similarly concurrent courses offered and tested for the same cohort of exam takers.

Funding: This research received no external funding.

Institutional Review Board Statement: The study was conducted according to the guidelines of the Declaration of Helsinki, and approved by the Institutional Review Board of Indiana University Purdue University at Indianapolis (protocol #: 2011678210 and date of approval: 25 November 2020).

Informed Consent Statement: Not applicable.

Conflicts of Interest: The author declares no conflict of interest.

References

1. CODA. *Accreditation Standards for Dental Hygiene Education Programs*; CODA: Chicago, IL, USA, 2018.
2. ADEA. ADEA Compendium of Curriculum Guidelines (Revised Edition). In *Allied Dental Education Programs*; ADEA: Washington, DC, USA, 2016.
3. Lyle, D.; Grill, A.; Olmsted, J.; Rotehn, M. Leading the transformation of the dental hygiene profession to improve the public's oral and overall health. In *American Dental Hygienists Association: National Dental Hygiene Research Agenda*; ADHA, CODA: Chicago, IL, USA, 2016.
4. Glass, A.L.; Sinha, N. Multiple-Choice Questioning Is an Efficient Instructional Methodology That May Be Widely Implemented in Academic Courses to Improve Exam Performance. *Curr. Dir. Psychol. Sci.* **2013**, *22*, 471–477. [CrossRef]

5. Momsen, J.; Offerdahl, E.; Kryjevskaia, M.; Montplaisir, L.; Anderson, E.; Grosz, N. Using Assessments to Investigate and Compare the Natureof Learning in Undergraduate Science Courses. *CBE Life Sci. Educ.* **2013**, *12*, 239–249. [CrossRef] [PubMed]
6. Dascalu, C.; Enache, A.; Mavru, R.; Zegan, G. Computer-based MCQ assessment for students in dental medicine-advantages and drawbacks. *Procedia Soc. Behav. Sci.* **2015**, *187*, 22–27. [CrossRef]
7. Jacobs, B.B.; Lazar, A.A.; Rowe, D.J. Assessment of pathology instruction in U.S. Dental hygiene educational programs. *J. Dent. Hyg.* **2015**, *89*, 109–118.
8. Koçdar, S.; Karadag, N.; Sahin, M.D. Analysis of the Difficulty and Discrimination Indices of Multiple-Choice Questions According to Cognitive Levels in an Open and Distance Learning Context. *Turk. Online J. Educ. Technol.* **2016**, *15*, 16–24.
9. Lesage, E.; Valcke, M.; Sabbe, E. Scoring methods for multiple choice assessment in higher education—Is it still a matter of number right scoring or negative marking? *Stud. Educ. Eval.* **2013**, *39*, 188–193. [CrossRef]
10. Pande, S.S.; Pande, S.R.; Parate, V.R.; Nikam, A.P.; Agrekar, S.H. Correlation between difficulty & discrimination indices of MCQs in formative exam in Physiology. *South-East Asian J. Med. Educ.* **2013**, *7*, 45–50.
11. Zheng, M.; Bender, D. Evaluating outcomes of computer-based classroom testing: Student acceptance and impact on learning and exam performance. *Med. Teach.* **2019**, *41*, 75–82. [CrossRef]
12. ExamSoft. A Guide to Statistics (Legacy and Enterprise Portal). 2021. Available online: https://community.examsoft.com/s/article/A-Guide-to-the-Statistics-Legacy-and-Enterprise-Portal (accessed on 19 March 2021).
13. Ganzfried, S.; Yusuf, F. Optimal Weighting for Exam Composition. *Educ. Sci.* **2018**, *8*, 36. [CrossRef]
14. Sayin, A. The Effect of Using Relative and Absolute Criteria to Decide Students' Passing or Failing a Course. *J. Educ. Train. Stud.* **2016**, *4*, 2–16. [CrossRef]
15. Daggett, L. All of the Above: Computerized Exam Scoring of Multiple Choice Items Helps To: (A) Show How Exam Items Worked Technically, (B) Maximize Exam Fairness, (C) Justly Assign Letter Grades, and (D) Provide Feedback on Student Learning. *J. Leg. Educ.* **2007**, *57*, 391.
16. Quaigrain, K.; Arhin, A.K. Using reliability and item analysis to evaluatea teacher-developed test in educationalmeasurement and evaluation. *Cogent Educ.* **2017**, *14*, 1301013. [CrossRef]
17. Sim, S.M.; Rasiah, R.I. Relationship between item difficulty and discrimination indices in true/false-type multiple choice questions of a para-clinical multidisciplinary paper. *Ann. Acad. Med. Singap.* **2006**, *35*, 67–71. [PubMed]
18. Overman, P.; Gurenlian, J.; Kass, S.; Shepard, K.; Steinbach, P.; Stolberg, R. Transforming Dental Hygiene Education: New Curricular Domains and Models. In Proceedings of the American Dental Hygiene Association Annual Meeting, Las Vegas, NV, USA, 19 June 2014.
19. Yang, B.W.; Razo, J.; Persky, A.M. Using Testing as a Learning Tool. *Am. J. Pharm. Educ.* **2019**, *83*, 7324. [CrossRef] [PubMed]
20. Schultz, D.S. A Model for Using the National Board Dental Hygiene Examination Results as a Method of Outcomes Assessment. Ph.D. Thesis, Department of Teaching, Learning and Leadership, Western Michigan University, Kalamazoo, MI, USA, 2004.
21. Skakun, E.N.; Nanson, E.M.; Kling, S.; Taylor, W.C. A preliminary investigation of three types of multiple choice questions. *Med. Educ.* **1979**, *13*, 91–96. [CrossRef] [PubMed]
22. Sabri, S. Item analysis of student comprehensive test for research in teaching beginner string ensemble using model based teaching among music students in public universities. *Int. J. Educ. Res.* **2013**, *1*, 1–14.
23. Thompson, J.J. What Are You Measuring? Dimensionality and Reliability Analysis of Ability and Speed in Medical School Didactic Examinations. *J. Appl. Meas.* **2016**, *17*, 91–108.
24. Abdulghani, H.M.; Irshad, M.; Haque, S.; Ahmad, T.; Sattar, K.; Khalil, M.S. Effectiveness of longitudinal faculty development programs on MCQs items writing skills: A follow-up study. *PLoS ONE* **2017**, *12*, e0185895. [CrossRef]
25. Kheyami, D.; Jaradat, A.; Al-Shibani, T.; Ali, F.A. Item Analysis of Multiple Choice Questions at the Department of Paediatrics, Arabian Gulf University, Manama, Bahrain. *Sultan Qaboos Univ. Med. J.* **2018**, *18*, e68–e74. [CrossRef]
26. Sabato, E.H.; Perez, H.L.; Jiang, S.; Feldman, C.A. Elements of Undergraduate Education Related to Students' Academic Performance in the First Year of Dental School. *J. Dent. Educ.* **2019**, *83*, 510–520. [CrossRef]
27. Williams, K.B.; Schmidt, C.; Tilliss, T.S.; Wilkins, K.; Glasnapp, D.R. Predictive validity of critical thinking skills and disposition for the national board dental hygiene examination: A preliminary investigation. *J. Dent. Educ.* **2006**, *70*, 536–544. [CrossRef] [PubMed]
28. Bianchi, S.; Bernardi, S.; Perili, E.; Cipollone, C.; Di Biasi, J.; Macchiarelli, G. Evaluation of effectiveness of digital technologies during anatomy learning in nursing school. *Appl. Sci.* **2020**, *10*, 2357. [CrossRef]

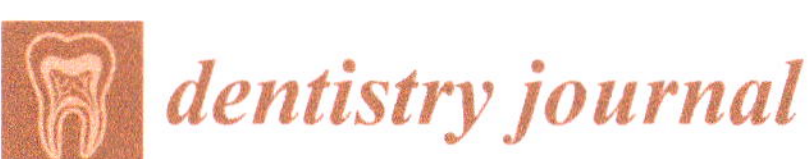

MDPI

Case Report

Epi-Mucosa Fixation and Autologous Platelet-Rich Fibrin Treatment in Medication-Related Osteonecrosis of the Jaw

Antonio Cortese [1,*], Antonio Casarella [1], Candace M. Howard [2] and Pier Paolo Claudio [3,*]

1 Unit of Maxillofacial Surgery, Department of Medicine and Surgery, University of Salerno, 84084 Fisciano, Italy; a.casarella1@studenti.unisa.it

2 Department of Radiology, University of Mississippi Medical Center, Jackson, MS 39216, USA; chowardclaudio@umc.edu

3 Department of Biomolecular Sciences, Maxillofacial Surgery, University of Mississippi, Jackson, MS 39216, USA

* Correspondence: ancortese@unisa.it (A.C.); pclaudio@umc.edu (P.P.C.)

Abstract: Medication-related osteonecrosis of the jaw (MRONJ) frequently affects patients after treatments with bisphosphonates or denosumab, especially with high doses in patients with bone osteoporosis, neoplastic metastases, or possibly anti-angiogenic treatment for cancer. The aim of this article was to show a new treatment planning for stage 2 and stage 3 MRONJ using platelet-rich fibrin (PRF) at the surgical field to enhance healing in association with a new epi-mucosal fixation technique to prevent or treat mandibular fracture. Two cases were treated by epi-mucosa fixation and autologous PRF use for prevention of mandibular fracture risks related to necrotic bone resection or a narrow fracture reduction. Both cases were successfully treated by this new technique of epi-mucosa fixation combined with autologous PRF and achieved good results and good quality of life. Ability to wear prosthesis with good mastication in the absence of side effect such as infection, plate and screw mobilization, pain, and other disabilities or extension of necrosis was reported. After surgical removal of necrotic bone, no infection was detected without any extension of the necrosis.

Keywords: medication-related osteonecrosis of the jaw; fracture; mandible; osteonecrosis; bisphosphonates

Citation: Cortese, A.; Casarella, A.; Howard, C.M.; Claudio, P.P. Epi-Mucosa Fixation and Autologous Platelet-Rich Fibrin Treatment in Medication-Related Osteonecrosis of the Jaw. *Dent. J.* **2021**, *9*, 50. https://doi.org/10.3390/dj9050050

Academic Editors: Marco Tatullo and Božana Lončar Brzak

Received: 1 March 2021
Accepted: 29 April 2021
Published: 30 April 2021

Publisher's Note: MDPI stays neutral with regard to jurisdictional claims in published maps and institutional affiliations.

1. Introduction

Medication-related osteonecrosis of the jaw (MRONJ) is an adverse effect of treatment with denosumab or bisphosphonates (especially with high doses to prevent skeletal events in patients with bone and neoplastic metastases) or possibly anti-angiogenic treatment for cancer. Preventive measures in recent years have reduced the risk of MRONJ in patients with bone metastases due to cancer, particularly by avoiding trauma or invasive therapies and preventing or treating dental infections before and during therapy with denosumab or bisphosphonate. If MRONJ is developed, conservative medical treatment (non-surgical) can provide improvement, but the achievement of mucosal closure remains challenging. Symptoms management and mucosal healing are the ultimate goals of therapy but, after the failure of conservative treatment, a surgical approach may be beneficial. Overall, a multidisciplinary and pragmatic approach to MRONJ should be adopted, giving priority to quality of life and management of the patient's malignant skeletal disease.

The stage of MRONJ at presentation is prognostic for the success of conservative (non-surgical) treatment, with only a very low likelihood of healing in patients who have higher stages of the disease [1]. Notwithstanding the disputes in the classification, we can distinguish three stages in the classification of MRONJ:

- Stage 1—In stage 1 the upper or lower jaw bone is exposed in the absence of symptoms; in this stage the treatment is conservative: Improve oral hygiene by actively treating dental and periodontal diseases; rinses with topical antibiotic. Surgical treatment is considered only to remove necrotic bone.

- Stage 2—In this stage we have exposed bone associated with pain and inflammation, swelling, or infection of adjacent soft-tissue. Treatment is like that in stage 1 with the addition of systemic antibiotic to treat any infection and symptomatic therapy.
- Stage 3—In the third stage we have same staging criteria of stage 2 plus at least one of these: Pathological fracture, extra-oral or oroantral fistula and radiographic evidence of osteolysis extending to inferior border of mandible or floor of maxillary sinus. Treatment is like that in stage 2 with administration of systemic antibiotics. However, in extended cases we consider a surgical resection of the jaw and reconstruction.

Although osteonecrosis of the jaw (ONJ) is typically diagnosed clinically, the use of orthopantomography, CT, and/or MRI are necessary. Another problem that should be considered in the staging of MRONJ is the lack of dimensional criteria; currently the disease affecting an entire quadrant can be staged in the same way as a lesion with a diameter of less than 1 cm, even if the probability of favorable outcome can be totally different.

Clinical observation has shown an association between the onset of MRONJ and dental extractions and infection, although the underlying mechanism of how these events lead to osteonecrosis remains poorly understood, and high-quality evidence is required. Other factors that negatively influence MRONJ have been reported in the literature as being associated with its accelerated development and an increase in the severity of the condition, but their causal association is not clear [1,2]. These negative factors include:

- Use of corticosteroids;
- Presence of diseases or concomitant conditions (e.g., pre-existing dental infections, anemia, diabetes mellitus and immunosuppression, or renal failure);
- Poor oral hygiene and smoking [1].

AAOMS emphasizes that priority should be given to cancer treatment for patients with cancer and bone metastases at risk of developing MRONJ [1]. We need to balance the risk of MRONJ with the benefit of bisphosphonates or denosumab in reducing the substantial risk of SREs [1].

A combination of preventive measures taken both before and during treatment with denosumab or bisphosphonates can significantly reduce the risk of MRONJ1 [1,2].

The aim of the work is to show new procedure and new planning for second-third stadium (heavy stadium) for medication-related osteonecrosis of the jaw (MRONJ), which is most conservative as possible and also effective in preventing mandibular fracture in risky cases or in a fractured affected case. In these cases, because of published evidence that osteonecrosis of the jaw is related to surgical aggressive therapies, there is a contradiction between etiology of the MRONJ and the most effective treatment with surgical procedure. To solve this problem, we developed this new therapeutic planning using an epi-mucosal fixation technique from our experience in orthognathic and orthopedic maxillofacial surgery. In this way, close reduction of the fracture and close stabilization of the fracture was achieved, minimizing surgical approach and surgical effect impact on the affected bone area. Stabilization of the affected bone segment can be achieved by fixing the plate using self-locking screws in the affected bone segment through the epi-mucosal technique without any need for periosteal elevation or mucosa incision. Autologous platelet-rich fibrin (PRF) was used, combined with fixation to improve the healing abilities of the bone segment and the mucosa after bone sequestrum removal and shaving of the sharp bone borders of the affected area.

Many studies have shown that PRF is a healing biomaterial with great potential. PRF stimulates bone and soft tissue regeneration, without inflammatory reactions, which can be used alone or in combination with bone grafts, promoting hemostasis, bone growth, and maturation [3,4]. PRF consists of a fibrin matrix rich in platelets and autologous leukocytes with a tetra-molecular structure, with cytokines, platelets, and stem cells inside. Therefore, it acts as a biodegradable scaffold improving micro-vascularization and is also able to guide the epithelium in cellular migration on the surface [3,4]. The routine use of such an inexpensive and affordable autologous grow factor delivery system certainly offers an interesting option for the treatment of horizontal defects [3–6].

The aim of this study was to develop a protocol for the treatment of stage 2 and stage 3 MRONJ with extensive bone necrosis causing segment fracture or high-risks for fracture. We combined the advantages of using PRF with the advantages of surgical removal of the necrotic bone and stabilization of the pathologic fracture of the necrotic bone segment that prevents fracture risks of the affected segments after resections or sequestrectomy. To avoid periosteum elevation during rigid bone fixation, we adopted a new technique for rigid fixation: The epi-mucosal fixation. This technique was already validated and published for jaws reducible fractures: It was the first time it was adopted in MRONJ cases, hence the scientific relevance. The study follows the rules of our Ethical Committee.

2. Materials and Methods

Two cases are described in this study.

Both cases were examined by X ray panoramic and CT scan pre-operatively and in the short post operatively time.

The first case was a 72-years-old woman of Caucasian origin, who was referred to the maxillo-facial unit of the University Hospital of Salerno complaining of pain in the region of the left side of the mandible. The patient had received a mastectomy in 2013 in another hospital for a primitive breast cancer. Since 2014 she was treated with denosumab for bone metastases secondary to a primitive cancer.

Surgery was performed under general anesthesia. We proceeded to the superficial removal of damaged tissues in the site of the osteonecrosis outbreak to avoid extension of the necrosis and to enhance healing abilities. We eliminated all the necrotic tissue, saving healthy tissue at the excision border to preserve as much as possible mandibular contour aesthetic and function. To stabilize the bone segment, an epi-mucosal fixation was performed using SMART Lock screws and plates without elevation of the mucoperiosteal flap, therefore avoiding any new bone necrosis risk (Figure 1C).

The self-locking screws and plate were inserted before the necrotic bone area resection or sequestrectomy by epi-mucosa plate modelling, positioning and fixing with trans mucosa screw insertion. No need for mucosa incision or periosteal elevation was required at this step of the procedure; the self-locking screws and plate acted as a rigid external fixation system.

Next, we proceeded to the preparation of autologous PRF to be used as a regenerating and healing stimulating material by collecting 40 mL of peripheral blood from the patient at the time of surgery. Blood samples were collected in 8.5 mL tubes without any anticoagulant and immediately centrifuged at 2700 rpm for 12 min to prevent activation of the coagulation cascades. A model Hettich® (Westphalia, Germany) EBA 20 of centrifuge with a fixed eight-point angular rotor was used for the procedure. Centrifugation time changed according to the consistency required for the PRF; the longer the centrifugation time, the harder the consistency of the PRF sample. After centrifugation, a PRF from the center of the tube was obtained; the centrifuged red blood cells at the bottom and the acellular plasma at the top were discarded. The PRF was inserted directly into the osteotomy slot after sequestrectomy and sharp bone trimming. Several studies have assessed the efficacy of PRF in intra-osseous and mandibular grade 2 MRONJ defects and found a positive clinical and radiographic outcome [7,8].

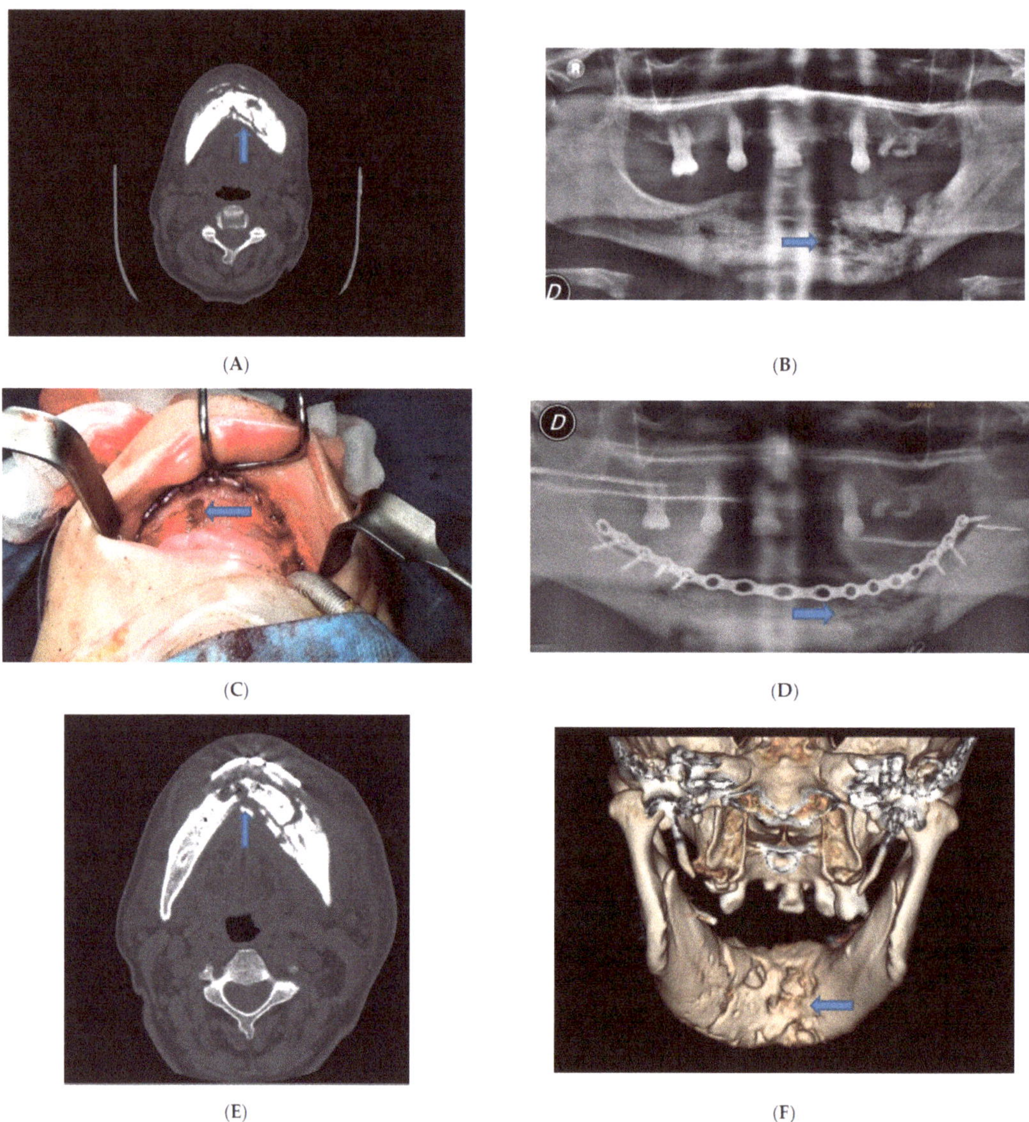

(A) (B) (C) (D) (E) (F)

Figure 1. Patient 1. (**A**) Pre-operative CT scan image showed lithic area in the mandibular horizontal branches, which appeared subverted and fractured on the left side. (**B**) Pre-operative panoramic X-ray image of the dental branch revealed lithic area. (**C**) Epi-mucosal fixation performed using SMART Lock screws and plates without elevating the mucoperiosteal flap. (**D**) Post-operative panoramic X-ray image of the dental branch. (**E**) Post-operative CT scan image. (**F**) Post-operative CT scan 3D reconstruction.

A vicryl polyglactin (91, 3/0) absorbable suture was used to close the flap.

The postoperative course was without complications. Postoperative therapy comprised oral hygiene instructions, rinsing with 0.2% chlorhexidine solutions twice a day, and an evening application of 0.2% chlorhexidine gel upon the sutured incision lines, as well as the administration of a non-steroidal anti-inflammatory aid (Ketoprofen 80 mg) for five consecutive days. The patient was also administered antibiotic therapy in the perioperative phase, starting the night before surgery for 4 days, using 500 mg of Amoxicillin and

Clavulanate every 8 h. The patient was examined for the first time one week later and then 3 and 6 months after surgery (Figure 1D–F).

The second case was an 80-years-old woman of Caucasian origin who referred bilateral pain in the mandibular body. The patient was treated with continuous therapy with bisphosphonates.

In this second case, despite the absence of fractures, it was decided to intervene and apply an epi-mucosal fixation because of the very high risk of pathologic fracture due to the osteonecrosis outbreak. Surgery was performed under general anesthesia. After the debridement and removal of the necrotic bone with sequestrectomy and bone trimming, also in this case we proceeded to an epi-mucosal fixation performed using SMART Lock screws and plates without elevating the mucoperiosteal flap (Figure 2C). As in the first case, we proceeded to the preparation of autologous PRF with the application of the PRF directly to the site of intervention. A vicryl polyglactin (91, 3/0) absorbable suture was used to close the flap.

Postoperative course was without complications. Postoperative therapy comprised oral hygiene instructions. Application of 0.2% chlorhexidine solutions twice a day, an evening application of 0.2% chlorhexidine gel upon the sutured incision lines, and administration of a non-steroidal anti-inflammatory aid (Ketoprofen 80 mg) for five consecutive days. Even in this case, antibiotic therapy was administered in the perioperative phase, starting the night before the surgery and up to 4 days after, using 500 mg of Amoxicillin and Clavulanate every 8 h. The patient was examined for the first time one week later and then 3 and 6 months after surgery (Figure 2D–F).

Post-operative pain was assessed with the VAS score. The VAS score is a tool for measuring the subjective characteristics of pain experienced by the patient. The scale consists simply of a strip of 10 cm paper at the ends presenting two "end points" that are defined as "no pain" and the "worst pain that I can imagine". The patient is asked to mark the pain at a point on the scale as perceived at that moment. The interval between the two ends (end points) is marked every centimeter and allows us to assign a value to the pain perceived by the patient. The initial score can be used as a subjective assessment of the pain experienced by the patient. The subsequent measurements required allow health professionals to understand if the pain is actually reducing and to what extent.

Ability to wear a prosthesis was possible also using the epi-mucosal fixation devices for stabilizing the dental prostheses, with the miniplates and self-locking screws acting as a bar supporting the prostheses.

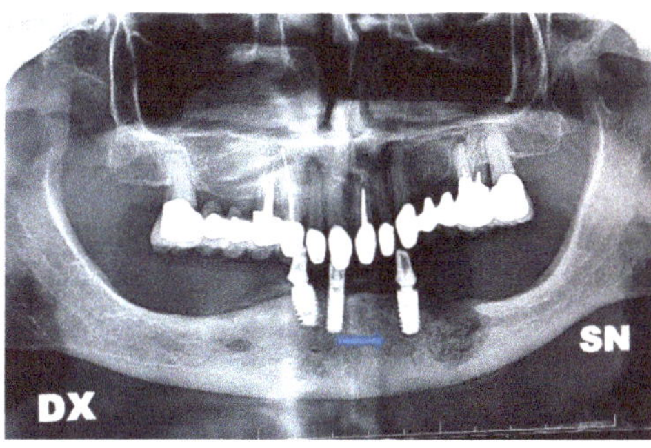

(A)

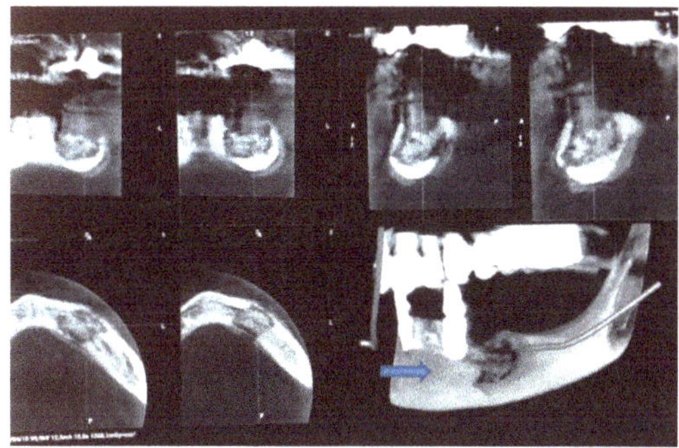

(B)

Figure 2. *Cont.*

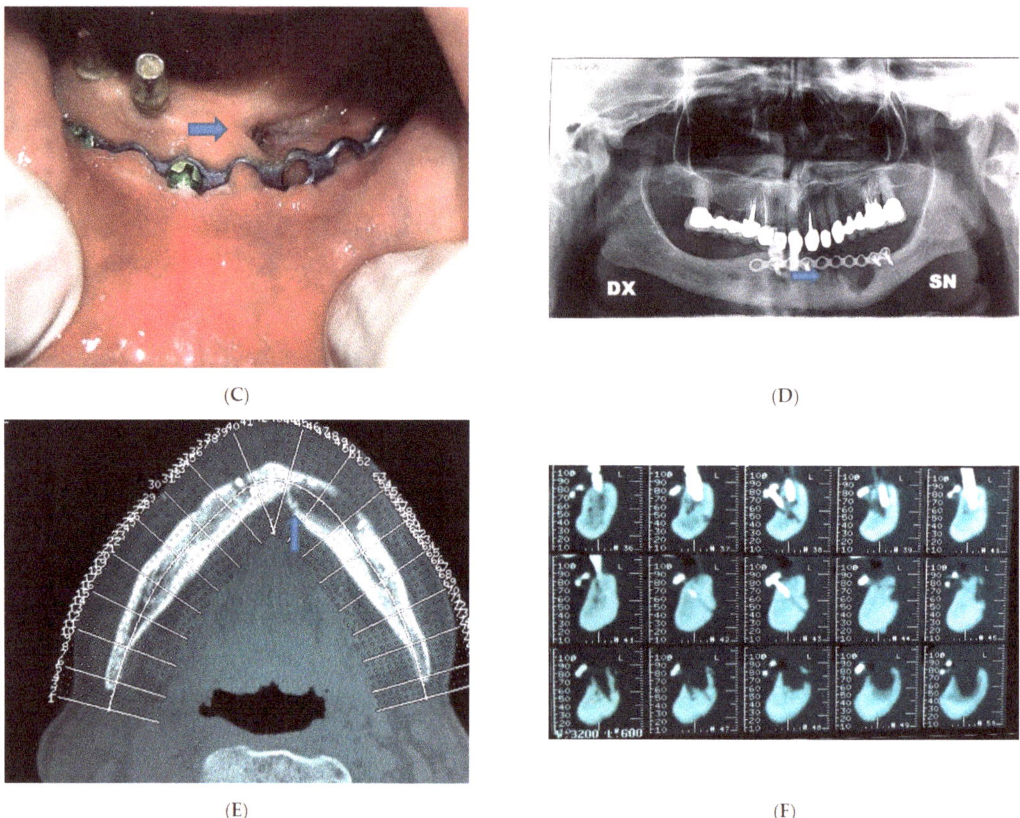

(C) (D)

(E) (F)

Figure 2. Patient 2. (**A**) Pre-operative panoramic X-ray examination showed no fractures, but there was a subversion of the normal organization of the bone. (**B**) Pre-operative X-Ray image showed lithic area in the lower branch. (**C**) Epi-mucosal fixation performed using SMART Lock screws and plates without elevating the mucoperiosteal flap. (**D**) Post-operative panoramic X-ray image of the dental branch revealed lithic area. (**E**) Post-operative CT scan Image. (**F**) Post-operative X-ray image.

3. Results

For case one, patient physical examination showed no obvious swelling of the face. CT examination showed a lithic area in the mandibular horizontal branches, which appeared subverted and fractured on the left side (Figure 1A). A panoramic X-ray image of the dental arches has revealed the same characteristics (Figure 1B). The alteration was bilateral but particularly accentuated on the left. An additional bone lysis area was also appreciated at the D8 body level. A pathological fracture with radiographic evidence of osteolysis extending to the inferior border of the mandible was compatible with a diagnosis of stage 3 MRONJ caused by the continuous use of denosumab for three years (administration of 1 vial subcutaneous every six months). Additionally, fistulas were present at the lower border of the mandible.

For case two, patient physical examination showed no obvious swelling of the face. Oral examination showed no irregularities.

CT examination showed that there was a lithic area in the lower branch of the mandible. Although there were no fractures, the subversion of the normal organization of the bone exposed the patient to a high-risk for pathological fracture. Radiographic evidence showed an extensive osteolysis compatible with stage 3 MRONJ (Figure 2A,B).

In both the presented cases treated by our protocol associating surgical removal of the necrotic bone outbreak by surgical drilling and smoothing of sharp edges in the affected segment followed by application of autologous PRF we achieved good results. Post-operative clinical conditions were evaluated by analyzing the following results:

- Mucosal integrity: Absence of necrotic bone exposure;
- Absence of residual infection: Absence of purulent exudate and reduction of swelling;
- Pain reduction: Evaluation of the VAS score.

We achieved good bone healing with absence of necrotic bone exposure, mucosa healing with complete necrotic site closure, and absence of residual infection without any swelling or residual fistulas.

Patients were able to wear a dental prosthesis without any referred pain at rest or during soft diet mastication.

We followed the first patient with periodic controls at one, three, and six months. In the post-operative controls, we could detect a progressive healing of the mucosa up to a final result, with complete mucosa healing without any signs of necrosis or infection. A significant reduction in pain was assessed by the VAS scale. Before the operation she reported a pain score on the VAS scale between 9 and 10, with the need to use painkillers. A few days after the operation, she had already reduced the use of painkillers. In the three-month post-operative control, she completely eliminated the use of painkillers, having a score on the VAS scale of 0, with no pain. The patient died two years after the operation as a result of breast cancer general complications.

In the second case, after the operation, we also followed the patient with periodic controls at one, three, and six months. In post-operative controls we observed that there was a progressive healing of mucosal integrity and infection. In this second case too, the patient had a progressive reduction of pain and no signs of necrosis or infection. Before the operation she reported a pain score on the VAS scale of about 8, with the need to use painkillers. Shortly after the operation she reduced the use of painkillers. In the one-month postoperative checkup she eliminated the use of painkillers, having a score on the VAS scale of zero with no pain.

4. Discussion

Both cases were treated with our new protocol, consisting of the combination of a well-demonstrated conservative treatment by autologous PRF and surgical removal of the necrotic bone area combined with epi mucosa mandibular fixation in case of fracture risks or conclamant fracture in the necrotic bone segments. By our new original epi-mucosal fixation technique it was possible to achieve close fixation of the segment, avoiding large periosteal elevation in the affected area of the jaws.

In the scientific literature, high doses of bisphosphonates or denosumab are associated with an increased risk of MRONJ compared to low dose regimens [1].

For patients who received continuous denosumab during the blinded treatment phase plus the open-label extension phase, the incidence of confirmed MRONJ, adjusted for years of patient follow-up, was 1.1% during the first year of denosumab treatment, 3.7% in the second year, and 4.6% per year thereafter. The median cumulative exposure to denosumab was 43.0 months for those patients with breast cancer (n = 318) and 36.9 months for those with prostate cancer (n = 147) [1].

Denosumab does not become physically bound to the bone matrix and consequently is associated with low levels of accumulation compared with bisphosphonates, which may remain covalently bound to the bone for many years due to its mode of action. The effects of denosumab are reversed faster on suspension of treatment [1].

Tooth extractions in patients receiving denosumab or bisphosphonate treatment, especially in the oncological setting, should be performed under antibiotic prophylaxis (e.g., amoxicillin/clavulanic acid) and accompanied by smoothening of sharp bony edges and closure of the wounds, and then monitored until complete mucosal healing is achieved.

In general, well-designed prospective clinical trials and non-interventional studies that investigate MRONJ management approaches in patients with cancer and bone metastases are lacking. Furthermore, inconsistent outcome measures (e.g., patient QoL scales, mucosal healing, and symptom improvement) are used in all studies [1]. This means that it is difficult to reach a consensus on the most effective MRONJ management approaches available. Patients who develop MRONJ should be referred to a maxillofacial surgeon or an oncologist [1]. A pragmatic approach to the management of patients with MRONJ should be adopted, with the management of malignant skeletal disease at the forefront of the care of each patient. Conservative management is recommended for the AAOMS I MRONJ stage, supplemented with appropriate surgical approaches for the most severe cases.

The current AAOMS guide recommends soft tissue debridement to treat irritation and infection in association with necrotic bone removal in stage 2, while bone resection at the necrotic area is considered in stage 3 [1]. The main problems related to surgery will consist of: temporary decrease in quality of life during convalescence, risks of relapse with extension of the necrosis with a second stage surgical need, possibility of complications (e.g., risk of infection or fracture), need for extended hospitalization, uncertain implications of interruptions necessary to chemotherapy and any cost per patient, and final treatment failure.

In our study, we developed a new protocol for the treatment of patients in stage 2 and stage 3 MRONJ causing segment fracture or showing high-risk for fracture. In MRONJ treatment there is a contraposition between two requirements: One is to remove the necrotic bone area, the other one is to prevent new necrosis by avoiding periosteal elevation in affected the area. To solve these two opposite requirements, we developed a new technique where bone resection was performed and fixation of the fractured bone segments in the affected area or preventive fixation of the resected area at risk of fracture was performed by our epi-mucosa fixation technique. This technique was already validated and published for jaw reducible fractures; because of the similar condition for reducible jaw fractures in MRONJ cases and in non-affected patients, we adopted this technique in the two reported cases. It was the first time the technique was adopted in MRONJ cases, hence the scientific relevance. In this way, it was possible to avoid periosteal elevation with a subsequent bone nutrition impairment and necrosis extension risk. In this new technique, the fixation is performed in closed surgery by fixing the bone plates over the mucosa using self-locking screws, as in an external fixation system. Conservative treatment by autologous PRF is also used in combination, to enhance and promote soft tissue and exposed bone area healing.

We developed the epi-mucosal fixation technique for reducible or well aligned fractures of the jaw; in these cases, fixation of the two bone segments is performed after close reduction of the fracture, avoiding surgical trauma and periosteal elevation, thereby preserving bone nutrition. In this way, we can ensure less surgical trauma with earlier healing of the lesion for the patient.

As shown in our previous study, the main indications for this technique were in well aligned fractures of the jaws (especially in elderly edentulous patients when minimally invasive techniques are needed) or in dislocated jaw fractures that can be reduced by closed manipulation without any incision. Particular indication for this technique is in case of multi segmented fractures with high risks for bone resorption and infection in case of periosteum elevation because of lack of nutrition of the bone fragments [9]. Long threaded-necked screws and plates are used, avoiding plate compression on the muco-periosteum and bone fragments, thus using a self-locking screws and plates system like external fixers. The bone fractures are fixed in position, after the reduction, by a rigid fixation system without compression that joins the insertion of the screw into the bone fragment on one side and the insertion of the thread screw neck in the holes of the plates on the other, obtaining a three-dimensional rigid system without any incision [8,10].

The main advantages of this technique are the minimum surgical trauma suitable for elderly patients, avoiding the risk of devascularization of the fragment even in comminuted or multifocal fractures; in this way, the quality and speed of the healing process is improved [9].

Other advantages are an easier removal of fixing devices, avoiding further surgical time, unlike in current techniques with sub-periosteal miniplates and screws, and no risk of periodontal damage, unlike in ferule methods, with lower costs and greater benefits of results [9,11]. It is conceivable to develop this technique and apply a double-plate fixation system for each fracture line in case greater stability is required, such as in unfavorable jaw line fractures, particularly in larger fractured areas [9].

With the use of this new epi-mucosa fixation technique, we were able to shorten the healing time with minimal surgical impact on the patients affected by MRONJ with fractured or weakened bone segments. In conclusion, the intraoral epi-mucosal fixation system is comparable to external fixation devices, with the advantages of avoiding trans-cutaneous pins or cumbersome devices with aesthetic and functional impairment. For the minimum device size, intraoral placement of the system is also possible for the molar areas using a ratchet screwdriver and contra-angle tips. Particular attention must be paid to the selection of the screw insertion sites in the interalveolar bone septa, avoiding damage to the dental roots.

5. Conclusions

Analyzing the result of the two cases treated by our technique, it was possible to achieve good results, combining the most effective treatment, even for advanced cases of MRONJ (stage 3). Excellent results were obtained, limiting risks and disadvantages, also in cases with high-risk for bone fracture or cases of effective fractured segment in necrotic bone segments.

The advantages are: Non-invasive surgical procedure; ability to stabilize a bone segment at risk for pathologic fracture; limited risks for necrosis extension; ability in solving pain and necrosis related symptoms achieving mucosa healing.

In our cases, we did not find any complications related to pain during plate and screw fixation, and there was no infection around the sites of screw insertion and no screw weakening or plate mobilization.

Even if the epi-mucosal fixation procedures are already used in close reducible max-illofacial fractures, the number of cases was limited, and additional studies with a larger number of cases are needed to finally assess the reliability and effectiveness of this proce-dure in MRONJ patients, even if showing promising results in our cases.

Author Contributions: Conceptualization, A.C. (Antonio Cortese); Data curation, A.C. (Antonio Cortese); Formal analysis, A.C. (Antonio Cortese), A.C. (Antonio Casarella), C.M.H. and P.P.C.; Writing—original draft, A.C. (Antonio Cortese), A.C. (Antonio Casarella), C.M.H. and P.P.C.; Writing—review & editing, A.C. (Antonio Cortese), A.C. (Antonio Casarella), C.M.H. and P.P.C. All authors have read and agreed to the published version of the manuscript.

Funding: Candace M. Howard is partially supported by the National Institute of General Medical Sciences of the National Institutes of Health under Award Number 1U54GM115428. The content is solely the responsibility of the authors and does not necessarily represent the official views of the National Institutes of Health.

Institutional Review Board Statement: The study was conducted according to the guidelines of the Declaration of Helsinki, and was approved by the Comitato Etico dell' Universita' di Salerno (38/06, 14 April 2006).

Informed Consent Statement: Informed consent was obtained from all subjects involved in the study.

Data Availability Statement: Data is available upon reasonable request.

Conflicts of Interest: The authors declare no conflict of interest.

References

1. Otto, S.; Pautke, C.; Van den Wyngaert, T.; Niepel, D.; Schiødt, M. Medication-related osteonecrosis of the jaw: Prevention, diagnosis and management in patients with cancer and bone metastases. *Cancer Treat. Rev.* **2018**, *69*. [CrossRef]
2. Otto, S. *Medication-Related Osteonecrosis of the Jaws*, 1st ed.; Springer: Berlin/Heidelberg, Germany, 2015.
3. Cortese, A.; Pantaleo, G.; Caggiano, M.; Amato, M. Platelet-rich fibrin (PRF) in implant dentistry in combination with new bone regenerative technique in elderly patients. *Int. J. Surg. Case Rep.* **2016**, *28*, 52–56. [CrossRef] [PubMed]
4. Cortese, A.; Pantaleo, G.; Ferrara, I.; Vatrella, A.; Cozzolino, I.; Di Crescenzo, V.; Amato, M. Bone and soft tissue non-Hodgkin lymphoma of the maxillofacial area: Report of two cases, literature review and new therapeutic strategies. *Int. J. Surg.* **2014**, *12*, S23–S28. [CrossRef]
5. Dohan, D.M.; Del Corso, M.; Charrier, J.B. Cytotoxicity analyses of Choukron's platelet-rich-fibrin (PRF) on a wide range of human cells: The answer to a commercial controversy. *Oral Surg. Oral Med. Oral Patholog. Oral Radiol. Endod.* **2007**, *103*, 587–593. [CrossRef]
6. Kang, Y.H.; Seon, S.H.; Park, J.H.; Choung, Y.H.; Choung, H.W.; Kim, E.S.; Choung, P.H. Platelet-rich fibrin is a Bioscaffold and reservoir of growth factor for tissue regeneration. *Tissue Eng. Part A* **2011**, *17*, 349–359. [CrossRef] [PubMed]
7. Shin, W.J.; Kim, C. Prognostic factors for outcome of surgical treatment in medication-related osteonecrosis of the jaw. *J. Korean Assoc. Oral. Maxillofac. Surg.* **2018**, *44*, 174–181. [CrossRef] [PubMed]
8. Cano-Duran, J.A.; Pena-Cardelles, J.-F.; Ortega-Concepcion, D.; Paredes-Rodriguez, V.M.; Garcia-Riart, M.; Lopez-Quiles, J. The role of Leucocyte-rich and platelet-rich fibrin (L-PRF) in the treatment of the medication-related osteonecrosis of the jaws (MRONJ). *J. Clin. Exp. Dent.* **2017**, *9*, e1051–e1059. [CrossRef] [PubMed]
9. Cortese, A.; Savastano, G.; Amato, M.; Pantaleo, G.; Claudio, P.P. Intraoral epimucosal fixation for reducible maxillary fractures of the jaws; surgical considerations in comparison to current techniques. *J. Craniofac. Surg.* **2014**, *25*, 2184–2187. [CrossRef] [PubMed]
10. Cortese, A.; Savastano, M.; Cantone, A.; Claudio, P.P. A new palatal distractor device for bodily movement of maxillary bones by rigid self-locking miniplates and screws system. *J. Craniofac. Surg.* **2013**, *24*, 1341–1346. [CrossRef] [PubMed]
11. Cortese, A.; Savastano, M.; Savastano, G.; Claudio, P.P. One-step transversal palatal distraction and maxillary repositioning: Technical considerations, advantages, and long-term stability. *J. Craniofac. Surg.* **2011**, *22*, 1714–1719. [CrossRef] [PubMed]

MDPI
St. Alban-Anlage 66
4052 Basel
Switzerland
Tel. +41 61 683 77 34
Fax +41 61 302 89 18
www.mdpi.com

Dentistry Journal Editorial Office
E-mail: dentistry@mdpi.com
www.mdpi.com/journal/dentistry

www.ingramcontent.com/pod-product-compliance
Lightning Source LLC
LaVergne TN
LVHW070140170726
843515LV00007B/1836

9783036531113